Autism Services Across America

Autism Services Across America

Road Maps for Improving State and National Education, Research, and Training Programs

by

Peter Doehring, Ph.D.
ASD Roadmap
with invited contributors

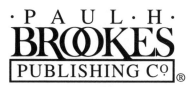

·P A U L·H·
BROOKES
PUBLISHING C⁰ ®

Baltimore • London • Sydney

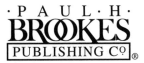

Paul H. Brookes Publishing Co.
Post Office Box 10624
Baltimore, Maryland 21285-0624

www.brookespublishing.com

Typeset by Apex CoVantage, LLC, Herndon, Virginia.
Manufactured in the United States of America by
Sheridan Books, Inc., Chelsea, Michigan.

The individuals described in this book are composites or real people whose situations are masked and are based on the authors' experiences. In all instances, names and identifying details have been changed to protect confidentiality.

As applicable, cover photos used by permission of the individuals pictured and/or their parents/guardians. Cover photos © istockphoto/bibikoff, © 2013 Jupiterimages Corporation, and © Venture Photography. Map cover Image © iStockphoto.com/meshaphoto.

Library of Congress Control Number: 2013940478

ISBN-13: 978-1-59857-095-3; ISBN-10: 1-59857-095-1

2017   2016   2015   2014   2013

10   9   8   7   6   5   4   3   2   1

Contents

· ·

I   Understanding the Scope

II   Exemplary Regional, Provincial, and Statewide Programs

About the Author

· ·

After completing his doctoral training as a clinical and research psychologist in Canada, Peter Doehring, Ph.D., began his career developing autism spectrum disorder (ASD) screening and early intervention programs within a regional psychiatric hospital in Montreal. He then served as Statewide Director for the Delaware Autism Program (DAP), the largest specialized public school program of its kind in the United States. He led DAP through an unprecedented period of growth and change that doubled the number of students served and the number of school districts operating affiliated programs, that included the development of programs of training and oversight for ASD identification and behavior support, that revitalized a specialized postgraduate certificate for teachers of students with ASD, and that reorganized a program of residential and respite services unique within the public school system.

As Director of Regional Programs at the Center for Autism Research (CAR) at the Children's Hospital of Philadelphia and the University of Pennsylvania, he then initiated a wide range of hospital- and community-based training programs. In this role, he served as Autism Training Director for the hospital's Leadership Education in Neurodevelopmental and Related Disabilities (LEND) program, helped to establish a regional consortium for training, services, and research, and obtained funding from the National Institutes of Health to begin a regional research registry.

As Director of Autism Services for Foundations Behavioral Health, he led the development of a new inpatient treatment program for children and adolescents with ASD in behavioral crisis. This program was designed as a model for others to be disseminated by the parent company Universal Health Services, the largest provider of behavioral health services in the United States.

Via his consultation services—ASD Roadmap—he now provides training and strategic support to families and agencies struggling to organize, expand, and improve services and programs. Throughout his career, he has actively championed the role of research in improving practice and in 2011 edited a volume reviewing evidence-based treatments for autism. Peter is also the father of three children, including a daughter with multiple and complex developmental disabilities.

Contributors

Barbara Becker-Cottrill, Ed.D., BCBA
Executive Director, The West Virginia
Autism Training Center
Marshall University
Huntington, West Virginia

Jennifer Bogin, MS.Ed., BCBA
Association of University Centers on
Disabilities
Silver Spring, Maryland

Matthew E. Brock, M.A.
National Professional Development Center
on Autism Spectrum Disorder
Frank Porter Graham Child Development
Institute University of North Carolina at
Chapel Hill
Chapel Hill, North Carolina

Paul S. Carbone, M.D.
Associate Professor of Pediatrics
University of Utah
Salt Lake City, Utah

Lana L. Collet-Klingenberg, Ph.D.
University of Wisconsin–Whitewater
Whitewater, Wisconsin

Ann W. Cox, Ph.D.
Director, National Professional
Development Center on Autism Spectrum
Disorder
Frank Porter Graham Child
Development Institute
University of North Carolina at Chapel Hill
Chapel Hill, North Carolina

Ellen L. Franzone, M.S., CCC-SLP
Program Coordinator
Allies in Autism Education CESA 6
Oshkosh, Wisconsin

Sarah Hoffmeier, LMSW
Family Service & Training Coordinator
TASN Autism & Tertiary Behavior Supports
Kansas City, Kansas

Judith M. Holt, Ph.D.
Co-Director, Utah Regional
Leadership Education in
Neurodevelopmental
Disabilities Program
Utah State University
Logan, Utah

Sue Lin, M.S.
Maternal and Child Health Bureau
Health Resources and Services
Administration
Washington, D.C.

Michael Miklos, M.S., BCBA
Lead Educational Consultant
PaTTAN Autism Initiative
Harrisburg, Pennsylvania

Samuel L. Odom, Ph.D.
Director Frank Porter Graham Child
Development Institute
University of North Carolina
Chapel Hill, North Carolina

Georgina Peacock, M.D., MPH
Centers for Disease Control and
Prevention
National Center on Birth Defects
and Developmental Disabilities
Atlanta, Georgia

Cathy Pratt, Ph.D., BCBA-D
Director, Indiana Institute on
Disability and Community
Indiana University
Bloomington, Indiana

Harper Randall, M.D.
Medical Director
Utah Department of Health
Division of Family Health and
Preparedness
Salt Lake City, Utah

Jo-Ann Reitzel, Ph.D.
Clinical Director
Autism Intervention Program
McMaster Children's Hospital
Hamilton, Ontario, Canada

Cheryl Rhodes, M.S., LMFT, LPC
Director, Case Management
Marcus Autism Center
Atlanta, Georgia

Sally J. Rogers, Ph.D.
Professor of Psychiatry, MIND Institute
University of California–Davis Medical
Center
Sacramento, California

Cathy Scutta, OTD, OTR/L, BCBA-D
The Competent Learner Model (CLM)
PaTTAN Autism Initiative
King of Prussia, Pennsylvania

Lee Stickle, M.S.Ed.
Kansas State Department of Education
Technical Assistance Systems Network
(TASN)
Kansas City, Kansas

Lisa H. Sullivan, Ph.D.
Educational Researcher
University of California–Davis
Davis, California

Jane Summers, Ph.D.
Psychologist, Autism Intervention Program
McMaster Children's Hospital
Hamilton, Ontario, Canada

Peter Szatmari, M.D.
Professor, Department of Psychology
McMaster University
Hamilton, Ontario, Canada

Katherine Szidon, M.S.
Special Education Developmental
Disabilities

Professional Development
Specialist, Waisman Center
University of Wisconsin–Madison
Madison, Wisconsin

Linda Tuchman-Ginsberg, Ph.D.
Program Director for Early
Childhood and Education Professional
Development, Waisman Center
University of Wisconsin–Madison
Madison, Wisconsin

Nina Wall-Cote, M.S.S.
Bureau Director
Bureau of Autism Services
Pennsylvania Department of Public
Welfare
Harrisburg, Pennsylvania

Erica Wexler, M.S.
Senior Communications and Training
Coordinator
Bureau of Autism Services
Pennsylvania Department of Public
Welfare
Philadelphia, Pennsylvania

Sarah Winter, M.D.
Associate Professor
University of Utah
Salt Lake City, Utah

Vincent Winterling, Ed.D.
Statewide Director
Delaware Autism Program
Christina School District
Newark, Delaware

Rebecca B. Wolf, M.A.
Team Leader
Learn the Signs. Act Early.
Prevention Research Branch
Division of Birth Defects and
Developmental Disabilities
Atlanta, Georgia

Foreword

. . . .

It has been 70 years since Kanner's classic description of the syndrome of "infantile autism" (Kanner, 1943). Over this time very significant change has occurred in our understanding of autism, its etiology, and its treatment. Until the 1970s there was considerable confusion about autism. In part this reflected some "false leads" inadvertently suggested by Kanner in his otherwise remarkably accurate initial report. He initially speculated that children with autism had normal intellectual potential given their performance on some parts of IQ tests—particularly in the nonverbal area. However, as time went on it became clear that children had marked scatter in skills with strengths in some areas and profound weakness in other (verbal) ones and that overall many functioned in the "intellectually deficient" range (Ozonoff, Goodlin-Jones, & Solomon, 2005). Kanner also noted the high rates of parent education and success in his first families, but subsequent work made it clear that autism is found in all strata of society and that his initial impression was based on a referral bias in the ability of the earliest cases to get to him (Wing, 1980). His original impression was that autism was not associated with other medical disorders; subsequently it became clear that there were some conditions (notably some genetic conditions) associated with autism and that over time many individuals with autism developed seizures (Volkmar & Nelson, 1990). His use of the word *autism*, meant by him to convey the profound social isolation experienced from the beginning of life, suggested to some a similarity with schizophrenia where the term *autism* had been used to describe self-centered thinking (Rutter, 1972). Finally, although he believed autism to be "inborn" and congenital, it did become clear that in a small number of cases the syndrome appeared to emerge after some period of normal development (Parr et al., 2011). On the other hand, his emphasis on the key features of autism—the lack of engagement with the social world and an oversensitivity to the nonsocial world—was profoundly insightful and has stimulated decades of research (Volkmar & Pelphrey, in press).

During the 1950s and 1960s, intervention mistakenly centered around notions of parental psychopatholgy as a cause of autism. Although occasional voices of opposition were heard (Rimland, 1964), mothers ("refrigerator mothers") were in particular blamed for causing their child's difficulties, and removal of the child from the family or intensive psychotherapeutic treatment was recommended (Bettelheim, 1967).

During the 1970s, this situation began to change as several different lines of evidence became available. Longitudinal studies clarified that there was marked increase for development of epilepsy—particularly during adolescence (Volkmar & Nelson, 1990). Other data suggested the validity of autism apart from childhood schizophrenia—for example, it differed in terms of its early onset, clinical features and family history (Kolvin, 1971; Kolvin, Ounsted, & Roth, 1971; Rutter, 1972). The first follow-up studies of autism to appear (Kanner, 1971) suggested relatively poor outcome but other work emerging at the same time (Rutter, 1972) suggested that more highly structured programs were associated with better outcome than the unstructured psychotherapeutic approaches frequently in use and that the application of behavioral psychological principles to learning could lead to skills acquisition (Ferster, 1972). During this period, many of the independent schools and treatment centers for autism began to develop—often started by parents or, sometimes, in university settings. Both in the United States and in the United Kingdom, parents also began to organize with clinicians and researchers the various national advocacy groups that remain active today. On the biomedical side, the first twin study of autism (Kanner, 1971) demonstrated a very significant genetic contribution (Folstein & Rutter, 1977). Efforts to provide more formal diagnostic guidelines were also made (Rutter, 1978; National Society for Autistic Children [NSAC], 1978) and led to the formal, first, recognition of autism as a diagnostic category in *Diagnostic and Statistical Manual of Mental Disorders, Third Edition* (*DSM-III;* American Psychiatric Association, 1980).

With official recognition and a set of formal (if initially somewhat limited) diagnostic guidelines, research on autism began to increase dramatically. At the same time, there was a very important impact of legislation at the federal level. Public Law 94-142 had been passed by the U.S. Congress in 1975 and mandated that public schools that received federal funding provide an education to children with handicaps. For autism, this was a watershed event. Prior to PL 94-142 schools could (and did) refuse to provide educational services to children with autism who, as a result, often were placed in large state institutions, where their progress was minimal. This law also gave students with disabilities (including autism) some basic rights relative to due process and administrative procedures in the development of an intervention program. It mandated access to services, management, monitoring, and federal support. It also suggested that, whenever possible, the "least restrictive" educational settings should be used. This mandate was consistent with a growing body of work on the importance of exposure to typical peers for development of social and other skills (Strain & Carr, 1975).

The official recognition of autism in *DSM-III* in 1980 stimulated research in the least restrictive environment, or one that allows the maximum possible opportunity to interact with nonimpaired students. Separate schooling may only occur when the nature or severity of the disability is such that instructional goals cannot be achieved in the regular classroom. Finally, the law contains a due process clause that guarantees an impartial hearing to resolve conflicts between the parents of children with disabilities to the school system. At the same time, the mandate for educational services also raised some complexities for insurance based coverage of important and effective treatments.

Early treatment programs often were organized by parents who lacked access to services in public schools. As interest (and research) increased, university settings began to be involved in treatment research. This included the pioneering work of Lovaas at the University of California, Los Angeles (Lovaas & Koegel, 1972), as well as at various other programs around the country (see National Research Council, 2001, for a review). Initially these programs tended to be center based but, over time, many expanded to home and community settings (National Research Council, 2001). By 2001, when the National Research Council group surveyed existing programs in the United States, a number of different models were available. These ranged from more eclectic models, like the first state-wide program for autism at Division TEACCH in North Carolina (Schopler, Mesibov, & Hearsey, 1995), to more behaviorally focused programs like those of Lovass and colleagues, to more developmentally oriented intervention programs as exemplified by the Denver model (Rogers et al., 2006) and Floortime (Greenspan & Wieder, 2009) and to approaches which integrated key developmental principles in behavioral interventions, such as Pivotal Response training (Koegel & Frea, 1993). The National Research Council (NRC) report made an important contribution to the field in reviewing the many areas of consensus, and a few areas of difference, in approaches to intervention.

Since 1980, research in autism has increased dramatically. In that year, about 100 peer-reviewed papers were published on autism; by 1990 this had doubled, and by 2000 near 400 papers had appeared with key words of *autism* or *autistic disorder* in the title. By 2010 this number grew to over 1,600. This growth in research paralleled increased awareness on the part of the public and of private foundations and advocacy groups and support from the National Institutes of Health (originally from National Institute of Child Health and Human Development [NICHD] in the Collaborative Programs of Excellence in Autism and then by the multi-institute Studies to Advance Autism Research and Treatment [STAART] and angiotensin-converting enzyme [ACE] programs). Major advances have occurred in many areas including genetics (State & Levitt, 2011) and the neuropsychology/neuroscience of autism (McPartland & Pelphrey, 2012). At the same time, a review of the research literature reveals many interesting gaps (either relatively or absolutely defined) in coverage. For example, there is a large body of work on infants and young children with autism reflecting the many advances and gains made in work on early diagnosis, siblings at risk, and new approaches to assessment (see Chawarska, Klin, & Volkmar, 2008). As noted above, the body of work on early intervention has also increased, although as with all intervention research there is a great need for more empirical study and evidence-based treatments (see Reichow, Doehring, Cicchetti, & Volkmar, 2011). Work on neural mechanisms and genetics has also dramatically increased (e.g., see McPartland et al., 2011; State & Levitt, 2011) as has work in the area of psychopharmacology (Martin, Scahil, & Christopher, 2010).

Although there has been a growing awareness of the needs of children and adolescents, research and intervention programs focused on adults have been substantially lacking. Indeed, in many respects the outcome literature in autism has seemed to focus on young adulthood, as if older adults with autism don't exist. It is clear that they do and that even while, as a group, they are doing better than previously, a significant majority remain in need of service. Both the lack of access to services and the lack of basic knowledge (e.g., little or no work on aging in autism, on rates of employment in adults, and on comorbid conditions) means that treatments and treatment models are assembled (when available at all) on an ad hoc basis, and much of what is available is generalized from work with younger individuals.

Despite the many advances made and the federal mandates for service, the United States has, effectively, been conducting a series of state by state (and sometimes town by town) interventions. This has posed many challenges for parents, educators, and others who care for individuals with autism. The present volume addresses this problem in a very useful way. The first chapters give overviews of autism, the range of services needed, and the range of agencies involved. The second part of the book provides a series of chapters on noteworthy treatment programs in the United States and Canada. The final sections of the book focus on aspects of national planning and social policy. This book does a tremendous service in providing a framework for viewing both what we know and what we don't know about how research findings can be translated into practice and training and, in turn, be informed by practioners and educators. It will be of tremendous interest to parents, educators and other professionals, and social policy planners as we enter the eighth decade of research on this intriguing condition.

Fred R. Volkmar M.D.
Irving B. Harris Professor of
Child Psychiatry, Psychology and Pediatrics
Director, Yale University Child Study Center
Editor, Journal of Autism and Developmental Disorders

REFERENCES

American Psychiatric Association. (1980). *Diagnostic and Statistical Manual.* Washington, DC: APA Press.

Bettelheim, B. (1967). *The empty fortress: Infantile autism and the birth of the self.* New York: The Free Press.

Chawarska, K., Klin, A., & Volkmar, F. (Eds.). (2008). *Autism spectrum disorders in infants and toddlers: Diagnosis, assessment, and treatment.* New York: Guilford Press.

Ferster, C.B. (1972). Clinical reinforcement. *Semin Psychiatry, 4*(2), 101–111.

Folstein, S., & Rutter, M. (1977). Genetic influences and infantile autism. *Nature, 265*(5596), 726–728.

Greenspan, S.I., & Wieder, S. (2009). *Engaging Autism: Using the floortime approach to help children relate, communicate, and think.* Cambridge, MA: Da Capo Lifelong Books.

Kanner, L. (1943). Autistic disturbances of affective contact. *Nervous Child, 2,* 217–250.

Kanner, L. (1971). Follow-up study of eleven autistic children originally reported in 1943. *Journal of Autism & Childhood Schizophrenia, 1*(2), 119–145.

Koegel, R.I., & Frea, W.D. (1993). Treatment of social behavior in autism through the modification of pivotal social skills. *Journal of Applied Behavior Analysis, 26*(3), 369–377.

Kolvin, I. (1971). Studies in the childhood psychoses. I. Diagnostic criteria and classification. *British Journal of Psychiatry, 118*(545), 381–384.

Kolvin, I., Ounsted, C., & Roth, M. (1971). Studies in the childhood psychoses. V. Cerebral dysfunction and childhood psychoses. *British Journal of Psychiatry, 118*(545), 407–414.

Lovaas, O., & Koegel, R.L. (1973). Behavior therapy with autistic children. In Thoresen, C.E. (Ed). Behavior Modification in education, (Chapter 6), pp. 230–238. Chicago, IL: University of Chicago.

Martin, A., Scahil, L., & Christopher, K. (2010). *Pediatric Psychopharmacology: Principles and Practice* (2nd ed.). New York: Oxford.

McPartland, J.C., & Pelphrey, K.A. (2012). The implications of social neuroscience for social disability. *Journal of Autism and Developmental Disorders, 42*(6), 1256–1262.

McPartland, J.C., Wu, J., Bailey, C.A., Mayes, L.C., Schultz, R.T., & Klin, A. (2011). Atypical neural specialization for social percepts in autism spectrum disorder. *Social Neuroscience, 6*(5–6), 436–451. doi: http://dx.doi.org/10.1080/17470919.2011.586880

National Research Council. (2001). *Educating young children with autism.* Washington, DC: National Academy Press.

National Society for Autistic Children. (1978). National Society for Autistic Children definition of the syndrome of autism. *Journal of Autism & Childhood Schizophrenia, 8*(2), 162–169.

Ozonoff, S., Goodlin-Jones, B.L., & Solomon, M. (2005). Evidence-based assessment of autism spectrum disorders in children and adolescents. *Journal of Clinical Child & Adolescent Psychology, 34*(3), 523–540.

Parr, J.R., Le Couteur, A., Baird, G., Rutter, M., Pickles, A., Fombonne, E., . . . International Molecular Genetic Study of Autism Consortium, Members. (2011). Early developmental regression in autism spectrum disorder: Evidence from an international multiplex sample. *Journal of Autism & Developmental Disorders, 41*(3), 332–340.

Rimland, B. (1964). *Infantile autism: The syndrome and its implications for a neural theory of behavior.* New York, NY: Appleton-Century-Crofts.

Rogers, S.J., Hayden, D., Hepburn, S., Charlifue-Smith, R., Hall, T., & Hayes, A. (2006). Teaching young nonverbal children with autism useful speech: A pilot study of the Denver Model and PROMPT interventions. *Journal of Autism & Developmental Disorders, 36*(8), 1007–1024.

Rutter, M. (1972). Childhood schizophrenia reconsidered. *Journal of Autism & Childhood Schizophrenia, 2*(4), 315–337.

Rutter, M. (1978). Diagnosis and definition of childhood autism. *Journal of Autism & Childhood Schizophrenia, 8*(2), 139–161.

Schopler, E., Mesibov, G.B., & Hearsey, K. (1995). Structured teaching in the TEACCH system. In E. Schopler & G.B. Mesibov (Eds.). *Learning and cognition in autism (Current issues in autism)* (pp 243–268) xxi, 346.

State, M.W., & Levitt, P. (2011). The conundrums of understanding genetic risks for autism spectrum disorders. *Nature Neuroscience, 14*(12), 1499–1506. doi: http://dx.doi.org/10.1038/nn.2924

Strain, P.S., & Carr, T.H. (1975). The observational study of social reciprocity: Implications for the mentally retarded. *Mental Retardation, 13*(4), 18–19.

Volkmar, F.R., & Nelson, D.S. (1990). Seizure disorders in autism. *Journal of the American Academy of Child & Adolescent Psychiatry, 29*(1), 127–129.

Volkmar, F.R., & Pelphrey, K.A. (in press). Autism. In P. Blaney (Ed.), *Oxford textbook of psychopathology.* Oxford, United Kingdom: Oxford University Press.

Wing, L. (1980). Childhood autism and social class: a question of selection? *British Journal of Psychiatry, 137,* 410–417.

Acknowledgments

I would first like to thank Barbara Becker-Cottrill for her support throughout the completion of this book. Her boundless enthusiasm from the very outset of this project helped to fuel my own belief in the book, her feedback helped to assure me that I was on the right path, and her experience was instrumental to identifying potential contributors. I also think that Barbara's own understated but steadfast determination to improve the lives of people with autism spectrum disorder (ASD), and her recognition that success often depends on the careful cultivation of collaborations, provides a model for ASD leaders across the country.

Many of the lessons described in this book grew from the work I have undertaken since the mid-1990s, and I benefited from the opportunity to collaborate with many smart and dedicated colleagues and caregivers. The professionals at the Delaware Autism Program and its affiliated programs throughout the Delaware education system showed me that public schools can provide services that are high quality *and* specialized *and* accessible; this further spurred my interest in translating research findings into practical applications that potentially benefit everyone. My emphasis in this volume on the role of caregivers as advocates is inspired largely by the parents of Autism Delaware: They channeled their energies into developing not only great supports for Delaware families but also constructive collaborations with people concerned about ASD throughout Delaware and even new services complementing those already available in the state. These experiences prepared me to seek—and benefit from—other opportunities to develop new programs at Children's Hospital of Philadelphia and Foundations Behavioral Health and other collaborations with colleagues at Yale University and elsewhere. Without these experiences, I might never have learned of the provincial, state, and national programs I am privileged to showcase in this volume.

I learned perhaps the most important lessons from my daughter, Margot, who taught me that stubborn determination, curiosity, a healthy sense of humor, and a love of people can also contribute to some of the broad outcomes described in this book: the health and quality of life of the person with disabilities and those in his or her circle of care.

And of course Rebecca Lazo, my editor at Paul H. Brookes Publishing Co., deserves a special thanks for her constant encouragement, thoughtful direction, and infinite patience.

Introduction

· ·

There has been a tremendous increase in the interest in and awareness of autism spectrum disorder (or ASD) since the 1990s. For people affected by ASD—that is, the person with ASD, caregivers responsible for that person, and for other family members—this increased interest has been accompanied by increases in the services available to them and the research conducted to identify causes, characteristics, and effective treatments for ASD. This increased interest is important, because ASD continues to have a profound and lifelong impact on the people affected by it, despite our growing understanding of ASD and of the interventions that are likely to lead to better outcomes.

A tremendous opportunity lies ahead. Service professionals now have tools and techniques at their disposal to rapidly and accurately diagnose ASD before 3 years of age and have identified interventions to address many of their most debilitating features and accompanying conditions. Those in the field are increasingly aware of the challenges faced by families and the unique needs of adults with ASD. Benefit can be had from the insights offered by people with ASD themselves. Given all that is known, why are more people affected by ASD not able to benefit from this knowledge?

Since the 1990s I have struggled with these questions through my work in different settings and with many dedicated and talented colleagues, parents, and children. Throughout my career, I have been driven by the potential of science to solve the most important questions and problems surrounding ASD and to help people living with ASD live fulfilling lives and contribute meaningfully to their communities. I have worked directly with children and their families, developed and provided training to parents and professionals, conducted research on various aspects of ASD, and provided leadership at the local and state level with the goal of influencing policy. I have worked as a leader in schools, hospitals, and universities; in the public and private sectors; and across two states, two countries, and two languages. As a parent to a young girl with multiple and complex disabilities, I have been bewildered at times by the labyrinth that is the support system in the United States and delighted when these supports can help my little girl blossom in her own unique ways.

In each of these roles and each of these contexts, the complexity of the work compelled me to examine ASD and elements from up close: As a clinician, for example, I worked to create treatment plans to meet the evolving needs of each child and parent; as a researcher, I struggled to identify how to define precisely those emerging characteristics of ASD that might help to diagnose it earlier; as a leader, I sought to coordinate programs for diagnosis and intervention so that more children could be identified and helped more quickly, with evidence-based protocols used across settings. In each of these experiences and others, I found myself dogged by the same kinds of questions: As a clinician, I wondered what kinds of training I could seek and how research could help improve the work of clinicians; as a researcher, I wondered how the research community might take its growing understanding and disseminate it through training; as a parent and professional, I wondered what kinds of policy could support these kinds of changes.

Through these experiences and others, I came to perceive similar gaps, barriers, and sources of misunderstanding and frustration across disciplines and domains. These perceptions were echoed repeatedly by others around me. Parents demanded more help and support from professionals, and professionals blamed parents for not implementing everything the professionals recommended. Researchers wondered why clinicians could not develop or implement treatment programs that drew from their findings, and clinicians searched in vain for research that gave them useful and practical guidance. Physicians who turned to medication or other interventions to manage behavior were unable to evaluate its effects because school and community supports seem so chaotic, whereas school and community providers pinned their hopes on medication to manage behaviors that were spiraling dangerously downward. Policy makers under pressure lacked the research and data to support increasing budgets, and instead focused on increasing "efficiencies," while everyone else was buried by paperwork that seemed to grow at the same time as the resulting services and supports were shrinking. Commiserating with other professionals and parents who perceived similar barriers assuaged my frustration enough to allow me to bury myself again in the work at hand and trust that somewhere, somehow, someone could close these gaps.

My career choices reflect my conscious attempts to bridge these gaps and overcome these barriers through increased understanding and improved coordination across elements of services, training, research, and policy; across the domains of health, education, and community services; across the public and the private sector; and between parents and professionals. In each case, I have gained a greater appreciation of the potential for services, training, research, and policy to bring about dramatic change. I have come to believe the greatest potential now lies in bridging these gaps to create a new synergy rather than reinforcing the isolated silos of expertise and the boundaries between disciplines and domains. Yet I am concerned that in the competition for decreasing resources, individual agencies and organizations will become more driven to distinguish themselves from others and not coordinate with them.

I am also concerned that a parallel decrease in the range of experience sought by professionals will compound the increasing specialization of agencies. More people are dedicating themselves to the challenge of ASD every day, and these gaps and barriers will channel their incredible passion and emerging talent into increasingly narrow fields of interest, experience, and expertise. Although professionals may shift from one agency or organization to another, most spend the majority of their career focused primarily on one element (e.g., service, training, research, policy) and working in one domain (e.g., health, education, community services) and without the opportunity to assume a leadership role in which they were expected to implement systemic changes. As a result, professionals are even less likely to accumulate the experiences needed to acquire a broad perspective.

I believe that the greater barrier to improving the lives of all people affected by ASD is no longer just a lack of knowledge: it is the fact that too many concerned about ASD do not understand all of the elements involved (e.g., services, training, research, policy). Moreover, few understand the tremendous challenge of scaling up or of building capacity—how to efficiently and effectively translate this knowledge not on a local, program-by-program basis but at the regional, state, and/or national level. This need for a more comprehensive understanding extends to parents and advocates, who view the bewildering world of services, training, research, and policy through the lens of their own particular needs. My first hope is that readers begin to grasp the potential for a more integrated network, become excited by the possibility of scientifically based services being scaled up to meet the needs of even the most traditionally underserved populations, and become emboldened to look for new collaborations beyond their own particular discipline, field of interest, and agency. My second hope is that readers discover specific programs that can serve as models for their own growth.

SECTION I: UNDERSTANDING THE SCOPE

When I originally conceptualized this book, I realized that no single volume provided a succinct summary of the scope of services needed by people with ASD across the life span; the training, research, and policy underlying these services; and the panoply of agencies and organizations involved at the local, state, and national level. As I began to accumulate examples from model state and regional programs, it became apparent that readers might find it difficult to generalize beyond these examples—however excellent and innovative—to the needs in their own programs. I also realized that effective advocacy for expansion and improved coordination will require the education of many people beyond program leaders. I initially hesitated to expand the breadth of the topics and the target audience: I considered whether it might be more beneficial to draw from others with more specific expertise in each of these areas but realized that they too would struggle to quickly outline key features within the number of pages allotted, especially if they did not fully understand and embrace the broader goals of the book. So I set out to accomplish a simpler goal: to provide parents, practitioners, and policy makers with enough knowledge to begin to advocate for and implement needed change. The first section of this book seeks to provide such a summary and to begin to identify important, cross-cutting themes.

About Autism Spectrum Disorder (Chapter 1): The challenges that ASD presents to each family vary tremendously because of their complexity (e.g., as a spectrum disorder changing with development), their lifelong impact, and their prevalence. I describe how co-occurring conditions (e.g., intellectual disability [ID], problem behavior, other psychiatric and medical conditions) might offer more immediate avenues for intervention and cross-domain coordination. The goal here is to set the stage for the more detailed discussion of the role of local, regional, and national organizations in training, research, and policy, which constitute the remainder of the book. As discussed throughout this volume, the scope of this challenge is underestimated because most professionals have experience with only a very small slice of the range of needs (e.g., they may work only with a specific age range), whereas parents of a newly diagnosed young child may be too overwhelmed to even consider what services they might need for an adult with ASD. Likewise, professionals and parents may not have grasped that one young man with an ASD may have very intensive self-care and behavioral needs such that his parents may no longer be able to care for him, whereas a college-bound young man with an ASD may need specialized coaching and support to help him to live on his own. To this end, I introduce a number of cases that I return to in subsequent chapters of the book to invigorate the discussion by reminding the reader how ASD affects individuals and families from many different backgrounds, in many different ways, and with many possible outcomes.

Services for People with Autism Spectrum Disorder: What Can This Include? (Chapter 2): Many people living with ASD grow through a broad range of services and supports in health, education, and community settings. I focus on a subset of services grouped by domain (health, education, and community support) that are commonly needed, that are offered across domains, or that play a pivotal role in helping most people with ASD gain access to other key services or settings. In this context, I touch on other important elements: which professionals typically deliver these services, whether consensus- or evidence-based guidelines for the service have been developed, and whether the service is likely to be needed by other populations. By focusing on a subset of service needs (and their associated training, research, and policy in Chapter 3), we can better characterize the complex interplay of factors.

An Overview of the Training, Research, and Policy Supporting Systems of Services for People with Autism Spectrum Disorder (Chapter 3): The effective development and expansion of services described in Chapter 2 depends entirely on the availability of associated programs of training. I broadly discuss the depth and breadth of such training programs and the potential to utilize existing avenues of training (e.g., programs leading to licensure, postgraduate training, agency-specific training), and I offer some principles and examples of a more integrated and comprehensive approach. I organize the discussion of ASD research around several critical questions (e.g., identification, prevalence, evidence-based interventions, costs, barriers) and distinguish between different kinds of research (e.g., basic, intervention, other applied research). I offer recommendations about prioritizing research to help people with ASD now, to create a culture of data-based decision making, and to bridge the gap between research and practice. I outline some general policy principles (building awareness and momentum for change; assessing and evaluating current resources; and promoting the convergence of scientific, ethical, and legal standards and oversight to drive programs of services and training) and discuss these in the context of various policy initiatives.

How It Works: The Infrastructure of Local, Regional, State, and National Agencies That Support Services, Training, Research, and Policy (Chapter 4): Any significant expansion of services, training, or research also requires that professionals understand and leverage the infrastructure of agencies and organizations. Initially, I felt this was critical for readers from other countries, whose research, health, education, and social welfare services may be funded and structured quite differently from those in the United States. But I have since learned that at least some elements of the infrastructure of services, training, research, and/or policy remain mysterious to most people here in the United States. To deconstruct this infrastructure and its constituent agencies and organizations, I describe critical dimensions such as the sector (public or private), the level (local, regional, state, or national) of the agency, and other important elements (e.g., domain, funding, mandate, mechanisms for oversight). I also illustrate the intersection of all of these elements by describing examples of agencies and programs such as those referenced elsewhere in this book.

SECTION II: EXEMPLARY REGIONAL, PROVINCIAL, AND STATEWIDE PROGRAMS

I became engrossed by the challenge of developing and overseeing large programs when I assumed leadership in 1999 of the Delaware Autism Program (see Chapter 7). After meeting with other state leaders in the National Autism Training and Technical Assistance Programs (NATTAP), I realized that others struggled with these same issues: how to provide effective training on a large scale and a small budget, how to work collaboratively with other universities and state agencies, how to bridge the research-practice gap, and so forth. I had also realized that the inner workings of other statewide programs would not be addressed via a traditional academic journal: Many of the services and training programs described here are very challenging to research effectively, and the understanding of regional models of service and training needed is more arcane than academic. It seemed like a volume with contributors offered me the best opportunity to involve colleagues whose innovative work I have admired for many years. This book began to take a clearer shape after several discussions with leaders such as Barbara Becker-Cottrill (see Chapter 5) and with the inspiration of other volumes such as Harris and Handleman's series on programs for young children (Handleman & Harris, 2000, 2006).

The first working outline was simply a collection of detailed descriptions of model regional and state programs for services, training, research, or policy, authored by program leaders themselves, which included a brief description of their own structure and funding. These are gathered together in Section II and are summarized in Figure 1. Although it was impossible to capture the truly excellent work being done throughout the United States and elsewhere, I also realized that it would be too cumbersome to develop

The West Virginia Autism Training Center (Chapter 5)

- Based at Marshall University, projects address training/services (the Family Focus Positive Behavior Support, Autism Mentors, College Support Program for Students with Asperger Syndrome), and research/policy (Autism Registry).

Pennsylvania Statewide & Regional Autism Programs (Chapter 6)

- Led by programs in the Pennsylvania Departments of Education and Public Welfare, projects address services (Adult ASD Waivers), training (Autism Initiative Applied Behavior Analysis Supports, National Autism Conference, regional autism centers), research (Pennsylvania Autism Census and Family Needs Assessment), and policy (Autism Focus Group & Task Force, Bureau of Autism Services).

Delaware Autism Program (Chapter 7)

- Based in the Delaware public school system, projects address training (Educational Classification, Behavior Support, Teacher Certification) and services (Extended Education and Support Services).

Indiana Resource Center for Autism (Chapter 8)

- Based at Indiana University, projects address a variety of service, training, and policy initiatives.

Autism Spectrum Disorder Program at McMaster Children's Hospital (Chapter 9)

- Based at a regional hospital in Ontario (Canada), projects address services (Community-Based Intensive Behavioral Intervention Program, ASD Birth-18 Pathway Program, and School Support Program) and research.

ASD Systems of Care for Children with ASD in Utah (Chapter 10)

- Based at the University of Utah, projects address services and related training (Early Detection in the Medical Home, Satellite ASD Services).

Kansas Instructional Support Network (Chapter 11)

- Based at the Department of Education, projects focus on training (Autism Interdisciplinary Teams, Autism Diagnostic Teams, Intense Support Teams, Structured Teaching).

Figure 1. Summary of statewide and regional programs covered in Section II.

and apply a rubric to ensure that the programs described here yielded the best outcomes. I sought to include agencies and organizations that not only have taken leadership in developing innovative programs but also have captured the variety of programs available in terms of the types of populations addressed, the domains they represented (e.g., education, health, community settings), and where they were based (e.g., in schools, hospitals, state/federal agencies, universities). With this variation, I hope that readers can identify opportunities that fit with their own unique circumstances and interests and that the specific initiatives described by the various programs highlighted in this book will themselves be replicated elsewhere.

SECTION III: EXEMPLARY NATIONAL INITIATIVES

As work on the book progressed, I learned of statewide initiatives that were inspired and shaped by the efforts of national organizations. By following closely the work of the Autism and Developmental Disabilities Monitoring (ADDM) network, I learned how a federal agency such as the Centers for Disease Control and Prevention (CDC) can mobilize a program of research to respond to emerging data (reports of high ASD prevalence in Brick Township—see Chapter 12) that, if verified, would have very significant policy implications. I also had the privilege of participating in some of the Act Early Summits initiated by the CDC, in partnership with the Association of University Centers on Disabilities. I was also excited by the work of the National Professional Development Center on Autism Spectrum Disorder (Chapter 13), whose efforts illustrate the potential depth and breadth of a well-designed training program that builds capacity by leveraging local resources. At this point, I realized that the leadership of organizations such as these could bring about a national strategy and so altered the title of the book accordingly.

SECTION IV: FACING AUTISM NATIONALLY: HOW TO IMPROVE SERVICES THROUGH TRAINING, RESEARCH, AND POLICY

What We Have Learned: How to Create Integrated Networks That Improve Access, Increase Capacity, Develop Expertise, and Address Meaningful Outcomes (Chapter 14): Repeated examples offered throughout this volume illustrate how different elements of our network (e.g., services, training, research, policy) operate independently within different domains (e.g., health, education, community supports) and often for different groups of individuals (e.g., those with and without intellectual disabilities, children versus adults). One important consequence is that the agencies and professionals have focused on narrow outcomes pertinent to their interests and have failed to capture broader and more meaningful outcomes. I suggest how a refocusing of our efforts on such outcomes at both the individual level (e.g., broad measures of well-being for children and families) and system level (e.g., ability to gain access to pivotal services), and explicit efforts to support caregivers, may help meet needs across the life span while also building bridges across domains and elements. I also touch on other aspects in each of the components of the network not addressed thus far: the division of the population according to age and presence of intellectual disability, building advocacy and awareness, and the perpetuation of domain- and element-specific silos.

    I reexamine how the elements of the network (services, training, research, and policy) grow in different ways that sometimes support accelerated growth and that at other times create barriers. For example, the lack of training resources clearly limits the rate at which overall service capacity can be scaled up and the likelihood that research and policy initiatives will improve outcomes. I conclude by offering some principles that describe how these elements (services, training, research, and policy) interact with the level of the agency and organization (e.g., local, regional, state, national) to suggest the best strategies to build an integrated network that increases overall capacity. For example, the level at which services should be provided depends on the number of people needing the services and the intensity with which the service must be delivered. Likewise, the level at which training resources are most efficiently and effectively developed depends on these factors, plus the intensity of the training required by professionals.

Where We Can Start: Immediate Opportunities for Improving the Lives of People with Autism Spectrum Disorder (Chapter 15): In the final chapter of the book, I briefly recap some of the principal themes and then outline examples of programs that integrate service, research, training, and policy and that cut across traditional domains at the local, regional, and state level to address pivotal needs for people with ASD. This includes programs better suited for regions and states with a poorly developed infrastructure (e.g., ASD identification) and others better suited for regions with more developed infrastructure (e.g., multiple levels of behavior support). I also propose other programs that offer the greatest impact relative to effort (e.g., implementation of specialized training for child care providers, paraprofessionals, and teachers). I conclude by revisiting some critical themes: the central role of caregivers, how to use evidence-based practice as fulcrum for change, and the need to build bridges with the community of those living with intellectual disability.

OTHER CROSS-CUTTING THEMES

One of the challenges of this volume was the number of themes cutting across elements and domains. At times, each of these themes appeared worthy of its own chapter or section but ultimately were subsumed into the chapters outlined in the previous sections.

Collaborating Across Agencies, Domains, and Sectors

The heterogeneity and complexity of ASD pose unique challenges to scaling up because most people with ASD will depend on interventions from a broad range of professionals and settings. As a result, a breakdown in support from any one system of care can limit the impact of all the others: An impeccably designed school-based program to address classroom-based sources of anxiety may fall short if opportunities for pharmacological management are not fully realized, and vice versa. Similarly, few agencies are well positioned to significantly address multiple elements (services versus training versus research versus policy) or address the needs of children and adults across the full spectrum of functioning. From the perspective of the child and the family, the distinctions between different elements, agencies, and even domains do not reflect a natural demarcation of needs within the child or family. These distinctions are an artifact of the functions of the institutions that have grown to address the spectrum of needs and populations. From a structural and a funding perspective, these functions and institutions have evolved to be independent and not interdependent, to be fiercely territorial and not collaborative, and to constitute separate silos and not a coordinated network. Barring significant new investments in funding, service professionals should therefore anticipate, however, that immediate improvements will require a new level of cross-agency understanding and collaboration.

Integrating Specialized and Frontline Services

Variations in the features of ASD across individuals and the life span pose other challenges to professionals who want to help. On the one hand, professionals who do not specialize in ASD are more likely to be on the front lines and potentially can act and intervene more quickly; with the right training and support, for example, pediatricians and family practitioners can quickly screen children and identify who may need more intensive and specialized assessment. But these frontline professionals may lack the training to provide more specialized supports or lack the confidence because they are unlikely to quickly amass experience with these more specialized service needs. On the other hand, individual professionals who choose to specialize in developmental disabilities may require years of training and experience to amass the breadth of understanding needed to work more independently. The need for specialists exaggerates the silo effect noted previously, because expertise is often defined in terms of the depth and not the breadth of knowledge. As a result, individuals and organizations naturally grow in expertise by narrowing their scope, especially as funders increasingly value such expertise. The more that individuals and organizations invest in developing expertise, the less inclined they are to recognize and value the expertise of others, and there is nothing more frustrating than trying to build consensus among "experts" whose narrow-mindedness is matched only by their arrogance. In addition, funders focus on the trappings of expertise (e.g., more highly specialized programs, more grants, more publications) and not on the evidence of real, lifelong outcomes reported across the spectrum of families. Professionals must simply accept that no one agency or individual—whatever their "expertise"—can ever meet all these needs without collaborating with others, and so service professionals must always work as a team. In the last section of this volume, I discuss ways to build these strategies into the planning process.

Other Themes

- *Caregivers:* The task of coordinating care and filling in the gaps in service across these different agencies and professionals often falls on the person with the least relevant formal training—the caregiver. Caregivers live with their hopes and dreams for a better life for their child as they grow into adulthood and so can more quickly grasp a life span perspective that recognizes the person's right to a reasonable quality of life. Given their importance, it is tragically ironic that the support and training available to caregivers is wildly inconsistent from one region to another. And yet the cost of failure in one case—that is, those resulting from the need to place a person with an ASD outside of the home—is probably equivalent to the cost of effectively supporting several people with ASD to maximize their full potential to enjoy a quality of life that the rest of us often take for granted.

- *Evidence-based practice (EBP):* The increasing emphasis on evidence-based practice may help to reshape training and provide new opportunities for collaboration between researchers and service providers. It also reveals important gaps in service development and oversight.

- *Intellectual disability:* There are many instances in which people with intellectual disabilities may benefit from services and supports identified as effective for people with ASD, and I think this has caused people to overlook the potential synergy between programs designed for both populations, especially in rural regions.

REFERENCES

Handleman, J.S., & Harris, S.L. (2000). *Preschool education programs for children with autism* (2nd ed.). Austin, TX: PRO-ED.

Handleman, J.S., & Harris, S.L. (2006). *School-age education programs for children with autism.* Austin, TX: PRO-ED.

To Monique, Nicholas, Margot, and Lili
for their patience during the many months it
took to complete this book
and to Jean Doehring
for her undying love and support of her granddaughter Margot

I

Understanding the Scope

1

About Autism Spectrum Disorder

Peter Doehring

In this chapter I begin to orient the reader to the challenge of designing and delivering a network of services, training, research, and policy at the regional, state, and national level. Specifically, I seek to accomplish this in three ways. First, I introduce readers to the general characteristics of autism spectrum disorder (ASD). Although many readers will already be familiar with essential features of ASD, I recognize that others may not, and I cannot begin to address my central goal of this book—to improve services, training, research, and policy by acting at the regional and national level—without assuring at least a basic understanding of the characteristics and associated needs of people with ASD that these initiatives are intended to address. Even for readers familiar with ASD, this discussion may offer new perspectives as I shift to address the challenge of developing an integrated network of support. For example, I believe that systems of services and supports to address the core social deficit have been slow to develop because this deficit has not been traditionally emphasized in the training of any one profession or in the services provided in any one community-based setting. By describing some of the more specialized needs of a subset of the population of people with ASD, I hope readers will better appreciate the challenge of developing effective *and* accessible interventions in a cost-effective matter. I am also cognizant that a comprehensive review of all possible elements is a Herculean undertaking. The goal of this review is, therefore, to highlight several characteristics of the broad population of people with ASD that are especially important in determining the nature, implementation, and impact of these elements of services, training, research, and policy. Readers seeking an understanding of the etiology of ASD, or a more thorough review of the characteristics of ASD or the needs of individuals with ASD, can find this information elsewhere (e.g., Johnson, Myers, & Council on Children with Disabilities, 2007; Levy, Mandell, & Schultz, 2009).

Second, I orient readers to some of the other commonly co-occurring conditions or disorders (e.g., intellectual disability, challenging behaviors, other psychiatric or physical conditions). Although the capacity of practitioners to help people living with ASD has grown tremendously since the 1990s, this help has been delivered via a system of services, training, research, and policy originally designed to help these associated conditions (e.g., developmental disability services, behavioral/mental health, physical health) and not ASD. Any efforts to improve the lives of people with ASD must build, at least in the short term, on systems of supports not originally designed for ASD but for these other co-occurring conditions. I believe that this presents an opportunity and not a barrier: These co-occurring conditions may paradoxically both complicate the treatment of ASD (and at times have a greater impact on functioning than the ASD itself) and offer more immediate opportunities to improve the lives of people living with ASD. Some associated characteristics (e.g., anxiety) may be more responsive to intervention than the core features (e.g., deficits in reciprocal social understanding). Other associated characteristics (e.g., intellectual disability [ID]) respond to some of the behavioral interventions traditionally associated with ASD. This may open the door to new cross-population collaborations that may help to build capacity synergistically; for example, teacher training programs that integrate principles of applied behavior analysis (ABA) into the education of all people with IDs regardless of whether they also have ASD.

Finally, I orient readers to the many different ways ASD can present itself across the life span, and the many different life circumstances faced by families living with ASD, via a series of case studies at the end of the chapter. These case studies put a human face to ASD and help counter the dry, detailed descriptions that, of necessity, make up much of this book. I also seek to convey the plight of people living with ASD across the United States and to inject the urgency needed to drive research and policy initiatives. I believe that if society is to ever decrease the tremendous disparities in access to quality education and health care the next wave of innovation must include not only the increasingly sophisticated and targeted interventions developed in traditional academic settings, but also programs to ensure that interventions already known to be effective are disseminated as broadly as possible. I elaborate on these case studies in subsequent chapters to express in human terms the impact of improvements to the network of support for people with ASD.

ESSENTIAL CHARACTERISTICS
OF AUTISM SPECTRUM DISORDER

Since the late 1990s there has been increasing convergence regarding the core features of ASD, with some exceptions. Relative to other disorders, there is much higher agreement that the prevailing taxonomies at the time this book was written—the criteria outlines in the *Diagnostic and Statistical Manual of Mental Disorders Fourth Edition, Text Revision* (*DSM-IV-TR*; American Psychiatric Association, 2000) and the International Statistical Classification of Diseases and Related Health Problems, *Tenth Edition* (*ICD-10*; World Health Organization, 2008)—capture the essential features of ASD.

Deficits in Social Interaction

All people with ASD demonstrate deficits in reciprocal social interaction, the specific nature of which varies somewhat from individual to individual (Carter, Davis, Klin, & Volkmar, 2005). These deficits include difficulties in using a variety of means to regulate interaction, immature peer relations, a failure to share interests and enjoyment, and a lack of social and emotional reciprocity. Infants often demonstrate delays and deficits in essential skills such as joint attention that may manifest during the first year of life. Other deficits in social and emotional understanding may also be evident very early on, including elements as varied as recognition of faces and of emotions. Together, these have a lifelong impact on the development of friendships and relationships, even among individuals who are otherwise very successful in their careers, and can contribute to the development of other disorders such as depression and anxiety. Although difficulties in any one of these areas are sometimes evident in a number of other disorders, it is the presence and the severity of multiple difficulties in social understanding and interaction that most clearly distinguishes ASD from other disorders.

Even though deficits in social skills are generally recognized as lying at the core of ASD, across the spectrum and the life span, society has been slow to develop effective systems of support for several reasons. Social deficits are the most subtle and the most difficult to assess because success or failure is not measured by knowledge but, rather, must be assessed by considering actual interactions with others across multiple contexts. Until recently, deficits in social skill have also been addressed indirectly; for example, communication training helps facilitate interaction, and the push for the inclusion of all children in typical community settings is based partly on the presumption that exposure itself facilitates social development. Since 2000, professionals have witnessed the development of training protocols for specific skills (e.g., joint attention), broad programs with an emphasis on social-emotional development (e.g., Relationship Development Intervention [RDI] and Social Communication, Emotional Regulation, and Transactional Supports [SCERTS] Model), and interventions that seek to use peers to facilitate training (Ferraioli & Harris, 2011). These advances have been spurred by the recognition that a relative lack of social skills may be one of the primary impediments to full community participation for adolescents and adults with Asperger syndrome (AS). Nevertheless, efforts to implement training in social skills are often fragmented because no single professional group or agency assumes leadership for developing such programs. Schools have not traditionally focused explicitly on social skills, and some professionals weave social skills into other group interventions more traditionally associated with their professions (e.g., speech pathologists may teach conversation skills, occupational therapists may teach peer play skills) (refer to Chapter 2 for a more thorough discussion).

Patterns of Unusual Interests and Behaviors

Most people with ASD present with a pattern of unusual interests and behaviors. This can range from interests that are odd in their focus (e.g., a fascination with ceiling fans or a preoccupation with hair) or in their intensity and persistence (e.g., a lifelong and exclusive interest in dinosaurs that pervades the person's play and conversation). Such preoccupations can interfere with the development of shared interests with peers or with integration into community settings when the individual seeks to avoid certain sensory stimuli (e.g., they become anxious in anticipation of the school's fire drill). Obsessions and compulsions, or a rigid adherence to nonfunctional routines, can be disruptive in the home or classroom and, in more extreme cases, can result in aggression or extreme anxiety when the attempt to act on the compulsion is blocked. Other behavior problems or social stigma can result from a preoccupation with the sensory qualities of objects—the way they look, smell, or feel. For example, a child fascinated with hair may approach strangers in a store to stroke their hair or to yank their hair.

The enigmatic variability in the types of unusual interests/behaviors and in their impact on functioning illustrates the need for highly individualized approaches, a need that makes the development of services and supports particularly challenging. For some individuals, the unusual interest or behavior may require the modification of educational or therapeutic approaches but will not fundamentally drive treatment. Some modifications may help limit the impact (e.g., a behavior plan may be needed to help a child stop playing a favorite video game) while other modifications can turn the interest into an opportunity (e.g., using the video game to reinforce appropriate behavior). For other children, the unusual interest can play a significant role in determining positive or negative outcomes. For example, a child with an unusual sensitivity to tactile stimuli may seek to continuously wrap him- or herself up in his or her arms or in the arms of a caregiver and may become extremely aggressive or self-injurious with this type of stimulation is interrupted (Freeman, Horner, & Reichle, 2002). Another child fascinated with busses and bus schedules may turn this interest into a career, providing information to callers seeking the best bus route. There is no assessment that can easily predict what the positive or negative impact of a given unusual interest or behavior might be. This places pressure on disciplines, professionals, and agencies to provide more comprehensive training.

Deficits in Communication

Many people with ASD also present with qualitative impairments in communication (Paul & Sutherland, 2005; Prizant & Wetherby, 2005). The pattern and severity of communication impairments depends in part on the developmental level of the child. Younger or more developmentally disabled individuals may manifest a lack of language together with a failure to compensate through nonverbal means (e.g., pointing or showing objects), and such deficits may prompt the parent to express concerns to a professional. More subtle deficits in pretend play and social imitative games (e.g., peek-a-boo) may become more prominent at a later age. Most children with ASD who acquire phrase speech nonetheless demonstrate other difficulties or unusual features. They may find it impossible to build conversations with others around topics of mutual interest. Their speech may also be characterized by unusual pitch, volume, or intonation or may include odd or repetitive phrases.

Communication deficits associated with ASD illustrate how effects can cascade if not addressed early and complicate the task of intervention if that intervention is not coordinated across professionals and settings. For example, people with ASD unable to communicate their essential wants, needs, and interests are at a higher risk for developing significant and associated behavior problems. These individuals essentially learn to "speak" through their behavior, conveying to a caregiver what he or she wants or does. The caregiver must partner with a behavior analyst or other professional to decipher the communicative function of the aggression, self-injury, or other challenging behavior, and then develop and implement a plan to replace the behavior with a functionally equivalent communication alternative. This may require the involvement of a speech pathologist to identify and begin to implement the best type of augmentative communication system (e.g., using signs, pictures, devices). Providing frequent and consistent opportunities to replace the problem behavior with its communicative equivalent requires coordination across home and school for the child to not revert to the established patterns of behavior that proved effective in communicating his or her needs in the past.

Other Key Characteristics

The Evolution of Autism Spectrum Disorder as a Spectrum Disorder   One of the most significant changes since the mid-1990s has been the recognition and acceptance of autism as a spectrum disorder. Across this field—and in this volume—authors now refer to an autism _spectrum_ with social deficits at its core but with considerable variability in the specific nature of the social deficits and the presence of other key features (i.e., impairments in communication and patterns of unusual interests and behaviors) from one person with ASD to another. These refinements are consistent with—if not informed by— the revised approaches to scoring instruments such as the Autism Diagnostic Observation

Schedule (ADOS; Gotham, Risi, Pickles, & Lord, 2007). Not all states recognize all ASDs as eligible for educational services or behavioral intervention; some focus primarily on autism and others exclude autism or ASD if not accompanied by ID. As the shift emphasizing a single spectrum disorder (with varying degrees of severity) continues to evolve, perhaps all states will someday recognize all levels of ASD as eligible for specialized supports and programs, as per the recommendation of the National Research Council (Committee on Educational Interventions for Children with Autism, 2001).

Autism Spectrum Disorder as a Developmental Disorder ASD is also a developmental disorder, such that the number and types of symptoms vary with the age and the level of functioning of the individual. While a core social deficit is always evident, the specific manifestation of this deficit—and of related deficits in communication and in the pattern of interests and behaviors—varies with development. ASD looks different in toddlers versus children versus adolescents versus adults, and in people with and without co-occurring IDs. As a result, additional training is needed for an individual to become a reliable diagnostician for all ages because one cannot simply generalize from experience with one age group to another. More important, different interventions are required for individuals at different ages and functioning levels, again necessitating additional training.

Autism Spectrum Disorder Across the Life Span Higher prevalence estimates for ASD are now widely accepted, and it seems likely that most children with ASD will grow up to be adults with ASD. The concept of a cure is at least unrealistic in the short term and perhaps undesirable in the long term for those who value their different-ness. In some states, the number of adults with autism is projected to increase by more than 600% between 2005 and 2015 (Lawer & Mandel, 2009). Parents and policy makers are now grappling with the reality that tens of thousands of adults will begin to require support. This growing need will soon outstrip the services that are now available, reveal the tremendous gap in the understanding of which interventions are effective for adults, and represent a competing interest in the attempt to prioritize changes in policy. On a more positive note, this will bring attention to one of the hardest-working but most neglected portion of the population—caregivers who elect to support their adult offspring in the home. The general increase of adults caring for other adults in the home may spur the development of new models of community supports. Adults on the spectrum and those who advocate for themselves also provide a new and compelling voice in the disabilities movement.

The Prevalence of Autism Spectrum Disorder Many of the discussions surrounding ASD since the 1990s have been informed—if not driven by—shifts in estimates of prevalence from the broadly accepted rates of 1 in 2,500 individuals in the 1990s to reports in 2010 that it exceeds 1 in 100. The popular and political response to the new scientific findings surrounding prevalence, and the factors contributing to it, has been unprecedented. Never have the pronouncements of researchers consistently garnered so much attention in the popular media, been so eagerly anticipated by advocates, or driven policy discussions at the local, state, and national level.

The popular interest in ASD and the ways in which research findings have begun to shape policy create new pressures on both scientists and policy makers. When disseminating their findings, scientists must now not only communicate with the technological precision demanded by academic journals but also try to prevent sensational overgeneralizations by the popular press. Scientists truly driven to achieve real change in their lifetimes will be excited by this challenge; will invest the energy needed to partner effectively with advocates, professionals, and policy makers; and perhaps help to usher in a new era of accountability. Other scientists will continue to seek refuge in the dusty halls of academia, comfort themselves with dry debates about arcane elements of methodology, and risk making their work increasingly irrelevant to the day-to-day struggles of real people living with ASD.

CO-OCCURRING AND ASSOCIATED CONDITIONS

With improvements in the identification of ASD and acceptance of higher-than-expected prevalence, researchers and clinicians have begun to recognize that some conditions that co-occur or are co-mingled with ASD merit closer attention (Levy et al., 2009). As I described earlier in this chapter, these conditions may be more debilitating than the ASD itself or be more amenable to intervention. Disentangling the contribution of ASD and these co-occurring conditions to the nature of the presenting problem, and then to the identification of the most effective intervention, can demand more intensive training and experience. But these interrelationships may also allow us to draw on techniques developed and then refined for other populations. I introduce some of the more important co-occurring conditions here and return in the final chapter of this volume to describe how regional, state, and national initiatives help to more rapidly disseminate emerging interventions.

Intellectual Disability

Perhaps the most common co-occurring condition is ID. Intellectual disability has been estimated to occur in 70%–75% of people with ASD (Committee on Children with Disabilities, 2001), but more recent reports suggest that this might need to be revised down to 50% (Yeargin-Allsopp et al., 2003). Compared to those with ID but not ASD, individuals with ID and ASD are more likely to have very uneven skill profiles with areas of relatively greater strength and greater weakness. For these individuals, estimates of overall ID derived from traditional cognitive tests may be less meaningful, and less accurate in predicting real-world performance. When ID is complicated by ASD, combining the cognitive assessment with measures of adaptive functioning can be more valuable in estimating overall needs and in targeting specific skills that impact day-to-day functioning (Tsatsanis, Saulnier, Sparrow, & Cicchetti, 2011).

Whereas the interrelationship between ASD and ID has yet to be elucidated, and the presence of the core deficits of ASD on top of ID clearly complicates education and treatment, many of the techniques, services, and supports developed to address the deficits in other academic skills and skills of daily life in people with ID are nonetheless relevant to people with ASD combined with ID. Moreover, some of the service needs of people with ID and ASD can arguably be better ascribed to the accompanying ID than the ASD per se. This overlap of ASD and ID presents important opportunities for developing local, regional, and national programs. For example, many programs and initiatives originally developed for people with ID at each of these levels can be—and often are—adapted to accommodate the need of the subset that also has ASD. Efforts to improve services for people with ASD can therefore begin by first considering how to build on services for people with IDs. Given that the percentage of people with ID is at least as great as that with ASD, considering both groups together yields a population whose local service needs are clearly too large to ignore. Services for people with ID may also benefit from the upsurge in interest in ASD. Such as upsurge may refocus and revitalize efforts to improve services and supports to the broader population of people with ID, efforts that seem to have lost some of the drive that helped pass the Individuals with Disabilities Education Act in 1990.

Problem Behaviors

Problem behaviors are also common in ASD. These can range from behaviors that are mildly stigmatizing (e.g., odd body movements) or disruptive (e.g., loud vocalizations) to behaviors that can be extremely dangerous to the individual (e.g., self-injury) or to others (e.g., aggression) (Powers, Palmieri, D'Eramo, & Powers, 2011). Some of these behaviors are common among people with ID, perhaps arising from the individual's inability to effectively communicate his or her basic wants and needs, to make sense of his or her world, or to enjoy a reasonable degree of independence and autonomy. Other behaviors may stem more directly from the pattern of unusual interests and responses characteristic of ASD: A toddler may be attracted to hair and pull it because of its unique sensory qualities, a school-age child may be petrified of fire drills in school because the sound is excruciating; an obsessive adult may become aggressive when he or she is blocked when trying to rearrange objects on a shelf. Sometimes the failure to naturally develop an understanding of and response to others may deprive the individual of the most natural incentives to behave—for example, to remain closely connected to the people around him or her.

Regardless of the etiology of these behaviors, their impact can be more significant than the ASD itself. In some cases, it is the problem behaviors and not the ASD that results in removal from the home and placement in highly specialized and costly programs for many years, if not for the rest of the individual's life. Now that evidence-based practices designed to prevent or reduce problem behavior are being identified (National Autism Center, 2009; Powers et al., 2011), professionals face the opportunity—and challenge—of implementation. In this regard, efforts to scale up services will have to draw on the new fields of translational research and technologies of implementation science. Given the cost of some of the services necessitated by more intense problem behaviors, failure comes at a very high price.

Other Psychiatric Disorders and Medical Conditions

The increased recognition of ASD, and the ability of individuals with ASD to communicate the source of their distress, has raised awareness of other mental health problems such as anxiety and depression. As with other challenging behaviors, these problems may have origins similar to those of other populations, or may derive some of their form and intensity from ASD itself. Anxiety is evident in a significant proportion of people with ASD (Towbin, Pradella, Gorrindo, Pine, & Leibenluft, 2005) and sometimes appears to stem directly from core ASD features (e.g., when the person is fearful of certain environments or social situations). Those with ASD may be at risk for depression or even suicide (Leyfer et al., 2006; Stewart, Barnard, Pearson, Hasan, & O'Brien, 2006), perhaps as a result of the challenges they face finding meaningful work or relationships. It is unclear whether co-occurring attention deficit-hyperactivity disorder (ADHD) has a common origin, although there are clearly cases of significant overlap in symptomatology (Holtmann, Bolte, & Poustka, 2007; Koyama, Tachimor, Osada, & Kurita, 2006).

Each of these co-occurring psychiatric conditions presents potential barriers to optimal outcomes and ready opportunities for improvement and collaboration. Professionals may have difficulty disentangling ASD from these related disorders, especially as the latter evolve over time. Take, for example, a school-age child with co-occurring ASD and anxiety who acts out in certain classroom settings: Does this reflect growing anxiety over increasingly difficult work, a behavioral response functioning to help the child escape from demands, or the interaction of both factors? Is the adolescent with ASD withdrawing from peers because he cannot navigate the high school culture, or is he depressed because everyone has a girlfriend but him? Community-based practitioners who hesitate to address some of these debilitating symptoms, because they lack expertise in ASD per se, may fail to recognize how they can help with medication or other therapies that specifically target these other psychiatric conditions.

Similar barriers and opportunities are evident with respect to co-occurring or comorbid medical conditions. People with ASD are at higher risk for a seizure disorder, with estimates as high as 38% for a sample of people with autism and intellectual disability who are now adults (Danielsson, Gillberg, Billstedt, Gillberg, & Olsson, 2005). Other problems of daily life common among people with ASD can be very taxing for the family and include such problems as chronic sleep, feeding, or gastrointestinal (GI) difficulties. As with the other mental health problems described earlier, many of these conditions can be effectively addressed via treatments that are not specific to ASD. The potential for training programs to address these co-occurring conditions has already been recognized in the Autism Treatment Networks, which are seeking to develop and disseminate best practice guidelines for sleep and GI problems.

✳ Case Studies

Here I describe several case studies that illustrate the range of skills and behavior problems that might characterize and accompany ASD and how these might vary over time. Each case is a collage combining my personal experiences and my experiences with different children, families, and programs with whom I have worked throughout the years. Each case is primarily a snapshot of a particular period in a child's life to set the stage for later discussions of how specific elements of service, training, research, and policy can have a critical impact on outcomes. I include these case studies for readers who may find some of the discussions of training, research, services, and policy that constitute much of this book too abstract or esoteric. But I hope that the case studies will help service professionals envision how their efforts can ultimately improve the outcomes and quality of life of people such as those described herein.

Asif's Story

Asif is a 2-year-old boy. His parents are graduate students who recently emigrated from an East Asian country and who live in the small capital of a Midwestern state with a large East Asian community. Two years ago Asif's parents brought his grandparents over to provide child care to him and his older brother while his parents completed their studies. Asif's parents had originally become concerned that Asif was not meeting his developmental milestones in language, and they expressed these concerns to their pediatrician at the scheduled well-child checkup. Their pediatrician had recently undergone training regarding the warning signs of ASD provided by the state chapter of the American Academy of Pediatrics (AAP) to disseminate new AAP standards, funded via a federal program established in response

the growing prevalence of ASD, and disseminated via a series of trainings in different regions of the state. The pediatrician determined via a standardized screening
checklist that Asif was at risk for ASD. The checklist also suggested that Asif had
a lack of response to other people, a complete lack of interest in peers, a lack of
language, and a fascination with cars. The pediatrician scheduled a separate visit
to conduct a more formal evaluation and he invited an advocate/translator from
a local East Asian community group (see the discussion later in the chapter) who
knew the family, because the grandparents did not speak much English. The pediatrician had previously reached out to this particular East Asian community because
it constituted a growing proportion of his practice. Anticipating specific questions
about ASD that the family might have in light of their culture and faith, the advocate
also joined subsequent meetings at which the pediatrician provided more guidance
regarding follow-up services.

The pediatrician confirmed a diagnosis of ASD, communicated some concerns
about Asif's overall development, and referred the family to the early intervention
(EI) agency in the county. The EI agency provided services locally through a contract
with three different providers: new referrals were posted on the EI agency website,
and a provider could pick up the case if he or she could ensure a rapid turnaround. By
encouraging private providers to move quickly to initiate services, the EI agency was
able to improve its ability to initiate EI within timelines specified in federal regulations
(its failure to do so had led to citations and the generation of an action plan following
an audit by the state developmental disability [DD] agency).

A psychologist with the EI agency administered standardized tests to confirm
mild developmental delays and establish Asif's eligibility for services. The EI agency
began 10 hours per week of generic in-home intervention with a paraprofessional
supervised by an early childhood educator and a speech language pathologist (SLP)
and occupational therapist (OT) who each provided 1 hour per week of therapy. Training provided by the SLP in the use of the Picture Exchange Communication System
(PECS) (which the SLP learned about by attending a 2-day workshop offered annually
in the region) helped to kick-start Asif's speech, while support from the OT helped the
parents adapt their play strategies and materials to Asif's needs.

The advocate/translator was partially funded by a pilot grant from a national advocacy organization to the East Asian community group. The community group also
benefited from training and other pilot funding provided by federally funded parent
information centers, and the combination of federal and private funding (from a local
foundation) was used to support a series of workshops to help parents of children
with ASD and ID advocate for services. Asif's parents have since participated in this
training, learning a lot about the characteristics of ASD. They became particularly
excited about the potential offered by EI programs that were more intensive and more
specialized in ASD, but they still did not understand where and how to gain access to
these and other important services. Asif's parents are especially interested because
they recently began to suspect that Asif can read, an ability that the paraprofessional
in the EI program has yet to recognize or tap into. Connections made through the
community group with other families in the community were also important: The family had grown increasingly isolated while struggling with their concerns about Asif's
development but had since found other families with children such as Asif with whom

they could comfortably socialize. The families worked together to help the preschool at their mosque accommodate the needs of their children.

Asif's pediatrician also referred his parents to a regional children's hospital when he became increasingly concerned that the lapses in Asif's responsivity may sometimes result from petit mal seizures. Careful questioning revealed that some of these lapses may result from episodes of reflux, and an evaluation by a gastroenterologist led to medication and dietary changes in an attempt to resolve the lapses. While a subsequent electroencephalogram (EEG) did not reveal abnormalities consistent with a seizure disorder, careful observation by the parents and EI services of specific episodes helped the family and neurologist determine that these were in fact seizures. Noticeable improvements were seen in Asif's engagement and a decrease in these episodes after seizure medication was carefully titrated up by Asif's pediatrician in consultation with Asif's neurologist.

Evan's Story

Evan is a 5-year-old Caucasian boy. He lives with his parents and an older brother in a rural region with very few specialized services. His parents' ongoing struggle to make ends meet was complicated by the lack of work in a flagging rural economy, and so each had often juggled multiple, low-paying, part-time jobs. Evan had been flagged by his physician with possible moderate developmental delay just before his third birthday (his physician had also considered referring Evan because of long-standing problems with aggression and activity levels). The physician referred the family to EI services, for which Evan was eligible until age 3 years. EI services were provided free of charge by a county agency for developmental disabilities, but were delivered by early educators (through a contract with a private regional agency) who traveled to the family's home.

Evan's physician was a recently graduated family practitioner who loved working in this small community. He had himself grown up in the same small town and returned to take over the practice of his own doctor. His decision was also influenced by a federal program that offered reduced interest rates on student loans for physicians who set up practice in rural regions. This physician soon appreciated the need for this program, because two practices in neighboring towns closed up when their physicians retired, and his own practice grew very quickly.

Evan's parents were already frequent visitors, trying to manage his chronic ear infections, which were initially thought to explain his long-standing sleep problems and which, in turn, were thought to contribute to severe and difficult-to-control tantrums. Evan's mother could not always rely, however, on Evan's physician for help: She resorted to a local, privately run walk-in emergency care clinic because Evan frequently became aggressive in the crowded reception area while waiting for his physician. Evan's parents had tried the emergency room at the regional hospital 40 miles away when a spike in his fever sparked more intense aggression, but the long drive (complicated further because the family had only one car), long wait, and subsequent battles with the insurance company to clear up billing issues had dissuaded them from using the emergency room again. In contrast, Evan's insurance readily reimbursed the local clinic. Evan's physician hesitated to provide markedly more extensive care for

Evan, in part because he did not receive any additional reimbursement for this kind of involvement. In fact, the walk-in clinic became so familiar with Evan that they adapted their practice to accommodate him, ushering him immediately into an exam room to prevent the crowded waiting room from precipitating aggression. The clinic was part of a regional chain that had learned to pay special attention to the needs of its clients when expanding into a new area. Evan's parents were particularly grateful for this service because their frequent absences from work required for Evan's care was jeopardizing their careers.

Following their physician's referral to EI services, a psychologist at the EI agency conducted a developmental assessment that identified significant delays and established Evan's eligibility for EI services. The EI agency referred the family to a case manager at the county's department of developmental disability service. Evan's case manager completed her training as a social worker 20 years prior, but had had begun to benefit from training in ASD offered by the county DD agency (12 hours in ASD training as part of its new employee orientation) and annual ASD conferences organized by the state department of education and the state department of public welfare (both agencies had recently received additional funding from the state legislature to increase ASD training). Evan's case manager helped his parents complete the paperwork needed to gain access to federal support (Supplemental Security Income [SSI]) and supplemental services and supports through the state. The case worker knew that respite was a supplemental (e.g., not a mandated) service covered by SSI, but the growing number of applicants together with shrinking state funding meant that Evan's parents were only allotted about $250 annually to help cover respite. Nonetheless, the case manager was able to direct the family to a resource from the state chapter of a national advocacy organization that provided an e-mail listing of respite providers. She also directed the family to community-based behavioral health and rehabilitation services (BHRS) for help with Evan's ongoing sleep and aggression. BHRS was provided by a series of private providers through contracts with the county DD services. BHRS services were undergoing significant expansion because the state had recently passed autism insurance legislation (providing more than $30,000 of additional support annually to eligible families) and was just completing the writing of regulations. Overwhelmed by the diagnosis, the meetings to start Evan's special education services, and the stress of his ongoing problems with sleep, aggression, and anxiety, the family did not, however, immediately pursue BHRS support. They were also discouraged because Evan lacked a diagnosis of ASD, which decreased access to some BHRS services.

When he turned 3 years old, Evan transitioned smoothly into special education services in his local school district. This transition was relatively seamless because it was facilitated by a series of meetings between EI and education services (as required by state and federal regulations) beginning 6 months prior to the transition. Although the special preschool program operated only 7 hours during 2 mornings per week (other, more affluent school districts offered 12.5 hours during 5 mornings per week), at least it provided transportation to and from school. Evan's preschool special education teacher had gone back to school to obtain a master's degree with a specialized certification in autism at a small regional campus of the state college. The campus had received many requests to offer a specialized ASD certificate after

the state and the school district recognized such certificates through pay increases
for teachers, but the campus lacked the resources to develop and support this level
of specialized training. Using autism teacher competencies recently adopted by a national professional organization, the state college created a curriculum that included
a mix and schedule of courses aimed at accommodating teachers who were already
working: introduction to ASD and to methods and curricula delivered traditionally by
on-site faculty during an intense summer institute, courses in specific behavioral and
educational teaching methods strategies delivered online during the spring and fall
semesters (to better accommodate working teachers), course credit for attendance
at an annual state autism conference, and a "practicum" including on-site and web-
based coaching combined with a series of day-long case conferences. The state legislature also offered reduced tuition for continuing education undertaken by public
school teachers, while the university integrated the ASD certificate into a master's
degree program.

   During her certificate coursework, Evan's teacher learned about the warning signs
of ASD and how to administer and score a screening instrument for ASD (this was part
of the national standards established for autism teacher competencies). The teacher
referred the parents to their physician for follow-up. While their physician shared
these concerns, he did not feel entirely comfortable diagnosing ASD without conducting a more thorough evaluation (he already had difficulty keeping up with families
after his partner retired) and hesitated to refer the family to the only developmental
pediatrician in the region (who was about 100 miles away and had a 10-month waiting list). After other families expressed similar concerns during the next 6 months,
the physician hired a practicing nurse practitioner (PNP) to finally ease the load. The
PNP eagerly assumed day-to-day management of children with developmental needs
because she had a brother with ASD. She gathered information via questionnaires
and observations, and, in consultation with the physician, assigned to Evan an ASD
diagnosis. The developmental pediatrician eventually saw Evan, confirmed the ASD
diagnosis, and provided feedback to Evan's nurse and physician to help them know
when this kind of consultation was needed. The developmental pediatrician provided
consultation even though it was not reimbursed because it helped to ease what were
becoming impossibly long waiting lists.

   Evan's nurse had completed an innovative training program in ASD diagnosis
targeting PNPs and funded by a state agency concerned about delays and disparities in ASD diagnosis. The training program was funded by the state's developmental
disability services as part of a state plan developed in coordination with the Centers
for Disease Control and Prevention, in an attempt to increase access to diagnosis of
ASD. The state agency had first funded research to identify pockets of potential underidentification (including Evan's region), and in the second phase funded targeted
training that encouraged the collaboration between experienced diagnosticians and
community-based practitioners.

   When the developmental pediatrician saw Evan, he also diagnosed him with an
anxiety disorder and recommended antianxiety medication. He felt that Evan's anxiety was inexorably intertwined with his aggression, toileting (occasional bowel ac-
cidents despite multiple attempts at toilet training, and occasional fecal play if he
was not changed immediately), and sleep problems. He had just read a review of

evidence-based practices suggesting that behavior interventions may be more successful than medication in the long-term management of anxiety, elopement, and toileting, and so he also urged Evan's nurse to push for behavior support in the school and community. He also specifically directed Evan's physician and nurse to a protocol under development that used a combination of simple behavioral interventions and a short-term medication regimen to reinstate normal sleep patterns. The development of this protocol occurred through an intervention research network initiated by a private national foundation and subsequently expanded through federal funding.

The nurse's increased involvement benefited Evan in other ways. After she joined the clinic to decrease the wait times for patients such as Evan and Evan's mother stopped relying on the emergency walk-in clinic, they were finally able to better manage Evan's ear infections. Evan's nurse began to implement the sleep intervention, and his sleep began to improve. In coordination with the developmental pediatrician, she was able to adjust his antianxiety medication. Once Evan began elementary school, his nurse also reached out to his school nurse in anticipation of questions she might have about his ASD and his behavior.

With the encouragement of his nurse, especially following his improvements in sleep, Evan's parents followed up on the case manager's recommendation to pursue community-based BHRS. The behavior specialist through the BHRS agency helped the family recognize how rigid Evan was in his routines and interests and how changes could trigger anxiety (especially when he was tired) and aggression (so that he would be left alone to retreat into the repetitive speech and flicking of string that seemed to calm him). The specialist helped Evan learn how to signal to his parents when he anxious, helped the parents recognize the calming effect of these repetitive behaviors, and helped to shape the flicking of string into the twisting of a rubber band he wore on his wrist. The addition of 10 hours of behavior support in the home helped Evan's parents become comfortable in implementing these interventions. The behavior specialist's earlier experience as a paraprofessional in a specialized school for those with ASD and the training she was completing to become a Board Certified Behavior Analyst (BCBA) helped her to target her recommendations.

Evan's parents became increasingly concerned with the start of elementary school in his neighborhood. Evan's public school program had little experience with ASD, and rarely did the school's behavior manager offer more than the completion of a cursory functional behavioral assessment and the development of a generic intervention plan (research reviews describing the need for a more comprehensive protocol had yet to be translated into practical protocols). This quickly changed during the first week of school when the school suspended Evan after he attacked a classmate. The suspension triggered an immediate meeting between the parents and the school (as required by state and federal regulations) during which the parents shared the behavior plan developed for the home, and the implementation of these interventions (plus several others) helped Evan to cope with these new routines. A classroom aide was assigned to Evan to help him to learn how to use and follow a schedule and to support his need for individual accommodations.

The parents reported to Evan's ID case manager that they had been unable to find an after-school program that accommodated children who still wore diapers, and the case manager encouraged the parents to renew their efforts to toilet train Evan.

Evan's parents called a meeting at the school, invited community-based behavioral support, and requested that toilet training be added as a goal for both school- and home-based services. The behavioral health provider initially responded that the school was barred by state regulations from providing "habilitative" services (e.g., toileting). Evan's case manager successfully argued that his inconsistent toileting represented a regression brought on by anxiety. The behavioral health provider concurred, and a simple program was developed that included a rich schedule of toileting, an intensive period of handwashing (which addressed a hitherto unrecognized source of anxiety for Evan—contamination from feces), and a rich schedule of reinforcement for "clean pants." While the behavioral health provider was clearing this change in policy with the national office, state regulations for autism insurance legislation was completed, clearing the way for reimbursement for these "habilitative" services. With overall reductions in anxiety, improvements in sleep, and collaboration between the classroom and the in-home behavioral support, Evan was quickly toilet trained. Within three weeks, he was out of diapers, his family initiated after-school care, and Evan's father returned to work.

Joshua's Story

Joshua is an 8-year-old African American boy. His parents are wealthy lawyers living in an affluent suburb of a large city. They already have a 14-year-old son, Mark, with classic autism, as well as a typical 11-year-old daughter. At age 5 years Joshua was originally diagnosed with ADHD by his pediatrician following a referral from his school's psychologist. Since then, Joshua's pediatrician (located in his community) and his psychiatrist (located in a psychiatric center in the city) had explored the effectiveness of various medications for ADHD, but with little success.

Joshua's teacher had attended a training workshop offered by a specialized ASD research clinic at a university in the city, and suspected that the extent of Joshua's social skill deficits and obsessive interests may be indicative of ASD in addition to, or instead of, ADHD. After consulting with the school psychologist, they shared their concerns with the family, cautioning that untangling ADHD and ASD can be difficult. The teacher also shared with the family that the specialized ASD research clinic offered free workshops through a local parent advocacy group to help families learn about EI and advocate for community-based resources. These free workshops were initially introduced by the research clinic as a condition of a federal grant it applied for (and subsequently obtained) to test a new intervention; the grant program had required that applicants provide education in related elements free of charge. The center continued the workshops even after grant ended because it helped the research clinic connect with the ASD community, increased interest in participation in research, and provided a new opportunity for interns to gain experience. The clinic also offered state-of-the-art evaluations free of charge as part of a study of siblings, and so Joshua's family elected to participate in the research. A formal and extensive evaluation of Joshua, conducted as part of the research, confirmed a diagnosis of AS because the research-based diagnostic protocol was able to disentangle ASD and ADHD.

This diagnosis helped crystallize several characteristics never fully explained by the diagnosis of ADHD: Joshua's extreme rigidity and reactivity to change, his difficulty reading social cues and situations, his above-average intelligence (especially his superior math skills), and his poor motor coordination. Through the advocacy workshop offered by the research clinic, Joshua's family learned about a speech pathologist in private practice who ran a weekly social skills training group. The speech pathologist had recently graduated from a training program at a regional college with a heavy emphasis on ASD; this emphasis was created when the faculty had specifically selected a new faculty member with specialized ASD doctoral training with the expectation that she would lead the development of ASD specific coursework and practica sites. The social skills training group helped reduce peer conflicts and ended the string of expulsions from various after-school programs. Deficits in social skills also contributed to Joshua's frustrating relationship with baseball: His prodigious knowledge of baseball (including a fascination with statistics) contrasted sharply with his clumsiness and his inability to "read" the game and anticipate the intentions of his teammates during the game. Joshua's parents were able speak with Joshua's coach to obtain some accommodations (e.g., additional time in drills to work on his ball handling) and suggestions for other resources (e.g., a DVD series describing different kinds of plays in baseball).

Even before the diagnosis of AS, Joshua's parents had successfully advocated for accommodations at his charter school, which specialized in serving children with mild learning disabilities. They had already sought out a progressive, overnight summer camp program in the region for typical children that offered additional camp counselor support for campers with special needs. This support was obtained through a work-study program designed to provide students at a local technical college, completing an associate degree in paraprofessional support, with fieldwork experience (credit for summer camp placement was also offered to students outside of this program working as camp counselors). These students participated in a week-long introductory training that was provided via a contract with a specialized regional autism center. The center had developed a training curriculum over several years, and then used psychology trainees to run the program as part of its postdoctoral clinical placement (in fact, the current trainee had herself been inspired to pursue graduate training in psychology following her experience as a summer intern). Although the camp was expensive, Joshua's parents knew that it met some of the requirements for his summer programming, and so they successfully advocated for one-half of the costs to be covered by the school district and the other half to be reimbursed via Medicaid. Joshua's parents also arranged for an additional 90-minute meeting with counselors prior to the start of camp to describe some of the accommodations that had worked at school.

The Asperger diagnosis also helped connect Joshua's parents with a local not-for-profit agency for children with disabilities that specialized (among other things) in helping children with disabilities practice calming techniques to decrease stressful experiences (e.g., getting a haircut, going to the dentist). This agency benefited from consultation provided by a local pediatrician and behavior analyst in identifying accommodations for children with ASD and creating opportunities to practice under less stressful conditions. Because of his general restlessness and his exquisite sensitivity to noises and crowds, attempts by Joshua's parents to take family vacations involving air travel had ended in utter disaster. The agency had recently arranged with air carriers and the local airport to conduct mock flights, including check in, passage through security, actual boarding of a flight, and deplaning. This practice, together with other individualized social and behavioral scripts developed by Joshua's speech pathologist, allowed Joshua and his father to take a short but highly successful trip to the national Baseball Hall of Fame.

Sofia's Story

Sofia is the 12-year-old daughter of illegal immigrants from Central America who have lived in an inner-city Hispanic community with extended family for the past 15 years. Sofia has tuberous sclerosis in addition to autism, which has resulted in severe ID. She has no language but pulls on adults or throws tantrums to indicate what she needs. Sofia also struggles with her weight (perhaps a side effect of the medication she takes in an attempt to control her head banging). Although the state in which Sofia lives recently passed autism insurance legislation, her parents juggle a variety of part-time jobs that pay the bills but do not provide consistent health care coverage.

Until recently, Sofia's educational needs have been largely met through a strong and supportive public school program. During her early childhood, Sofia was in a special class in a typical public school. When she turned 10, she was shifted into a special school operated by the city's school district, serving children with significant intellectual and physical disabilities. A dedicated classroom team served a mixed group of students, many of whom did not have ASD but all of whom had significant ID. The concentration of students with ID and ASD allowed the district to hire a behavioral consultant from a regional center to offer more in-depth functional behavioral assessments and intensive in-class support. This was instrumental in helping to identify that chronic constipation was a factor in significant spikes in Sofia's self-injury. In consultation with Sofia's physician (at a local, not-for-profit community health center), the school nurse was able to use laxatives, monitor her bowel movements, and reduce episodes of severe constipation and concomitant self-injury. The behavior consultant also identified that self-injury functioned to draw adults to Sofia, which sometimes led either to her needs (e.g., her boredom, her hunger) being more promptly addressed or to her demands being decreased. The school began to teach Sofia some simple signs to communicate her desire for attention and help, contributing to a decrease in her self-injury. As a result, Sofia's grandmother could continue to provide after-school care (even though her own health was fragile).

Unbeknownst to her parents or school, Sofia had recently developed several cavities: Her parents could only afford treatment at a local clinic that had little experience in children with ID, and so Sofia has had little dental care in her lifetime. The family and school attributed the rapid increase in her self-injury to her constipation and other family changes (Sofia's grandmother, who had provided after-school care while Sofia's mother worked, had recently fallen ill, and so Sofia's mother had to quit work). During the past month, the worsening of the self-injury together with staff injuries that resulted from a poorly executed attempt to physically restrain Sofia during a particularly severe episode, prompted the school to suspend Sofia pending a mandatory reevaluation of her behavioral support needs. Increased medication was unsuccessful in decreasing her negative behavior, although it caused her to fall asleep during the day, which then resulted in waking spells in the middle of the night. The increased attention and decreased demands resulting from her behavior became another factor increasing her self-injury. The periodic "respite" informally provided by the extended family and broader community also ended with the increase in self-injury.

Late one evening, Sofia's parents finally brought her to the emergency room of the local hospital. They were terrified that her self-injurious behavior (SIB) was causing brain injury and were desperate to obtain medical tests to clarify her worsening condition. The emergency room staff prematurely attributed her self-injury to her ASD, and did not conduct a thorough examination because they were concerned about provoking more behaviors. Following a series of disastrous admissions, the emergency room program had been developing a specialized triage and support system for people with developmental disabilities and had already engaged a nurse's aide (herself the mother of a young man with ASD) to provide direct support in the emergency room under the guidance of a staff psychologist. The aide was able to identify and implement some simple accommodations for Sofia that helped her to be more comfortable (e.g., moving Sofia into a single room), while emergency room staff began to call other possible placements. None of the traditional in-patient programs most commonly used in the immediate region had beds available.

The next morning, the emergency room team consulted with a hospital social worker regarding options. Although the social worker initiated a referral for residential services, she also confirmed that residential treatment programs did not have the capacity to respond in a crisis, and that recent cuts to the funding of such services by the state's developmental disability services prompted policy changes such that all in-state options must be exhausted before an out-of-state placement could be considered. The social worker recalled that a new in-patient treatment program specializing in ASD and related developmental disabilities was being developed at a local site of a national, private provider of behavioral health services. This provider had discovered that it was very difficult to adapt traditional psychiatric in-patient programs to also meet the needs of children and adolescents with ASD, and so identified a local site to pilot a new kind of service designed to address these shortcomings. The social worker confirmed that the program was open, and that beds were available.

Five days after Sofia's admission, the in-patient program had begun to isolate possible dental pain as a source of discomfort, and a dental exam with an experienced consultant revealed suspicious spots on Sofia's teeth. Arrangements were made at a specialized dental clinic for her cavities to be addressed under sedation the following week. At the same time, the in-patient psychiatrist was able to titrate her medication to below levels possible even prior to the likely onset of her cavities, because the management of her constipation combined with improved behavior support significantly decreased her self-injury. An interagency team meeting and visits by her school team to observe changes to her programming were sufficient to transfer her new program back to the community upon discharge. The request for a residential treatment program was withdrawn, and Sofia returned home.

Liam's Story

Liam is a 18-year-old Caucasian boy diagnosed with autism and borderline intellectual functioning. He lives at home with his unemployed single mother and older sister in a poor suburb of a large city. Liam's mother has a history of mental health and substance abuse problems that had resulted in referrals to child protective services for neglect. Liam is about to turn 18, and his mother has not sought legal guardianship of him.

Liam has done well in a special program in his high school, especially during the past 3 years during which he benefited from the support of a particularly dedicated teacher. The teacher had taken the initiative to expand vocational training opportunities for his class of students with varied disabilities as part of expanded transition planning he learned about through training provided by the state department of education. Through contacts made during this training, the teacher helped to promote a partnership between the local office of vocational rehabilitation and a local ASD nonprofit agency. The ASD agency had sought to move beyond advocacy to pilot services to address known gaps, and so developed a community-based vocational support program to supplement traditional sheltered workshops. The school district and the vocational rehabilitation agency now contracted with the ASD agency, which provided a job coach (supported by a vocational specialist) to bridge the gap between the final year of high school and the first year of adult services. Liam began to work at a grocery store restocking shelves and making coffee, and was soon beginning food preparation in the delicatessen.

It had seemed like transportation to work would soon become more of a challenge: Liam's older sister had coordinated her schedule of classes at a local community college to be able to drop him off and pick him up, but she just accepted a job that, upon graduation, would prevent this arrangement from continuing. Fortunately, Liam has always been fascinated by vehicles and schedules, and so it was thought that he would be able to tolerate public transportation. One board member of the grocery store chain was also active in the local ASD agency (he had a brother with Down syndrome), and he had lobbied for all stores to carve out jobs for those with disabilities. As a result, Liam was set to switch his work to a branch readily accessible via public transportation.

Liam struggled at times with his sexual maturation. Several years prior, he had begun to masturbate and then initiated this in the classroom. His teachers were able to incorporate sex education into his individualized education program (IEP) goals, and in this context assured his mother that this behavior was part of normal development. Liam's behavior prompted the school to reexamine sex education for all people with disabilities, and a new curriculum had been introduced after the special education director had engaged an expert in the state initially to provide consultation in some potentially litigious cases. The consultation had evolved into a short-term training program for all district teachers that continued through a contract with the expert. Liam's program included instruction to Liam regarding when and where it is and is not permissible to masturbate. More recently, Liam has begun making inappropriate sexual comments to girls at his school, resulting in several suspensions. Liam has a crush on another classmate who reported to the police that he had been "stalking" her. This escalated into a physical advance outside of school, for which Liam is now being prosecuted. Fortunately, the public defender's office recently participated in an ASD orientation in partnership with a center of excellence in developmental disabilities at the state university and is exploring whether a treatment program for Liam, including social skills and sex education, may help avoid incarceration.

Chloe's Story

Chloe is a 22-year-old Caucasian woman with ASD. She is in her second year of undergraduate studies in engineering at a small community college and excels academically. She continues to struggle with anxiety and panic attacks, which sometimes cripple her and make it impossible to live alone or in college residences. When the panic attacks first emerged in adolescence, Chloe was fortunate that her physician referred her to an experienced psychiatrist in the region who was able to ascertain that these were clearly the manifestation of both an autism spectrum and an anxiety disorder—the psychiatrist prescribed the appropriate medication for the latter. Chloe has developed a small circle of female classmates through her recent involvement in an Asperger self-advocacy group organized at her university. This pilot program was started with seed money from a state developmental disabilities agency to a member of the social work faculty. It included funding to support other college students as peer mentors to students with ASD.

Chloe's peer mentor helped her work out awkward social situations with others in her group. In fact, Chloe's relative lack of self-consciousness led her to share potentially embarrassing questions and concerns too readily with others, which led them to avoid her or to make fun of her. Chloe talked a lot about her unsuccessful attempts to find a boyfriend, which had left her depressed, angry, and confused. Her description of one incident led her mentor to conclude that Chloe had been a victim of "date rape" by a college freshman. The peer mentor helped Chloe gain access to cognitive-behavioral therapy for her depression through a college counselor. The support of her peer mentor and self-advocacy group also helped Chloe gain access to a rape crisis center and institute proceedings against the perpetrator.

Chloe lives with her grandparents but dreams of living on her own and learning to drive. She was raised by her grandparents following her removal from her parent's home by child protective services. The stability provided by her grandparents was critical to reversing the panic attacks that at one point left Chloe unable to leave the house. Her grandfather's recent diagnosis of Alzheimer's disease has, however, increased the pressure on Chloe's grandmother. Chloe's grandmother is now the sole caregiver and breadwinner, struggles herself with diabetes, and is trying to find a supported living arrangement for Chloe and some support for her husband so that she can continue working. While Chloe is excited by the idea of living with friends, both she and her grandparents wonder how she could create the daily supports needed to prevent the recurrence of her panic attacks, should another crisis arise.

A local advocacy group was recently approached by a local religious order interested in donating some of its land and buildings to help people with disabilities. The holdings are in a highly desirable location near the university and with access to public transportation. The advocacy group has convened a stakeholder group, including representatives of state agencies, the university, the city, people with disabilities (including Chloe), and a for-profit provider of behavioral health services. Their vision is to create a mixed-use development that includes apartments designed to mix college students and people with disabilities. This kind of support will become more important to Chloe when she begins to plan the difficult, but inevitable, move from her grandparents' household.

Common Threads

These case studies illustrate some of the factors discussed earlier in this chapter: the types of social, communication, and unusual interests/behaviors specific to ASD; how these vary as a function of the person's age and overall developmental level; and how these are affected by other co-occurring conditions. Readers less familiar with the struggles of people living with ASD may conclude that few cases are as complex as these. While I acknowledge some literary license in the creation of these cases, I have found that most families struggle to address multiple factors, and that the nature of these challenges changes dramatically with age. I have worked with many families facing challenges as complex as these and have lived some of them myself. Even researchers and practitioners who specialize in ASD underestimate their true complexity because their exposure to the totality of factors listed earlier is inevitably limited by the scope of their training, their professional responsibilities, the mandate of their agency, and by the lack of true multidisciplinary and multiagency collaboration. In Chapters 2 and 3 I provide a summary of key elements of services, training, research, and policy to help researchers, practitioners, and program leaders understand the true extent of the challenge. I continue this overview in Chapter 4 by trying to quickly summarize the infrastructure underlying services, training, research, and policy at the local, state, and national level.

From the outside, ASD is a fascinating enigma, a tantalizing puzzle, a mysterious, exciting, unfolding quest to understand the human mind. How is it that Asif can read and that Joshua knows so much about baseball, and yet they struggle to acquire fundamental social skills? From the inside—for most parents of children with ASD—its unfolding drama is anticipated with foreboding, not fascination, and its mystery is terrifying, not tantalizing. Through these case studies I try to convey the uncertainty with which people with ASD and their caregivers must often live: It is impossible to predict how ASD will present itself; no single, reliable cause or causes have been identified; few professionals can help families understand and successfully navigate the entire system of services and support; and few professionals can help families anticipate the next challenge lying just around the corner, let alone prepare them for long-term outcomes that might realistically range from group homes and sheltered workshops to the kind of independent and fulfilling life parents come to expect for their typical child.

I also acknowledge some literary license in the manner and likelihood with which these cases were resolved: In my experience, families are more often left with unanswered questions and unresolved problems. Unlike cases of ASD portrayed in the popular media, real-life stories do not always come to convenient and comfortable closure. Will Asif go to a regular school? Will Sofia get help for her dental problems and return home, or inflict increasingly serious self-injury, or be removed from her parents and placed in institutional care for the rest of her life? Will Liam go to jail? Will Chloe be able to live on her own, or will she struggle again with panic attacks that could jeopardize her education and career? In Chapter 14, I discuss how services, training, research, and policy must broaden to recognize the essential, irreplaceable role that caregivers play in the support of people with ASD, in some cases for the person's lifetime.

These case studies remind us that ASD does not render the person or their family immune to other challenges or remove the hurdles all people face as they age. Families from diverse racial, ethnic, and socioeconomic backgrounds encounter different opportunities and barriers in gaining access to services and supports in the community. Family members may themselves struggle with their own physical or mental health. I have found that these other factors, alone or in combination, can ultimately determine whether families sink, survive, or thrive in the face of the challenges that can accompany ASD. Helping all individuals affected by ASD will require that science shift from developing more increasingly specialized techniques that will reach a small and privileged percent of the population to efficiently disseminating simple, effective techniques to everyone affected by ASD.

Although I want readers to frankly acknowledge the potential burden of ASD, I also want them to recognize the many sources of hope. People with ASD engage us with their endearing idiosyncrasies and inspire us in their earnest struggle to acquire skills we take for granted. For some families, the uncertainty and trauma of ASD is transformative, helping them to identify new sources of strength and support and to approach the world with greater compassion, humility, and humor. More central to the purpose of this book are the many ways that individuals and programs at the local, regional, state, and national level can provide services, training, research, or policy that can make a real difference. In each of the cases presented previously, professionals sought additional training and support or reached beyond their traditional role to become better able to help someone they were concerned about. In a similar manner, agencies were able to look creatively beyond their traditional mandates to close a critical gap. I therefore take hope in the professionals reading this book who embrace new understanding, interventions, and collaborations as they seek to help their patients, clients, students, and constituents. And service professionals can take hope that their growing knowledge about effective interventions, in the hands of articulate advocates and informed leaders, can lead to enlightened policy. As professionals, we are at a watershed in the evolution of an integrated network of services, training, research, and policy, such that targeted and coordinated program development across local, regional, state, and national programs can help close some of the most significant gaps in relatively cost-effective ways.

REFERENCES

American Psychiatric Association. (2000). *Diagnostic and statistical manual of mental disorders* (4th ed.). Washington, DC: Author.

Carter, A.S., Davis, N.O., Klin, A., & Volkmar, F.R. (2005). Social development in autism. In F.R. Volkmar, R. Paul, A. Klin, & D. Cohen (Eds.), *Handbook of autism and pervasive developmental disorders: Vol. 1. Diagnosis, development, neurobiology, and behavior* (3rd ed., pp. 312–334). New York, NY: Wiley.

Committee on Children with Disabilities. (2001). Technical report: The pediatrician's role in the diagnosis and management of autistic spectrum disorder in children. *Pediatrics, 107*(5), e85.

Committee on Educational Interventions for Children with Autism. (2001). *Educating children with autism.* Washington, DC: National Academies Press.

Danielsson, S., Gillberg, I.C., Billstedt, E., Gillberg, C., & Olsson, I. (2005). Epilepsy in young adults with autism: A prospective population-based follow-up study of 120 individuals diagnosed in childhood. *Epilepsia, 46*(6), 918–923.

Ferraioli, S.J., & Harris, S.L. (2011). Treatments to increase social awareness and social skills. In B. Reichow, P. Doehring, D.V. Cicchetti, & F.R. Volkmar (Eds.), *Evidence-based practices and treatments for children with autism* (pp. 171–196). New York, NY: Springer.

Freeman, R.L., Horner, R.H., & Reichle, J. (2002). Functional assessment and self-restraint. In S.R. Schroeder, M.L. Oster-Granite, & T. Thompson (Eds.), *Self-injurious behavior: Gene-brain-behavior relationships* (pp. 105–118). Washington, DC: American Psychological Association.

Gotham, K., Risi, S., Pickles, A., & Lord, C. (2007). The Autism Diagnostic Observation Schedule: Revised algorithms for improved diagnostic validity. *Journal of Autism and Developmental Disorders, 37*(4), 613–627.

Holtmann, M., Bolte, S., & Poustka, F. (2007). Attention deficit hyperactivity disorder symptoms in pervasive developmental disorders: Association with autistic behavior domains and coexisting psychopathology. *Psychopathology, 40*(3), 172–177.

Johnson, C.P., Myers, S.M., & Council on Children with Disabilities. (2007). Identification and evaluation of children with autism spectrum disorders. *Pediatrics, 120*(5), 1183–1215.

Koyama, T., Tachimor, H., Osada, H., & Kurita, H. (2006). Cognitive and symptom profiles in high-functioning pervasive developmental disorder not otherwise specified and attention-deficit/hyperactivity disorder. *Journal of Autism and Developmental Disorders, 36*(3), 373–380.

Lawer, L., & Mandel, D.S. (2009). *Pennsylvania Autism Census Project: Final report.* Harrisburg: Bureau of Autism Services, Pennsylvania Department of Public Welfare.

Levy, S.E., Mandell, D.S., & Schultz, R.T. (2009). Autism. *The Lancet, 374*(9701), 1627–1638.

Leyfer, O.T., Folstein, S.E., Bacalman, S., Davis, N.O., Dinh, E., Morgan, J., et al. (2006). Comorbid psychiatric disorders in children with autism: Interview development and rates of disorders. *Journal of Autism and Developmental Disorders, 36*(7), 849–861.

National Autism Center. (2009). *The National Standards Project: Addressing the need for evidence based practice guidelines for autism spectrum disorders.* Randolph, MA: Author.

Paul, R., & Sutherland, D. (2005). Enhancing early language in children with autism spectrum disorders. In F.R. Volkmar, R. Paul, A. Klin, & D. Cohen (Eds.), *Handbook of autism and pervasive developmental disorders: Assessment, interventions, and policy* (3rd ed., pp. 946–976). New York, NY: Wiley.

Powers, M.D., Palmieri, M.J., D'Eramo, K.S., & Powers, K.M. (2011). Evidence-based treatment of behavioral excesses and deficits for individuals with autism spectrum disorders. In B. Reichow, P. Doehring, D.V. Cicchetti, & F.R. Volkmar (Eds.), *Evidence-based practices and treatments for children with autism* (pp. 55–92). New York, NY: Springer.

Prizant, B.M., & Wetherby, A.M. (2005). Critical issues in enhancing communication abilities for persons with autism spectrum disorder. In F.R. Volkmar, R. Paul, A. Klin, & D. Cohen (Eds.), *Handbook of autism and pervasive developmental disorders: Assessment, interventions, and policy* (3rd ed., pp. 925–945). New York, NY: Wiley.

Stewart, M.E., Barnard, L., Pearson, J., Hasan, R., & O'Brien, G. (2006). Presentation of depression in autism and Asperger syndrome: A review. *Autism, 10*(1), 103–116.

Towbin, K.E., Pradella, A., Gorrindo, T., Pine, D.S., & Leibenluft, E. (2005). Autism spectrum traits in children with mood and anxiety disorders. *Journal of Child and Adolescent Psychopharmacology, 15*(3), 452–464.

Tsatsanis, K.D., Saulnier, C., Sparrow, S.S., & Cicchetti, D.V. (2011). The role of adaptive behavior in evidence-based practices for ASD: Translating intervention into functional success. In B. Reichow, P. Doehring, D.V. Cicchetti, & F.R. Volkmar (Eds.), *Evidence-based practices and treatments for children with autism* (pp. 297–308). New York, NY: Springer.

World Health Organization. (2008). *ICD-10: International statistical classification of diseases and related health problems* (10th rev. ed.). New York, NY: Author.

Yeargin-Allsopp, M., Rice, C., Karapurkar, T., Doernberg, N., Boyle, C., & Murphy, C. (2003). Prevalence of autism in a US metropolitan area. *JAMA: The Journal of the American Medical Association, 289*(1), 49–55.

2

Services for People with Autism Spectrum Disorder

What Can This Include?

Peter Doehring

Many different kinds of services, training, research, and policy are relevant to the care and support of people with autism spectrum disorder (ASD). A thorough discussion of each is beyond the scope of a single book—let alone a single volume—and in fact, there are few authors who have successfully undertaken this for a professional audience (Volkmar, Paul, Klin, & Cohen, 2005a; Volkmar, Paul, Klin, & Cohen, 2005b). The rest of this section and the final section of the book therefore focus on a subset of service needs (this chapter), and their associated training, research, and policy (Chapter 3), instead of seeking to capture the entire spectrum of possible service needs. In writing this book, the contributors and I sought to select a variety of services that are commonly needed, that capture the range of needs across age and functioning level, and that address defining characteristics and accompanying conditions. Some of these services were also selected with knowledge of the programs presented in Sections II and III and in anticipation of recommendations to be offered in Section IV about which services could be most efficiently and effectively developed in most regions of the United States. Finally, we sought examples for which there have been recent and important changes in the understanding of the services needed and that illustrate the range of challenges in developing services.

The rest of Section I also focuses on describing specific examples of services, training, research, and policy in ASD and not on the potential interplay between them. The first goal is to map out the territory covered by these elements, because it is anticipated that most readers will have focused their work on a small area and neither appreciate the breadth of the challenge nor recognize the specific and important opportunities for growth outside of their particular sphere of interest and influence. This map will also help readers to understand how the different programs described in Sections II and III may be interrelated. The final section of the book reexamines interrelationships between these elements to review specific and persistent gaps and to propose opportunities for increasing system capacity. Focusing on a subset of services also helps readers envision how associated training, research, and policy might concretely and immediately improve the quality of life for people with ASD, through the stories of Asif, Evan, Joshua, Sofia, Liam, and Chloe, introduced at

Table 2.1. Case studies—general characteristics

Name	Age	Intellectual disability (ID)	Co-occurring conditions
Asif	2	Mild	Seizures; reflux
Evan	5	Moderate	Anxiety; aggression; toileting; sleep
Joshua	8	None	Attention deficit-hyperactivity disorder (ADHD)
Sofia	12	Severe	Tuberous sclerosis; constipation; cavities; self-injury
Liam	20	Borderline	Inappropriate sexual behavior
Chloe	22	None	Panic attacks; anxiety; depression

the end of the Chapter 1 (see Table 2.1) and specifically highlighted in case studies throughout the rest of Sections I and IV. As discussed in greater detail in Chapter 14, services and supports are a pivot point for system change: If changes to training, research, and policy are to have a real impact on the entire population of those living with ASD, it is almost always through improvements to services and supports. The interdependence of services, and their associated training, research, and policy impact, also becomes even more apparent in Chapter 4, which outlines the complex infrastructure of agencies and funding that supports all of these elements.

The rest of this section and the final section of the book frame discussions of services, training, research, and policy using the more traditional distinctions between different service domains (e.g., education, behavioral health) that demarcate the boundaries of agencies and organizations within the network, instead of the diagnostic features of ASD (e.g., social/communication deficits, unusual interests and behaviors) (see Figure 2.1). Grouping services by domain helps readers begin to align them with the agencies and organizations in the service infrastructure (discussed in greater detail in Chapter 4). In part, this simply acknowledges that improvements must often be built upon the existing network of agencies and organizations that provide or direct ASD services, training, research, and policy. This approach also acknowledges that any attempt to frame discussions of services, training, research, and policy using the diagnostic features of ASD may overemphasize the ways that ASD differs and lead professionals to miss ways that ASD resembles other conditions and that offer important opportunities for growth.

In anticipation of issues to be discussed later in the book, I include other information about each of these services. I highlight some of these services as pivotal because they regulate access to, or transitions between, other key services, supports, and environments and discuss these pivotal services in greater detail at the end of the chapter. Whenever possible, I identify areas for which standards or "best practices" have been identified that are consensus based (e.g., published position statements by public agencies or professional organizations) or evidence based (e.g., with reference to systematic reviews of available outcome research) (e.g., National Autism Center, 2009; National Professional Development Center on Autism Spectrum Disorders, 2011; Reichow, Doehring, Cicchetti, & Volkmar, 2011) specific to individuals with ASD. Whenever appropriate, I try to distinguish between

Cross-cutting services		
Health	Education	Community

Figure 2.1. Service domains.

those services more specific to people with ASD and those that are likely applicable to other populations and between those services that might be considered basic and those that are more specialized (because of the level of training required and/or the small proportion of people who require them). Whenever possible, I also offer estimates of the frequency which with different kinds of services might be needed or used based on the series of reports emerging from the Pennsylvania Autism Needs Assessment (see Chapter 6). Finally, I list the kinds of personnel likely to be delivering each of the services described next, in anticipation of more detailed discussions in Chapter 3 of their training and the types of agencies in which they might work.

CROSS-DOMAIN SERVICES

I begin with a number of services that cut across traditional domains and at the end of the chapter discuss how such cross-cutting services provide opportunities to break down barriers between traditional service silos (see Figure 2.2).

Identification of Autism Spectrum Disorders

I consider identification of ASD to be a pivotal service, because it is often necessary for gaining access to other specialized services and for determining eligibility for certain sources of funding (see Chapters 3 and 4).

Screening for Autism Spectrum Disorders Screening is the use of simple and cost-effective procedures to identify a subset of those who merit more extensive testing. Screening for ASD entails the use of brief checklists completed by a parent or a professional to flag children at high risk for ASD and to support a referral for formal diagnostic evaluation (Baron-Cohen et al., 2000). Screening is particularly important in the case of ASD because the professionals most likely to interact with people with ASD usually lack the time and/or the training to accurately diagnose them but can be provided with the training to accurately screen them. Screening is pivotal because of research suggesting the potential for very significant progress when intensive intervention begins early (Lovaas, 1987). Screening also offers great promise because research suggests that parents often have specific concerns about their child's development long before professionals. Although screening for ASD is not applicable to other populations, by definition it would be considered a basic service because it should not require highly specialized training. Finally, screening can conceivably be conducted by any properly trained professional, although most programs have promoted screening by community-based physicians and are ultimately limited by the access to diagnostic services.

Autism Spectrum Disorder (ASD) identification (screening & diagnosis)[a]	
	Behavioral intervention (including behavioral assessment and support)[a]
Social skills training	
Case management and planning[a]	Other therapies
Assessments of cognitive and adaptive functioning	Paraprofessional support[b]

Figure 2.2. Services cutting across domains.

[a]Pivotal service.
[b]Nonprofessional direct care in home, school, residential, in-patient, and other settings.

Given all of these factors, it is not surprising that recent guidelines have emphasized the importance of early screening of ASD (Johnson, Myers, & Council on Children with Disabilities, 2007). Compared to other services discussed in this volume, a significant amount of research has been conducted on screening instruments and protocols, their effectiveness, and their utilization by practitioners, and this has spurred various public agencies and professional organizations to adopt standards of practice. For example, there is evidence that instruments such as the Modified Checklist for Autism in Toddlers (M-CHAT) can help community-based practitioners accurately and efficiently identify a significant proportion of those with ASD at a relatively early age (Kleinman et al., 2008). Other research has suggested that training programs can greatly facilitate the effective coordination between community-based practitioners and more specialized diagnosticians (Warren, Stone, & Humberd, 2009). Other chapters in this volume describe innovative programs to implement screening in community settings (see Chapters 9 and 10), the most notable of which is the Learn the Signs. Act Early. program led by the Centers for Disease Control and Prevention (see Chapter 12).

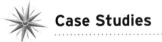 ## Case Studies

Screening by his pediatrician helped Asif gain access to early intervention services more quickly. Screening by Evan's preschool teacher helped him obtain the specialized support for his other behavior problems.

Despite the existence of powerful screening protocols and standards set by various agencies, there are still many opportunities to expand the knowledge and use of screening. Much of the work has focused on screening of very young children; it is still very common for individuals to be referred for a diagnostic evaluation later or only after other diagnoses have been made. Screening for ASD in older children, adolescents, and adults is not an established practice, although perhaps it should be given the likelihood of underidentification of ASD among older individuals. Whereas screening for ASD can potentially be accomplished by many different kinds of professionals and in many different settings, there is relatively little research on screening conducted outside of the physician's office.

Diagnosis of Autism Spectrum Disorders   The psychiatric and educational diagnosis is important to people with ASD for many reasons. The diagnosis helps to make sense of areas of strength and weakness and to anticipate potentially fruitful areas of intervention. In some cases, it establishes the person's eligibility for more specialized services and supports. The diagnosis also helps the individual's family to connect with a community of support and advocacy attuned to its needs. The psychiatric diagnosis is specifically helpful in disentangling ASD from related conditions and has helped to group individuals together in research seeking to identify common characteristics, genetics, neurological features, and environmental factors that may eventually explain underlying cause(s).

Case Studies

A basic diagnostic evaluation helped to speed Evan's and Asif's access to specialized services in their community. A specialized diagnostic evaluation helped to clarify that Joshua has ASD in addition to, or instead of, attention deficit-hyperactivity disorder (ADHD).

To assign a psychiatric diagnosis of ASD, the practitioner must establish whether the person demonstrates the pattern of features consistent with a disorder on the autism spectrum, as defined in the *Diagnostic and Statistical Manual of Mental Disorders, Fourth Edition, Text Revision* (*DSM-IV-TR*; American Psychiatric Association, 2000). (Many countries outside of North America also use the *International Statistical Classification of Diseases and Related Health Problems, 10th Edition* (*ICD-10*; World Health Organization, 2008). The psychiatric diagnosis can be assigned by a physician, licensed psychologist, or (in some regions) a practicing nurse practitioner (PNP). To assign an educational diagnosis (sometimes referred to as educational classification) of ASD, an educational diagnostician must establish whether the person demonstrates the pattern of features defined in state regulations. Whereas the diagnostic criteria for the different medical systems of classification have converged since the early 1990s, there is considerable variability across states in the categories and criteria for the educational classification of autism; specifically, whether it includes other disorders on the autism spectrum (e.g., pervasive developmental disorder not otherwise specified, Asperger syndrome), and whether it aligns with the medical diagnosis (see Chapter 7). The lack of experienced psychiatric diagnosticians has already contributed to long waiting lists for evaluations at many specialized centers that can negate the potential benefits of even the most ambitious screening programs, although educational regulations set limits in the length of time that families must await the completion of an educational evaluation.

Considerable research on the validity, reliability, and predictability of instruments such as the Autism Diagnostic Observation Schedule (ADOS; Lord, Rutter, DiLavore, & Risi, 1999) and the Autism Diagnostic Interview–Revised (ADI-R; Lord, Rutter, & Le Couteur, 1994) have set these as the gold standard for specialized diagnostic evaluations conducted in the context of research. Although the use of these instruments is central to many state guidelines and training programs (see Chapters 6, 7, and 11), in practice few community-based medical or educational diagnosticians have either the time or the training to use these instruments systematically (see Chapter 7 for an exception). In my experience, specialized diagnostic evaluations are important in disentangling ASD from some co-occurring conditions, especially in very young children in individuals with severe intellectual disability (ID). In practice, I have found that most practitioners outside of highly specialized hospital- or research-based settings rely on a basic diagnostic evaluation, consisting at most of informal observations and interviews, perhaps informed by the results of other checklists such as the Childhood Autism Ratings Scale (CARS)–Revised, or Social Communication Questionnaire (SCQ) (Rutter, Bailey, & Lord, 2003). I believe that the greater precision gained from specialized diagnostic evaluation is nullified by the delays in accessing early interventions when families faced long waiting lists, and I have promoted specific training of community-based practitioners in a basic diagnostic evaluation protocol, as long as this includes guidelines that help them to recognize when potential co-occurring or complicating conditions should prompt a referral for a specialized diagnostic evaluation.

Behavioral Intervention

One of the most significant movements in ASD has been the rise of applied behavior analysis (ABA). In many respects, ABA is naturally suited to addressing the challenges of ASD as outlined in this volume: As an applied science, scientific studies describing new methods always include some demonstration of their use in the real world; its use of single-case design (i.e., in which progress before and after intervention is graphed individually instead of being expressed as an average) is more suited to capturing the highly individualized responses of individuals with ASD; ABA has been used across a wide range of settings (e.g., in the home, at school, in the workplace); and ABA has been used effectively for people with ID and people with ASD. Some confusion surrounding ABA has arisen because of the use of a wide range of terms that address overlapping and/or nested elements (e.g., a broad field of study, a package of interventions, a discipline, a specific method, a specific treatment target). For example, I consider *ABA* to refer to the broad field of study and *Board Certified Behavior Analyst (BCBA)* to refer to the professional discipline for which certification criteria have been identified by a national body. Although ASD has become a predominant focus of the field of ABA—and by extension the work of BCBAs—ABA is applied to many different populations and includes many techniques beyond those covered here. Within the following sections, I try to deconstruct other overlapping terms and describe cognitive behavior therapy separately under "Other Therapies."

Behavioral Assessment and Support for Decreasing Problem Behaviors

The term *behavioral assessment and support* includes the systematic collection of information to identify the possible cause(s) of problem behaviors (e.g., aggression, self-injury, tantrums) that interfere with a person's success at home and in the community, and to prioritize interventions to reduce these behaviors. Behavioral support can include everything from interventions as simple as a behavior plan that emphasizes certain strategies to prevent or respond to the behaviors to the justification for the ongoing involvement of specialized professionals for consultation, training, or direct intervention and/or paraprofessionals for daily support. The term *behavior plan* as used here encompasses other terms commonly used elsewhere, such as *behavior intervention plan, behavior support plan,* and *behavior modification plan.*

Since the 1960s, practitioners and researchers within the field of ABA have sought to identify effective methods of assessment and intervention to reduce problem behaviors in people with ID and ASD. *Functional behavioral assessment* (FBA) refers to a package of assessment strategies (e.g., checklists, interviews, direct observation) that together help to identify the purpose or function of the behavior (e.g., to get access to or to escape from stimuli that include attention and tangible items). The purpose or function is often expressed as a hypothesis centered on an antecedent-behavior-consequence (ABC) chain: When Johnny is presented with a difficult task (antecedent), he hits the teacher (behavior), in order to avoid completing the task (consequence) (O'Neill et al., 1997). Functional behavioral assessment increasingly considers an expanded range of conditions (i.e., establishing/abolishing operations) that affect the direction and/or strength of the ABC chain; for example, the aforementioned hypothesis is especially likely when Johnny has not slept well the night before. In this context, other professionals may play a role in evaluating the presence or absence of these conditions. In addition, clinicians are increasingly combining FBA with person-centered, positive, and preventative strategies (including the previously described consideration of conditions), as contrasted with reactive strategies (e.g., various forms of punishment) (Bambara & Kern, 2005), as part of the broader movement of positive behavior support (Carr et al., 2002).

✳ Case Studies

Behavior support was critical to helping Evan (e.g., behavior plans to address toileting, sleep, and aggression), Joshua (e.g., designing accommodations to help with dental visits and air travel), and Sofia (e.g., identifying functions and triggers for her self-injury).

Behavioral assessment and support can be indispensable when problem behaviors potentially necessitate placement outside of the home, or treatment in a more restricted setting (e.g., separate classroom, separate school, other specialized program). All BCBAs receive specific training in behavioral assessment and support: In practice, other professionals, such as psychologists, are often involved in the assessment and design of plans, and the plans are largely implemented by those involved in day-to-day care (e.g., caregivers, teachers, paraprofessionals). The most successful behavior assessment and support is rarely done in isolation, but requires collaboration among multiple professionals: the physician prescribing medication for mood, the teacher identifying and implementing accommodations to the classroom routine, the speech pathologist recommending communication strategies, and so forth. Behavior assessment and support can also be provided within and across many different settings: a home-based plan developed by an early intervention or community-based behavioral support program, a school-based program developed by education-based teams (see Chapter 7), a plan developed for residential- or hospital-based settings, or plans specifically developed to cut across home and community settings (see Chapter 5).

There is considerable professional and scientific consensus regarding best practices in behavior assessment and support. Functional behavioral assessment is recognized as an evidence-based practice, as are a wide variety of interventions intended to reduce problem behavior among children with ASD (National Autism Center, 2009; National Professional Development Center on Autism Spectrum Disorders, 2011; Powers, Palmieri, D'Eramo, & Powers, 2011). The widespread adoption of FBAs combined with preventative behavior strategies by education-based agencies is particularly noteworthy. A number of state and federal laws mandate the use of FBAs when addressing problem behaviors in the public schools, especially when such behaviors have resulted in suspension or expulsion from school. This has been associated with a wave of state and federal programs centered on the use of positive behavior support (PBS) to help students both with and without disabilities in the public schools. I argue that behavior support is a pivotal service when problem behaviors are the primary factor limiting gaining access to a community-based service: a child moved from placement in a typical classroom to a special classroom because of tantrums, an adolescent hospitalized because of self-injury, or a young adult removed from his or her home to a residential program because of aggression. The rise of PBS also speaks to the applicability of behavior support to a broad range of populations. Most models of PBS also distinguish between more basic services required by a substantial minority of the overall population and more specialized services required by a small proportion (which I suspect includes a relatively high proportion of people with ASD).

Teaching Methods, Packages, and Programs for Increasing Skills   Parallel to their efforts to address challenging behaviors, practitioners and researchers within the field of ABA have also sought to identify effective teaching strategies for people with ID and ASD. Practitioners and researchers have promoted specific methods applicable to a broad range of skills—for example, including the use of reinforcement, prompting, shaping, fading, task analysis, and others (Cooper, Heron, & Heward, 2007)—that form the core of most behavioral intervention programs intended to increase skills or decrease behavior. There is considerable consensus that many of these core practices listed previously are evidence-based (National Autism Center, 2009). Sometimes these methods are combined into a package that addresses a subset of skills, as in the case of Pivotal Response Training (Koegel, Koegel, & McNerney, 2001) and Picture Exchange Communication System (Bondy & Frost, 2001). These methods have also combined with specific assessment tools and curricula into comprehensive educational programs. Lovaas and his colleagues reported that almost one-half of young children with autism who received 2 years of his program of early and intensive behavioral intervention (EIBI) were indistinguishable from their colleagues (had "recovered" from their ASD) by the time they reached kindergarten (Lovaas, 1987). Verbal behavior approaches combine a structured curriculum with a range of ABA-based techniques that emphasize more naturalistic teaching strategies and that more systematically address the full range of communicative functions (Partington & Sundberg, 1998). Behavior plans based on increasing appropriate alternative skills for addressing the same function as the problem behavior—as in the case of Functional Communication Training (Mancil, 2006)—draw on many of the same core teaching methods described earlier.

Social Skills Training

Social skills training is primarily designed to improve social understanding and increase effective social interaction. Together with screening and identification, it is one of the few interventions more specifically applicable to people with ASD. I recognize that many skills contribute indirectly to social understanding and interaction—improved language can perhaps contribute to improved conversation, increased solitary pretend play can perhaps contribute to interactive play, decreased aggression may increase opportunities for peer interaction, and so forth—but I focus here on those interventions that specifically and directly target social understanding and interactions. Although social skills training is not as commonly used as other interventions described here, the fact that it targets deficits more specific to ASD and includes many specific interventions recognized as evidence-based (see discussion later in the chapter) warranted its inclusion here.

✳ Case Studies

Joshua benefited from social skills training provided privately by a speech pathologist, while Chloe benefited from social skills training provided by peer mentors at her college.

Social skills training includes a variety of treatment methods and targets. For example, joint attention training helps adults (especially caregivers) support the emergence of a shared focus (e.g., pointing, gaze following, commenting), usually in the context of naturalistic play (Whalen, Schreibman, & Ingersoll, 2006). Imitation training helps adults and peers to increase imitation in the context of play and social interaction (Ingersoll, Lewis, & Kroman, 2007). Research in these strategies and others primarily targeting early social skills (e.g., video modeling, peer training) has established many that are evidence based (Ferraioli & Harris, 2011; National Autism Center, 2009; National Professional Development Center on Autism Spectrum Disorders, 2011). Social skills interventions likely to be used with older children include Social Stories and various social skills training packages, a number of which constitute emerging evidence-based practices (Ferraioli & Harris, 2011; National Autism Center, 2009; National Professional Development Center on Autism Spectrum Disorders, 2011; Wood, Fujii, & Renno, 2011), while peer mentor programs are becoming an increasingly popular way to help college students with Asperger syndrome (AS) navigate complex academic and social expectations (see Chapter 4).

I have observed social skills training that occurs across a variety of settings using different professionals. In my experience, efforts to provide social skills training have been most often led by speech pathologists, psychologists, and teachers, and at other times by professionals such as social workers, occupational therapists, behavior analysts, and so forth. Similarly, I have observed social skills training provided by public schools, private for- or nonprofit agencies, university-based clinics, and hospital programs. The fact that social skills training has not been identified as the mandate of any one professional group or agency has in some contexts helped it grow freely when providers step forward, but is more often ignored by providers reluctant to expand their programs beyond their core mission.

Other Therapies

Speech and Occupational Therapies   A number of other therapies are available across a variety of settings. Speech and occupational therapies are commonly used for young children across a range of school, hospital, and community-based agencies. Speech therapists are generally recognized as the experts in 1) verbal and nonverbal language assessment, 2) the identification and implementation of augmentative and assistive speech technologies, and 3) the diagnosis and treatment of many feeding and swallowing disorders. Occupational therapists are generally recognized as the experts in assessment and intervention related to motor skills. Both of these professional groups have expanded their areas of expertise and intervention in response to the specific needs of children with ASD: Some speech pathologists have developed innovative programs to address the social, play, and emotional skill development critical to childhood (Prizant, Wetherby, Rubin, Laurent, & Rydell, 2006); many occupational therapists promote the use of sensory integration and related strategies, become involved in the development of play skills, and may lead or contribute to feeding programs centered on oral sensitivity and oral-motor coordination. Both speech and occupational therapists conduct discipline-specific assessments, may implement various combinations of individual and group therapies, provide consultation and support to educators and paraprofessionals working directly with children, and (with the exception perhaps of sensory integration) apply many of these techniques to other populations.

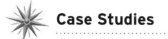 **Case Studies**

Asif benefited from speech and occupational therapy as part of his early intervention (EI) program. Cognitive-behavioral therapy (CBT) offered by a college counselor helped Chloe with her depression.

Despite the widespread reliance on speech and occupational therapies, there is not the same level of professional and scientific consensus regarding best practices as there is, for example, regarding the identification of and behavior support for ASD. With respect to speech therapy, some specific assistive and augmentative communication strategies such as Picture Exchange Communication System (National Autism Center, 2009; National Professional Development Center on Autism Spectrum Disorders, 2011; Prelock, Paul, & Allen, 2011) have been recognized as evidence-based, while the American Academy of Pediatrics has adopted strong position statements challenging the efficacy of other strategies, such as facilitated communication and auditory integration training (American Academy of Pediatrics, 1998). With respect to occupational therapy, there is consensus that people with ASD often present with specific difficulties in their motor skills and sensory responsiveness, and that intervention programs should include therapies to address these needs (Committee on Educational Interventions for Children with Autism, 2001). Nonetheless, scientifically based reviews have failed to conclude that there is sufficient evidence to clearly recommend the use of specific therapies such as sensory integration (National Autism Center, 2009; National Professional Development Center on Autism Spectrum Disorders, 2011), although the number of studies with more promising designs and results has been growing (Schaaf, 2011).

Cognitive-Behavioral Therapy Professionals have also become increasingly excited by the potential of cognitive-behavioral therapy (CBT). Recent reviews that suggest that CBT is a promising evidence-based practice for treating a range of problems such as anxiety, social skills, and so forth (Wood et al., 2011) become more compelling given that many such techniques are already well established as evidence based in the treatment of anxiety, depression, phobias, and other related disorders in more typical individuals (Hollon & Ponniah, 2010). Cognitive-behavioral therapy can include a range of short- to medium-term group or individual therapies, sometimes supplemented by parent training. Despite the emerging evidence regarding its effectiveness, I have not found CBT for people with ASD to be readily available, perhaps because it is most effectively utilized by doctoral-level clinicians with specific training both in ASD and CBT. I believe that CBT can sometimes be effectively used in specific applications by master's-level clinicians, with the right training and supervision, in more specialized settings.

Paraprofessional Support

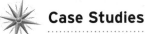 **Case Studies**

Paraprofessionals provided critical support to Asif at home, to Evan at school, to Joshua at summer camp, to Sofia in the emergency room, to Liam on the job, and to Chloe in college.

Paraprofessional support refers to the nonprofessional, direct-care staff who provide the intensive, day-to-day support critical to the success of a significant proportion of people with ASD across the full range of settings. This includes categories such as teaching assistants, residential assistants, mental health technicians, day care/after-school assistants, camp counselors, health aides, job coaches, in-home assistants providing intensive early intervention or wraparound services, peer mentors, and others. Paraprofessional support is provided for the full range of social, communication, academic, self-care, vocational, community, and leisure skills. In all of these cases, however, paraprofessionals work under the direct supervision of a professional (e.g., teacher, nurse, residential advisor, vocational specialist) who sets goals and methods and evaluates progress. Although paraprofessionals do not offer a specific area of expertise, they typically provide more direct intervention than any professional per se, and are therefore indispensable. Nonetheless, there is no clear standard of care for paraprofessionals, and relatively little effort is invested in tailoring training programs to their needs (for an exception, see Chapter 4).

Case Management and Planning

Case management and planning is used here to refer to a broad range of activities that all facilitate at least access to, if not coordination across, multiple agencies and/or providers.

The scope of case management varies from one context to another. In most cases, case management is restricted to facilitating access (e.g., by helping the family to complete the forms needed to initiate services in different agencies) or helping lead the development if not the implementation of a plan (e.g., by facilitating interagency meetings). Multiagency coordination can also occur during the transition from one set of services to another. For example, state and federal guidelines set standards regarding the management of the transition from early intervention (from birth to age 3 years) services to education services (from age 3 to 21 years), and from education services to adult (age 21 and older) services. Forward-thinking policy with respect to the post-21 transition in particular requires planning to bring together partners from multiple agencies to consider long-term outcomes across all aspects of life. The West Virginia Family Focus Positive Behavior Support model (see Chapter 5) enhances this approach by promoting a common vision across team members through a uniform training curriculum provided to all team members and a structured planning process. I do not know, however, of any examples in which the case manager has a more decisive role in actively directing the selection and allocation of services. As noted in Chapter 14, most parents assume this "case management" role by default for at least some (but often all) of their child's lifetime. Although case management is provided for other populations, I argue that people with ASD are in greater need of case management because of the range of medical, behavioral, and other issues that complicate their treatment. For this reason, I have designated case management and planning as a pivotal service.

Case Studies

Case management helped Evan's parents gain access to financial support and coordinate clinical services. Transition planning by Liam's teacher was critical in coordinating vocational services across school and community agencies.

The professionals who undertake case management, and the extent of their involvement, also varies from one situation to another. Sometimes case management is the principal role played by the professional in the life of the child (e.g., a social worker in a developmental disabilities agency who helps the family apply for services through various agencies) or at a particular moment in the child's care (e.g., a discharge coordinator who helps the family to transition back in school and community placements following hospitalization). In these cases, those with a background in social work are perhaps the most likely professionals to assume this role. More often, case management is a relatively small part of a professional's work with the child: a nurse who helps to coordinate medical care between the home, the school, and the physician; a teacher leading the post-21 transition planning process by coordinating meetings to prepare a long-term vocational or a residential plan; or a social worker facilitating an interagency phone conference to help the biological family, therapeutic foster family, and school family confer regarding the need for a possible residential placement. Given the many different contexts in which case management occurs and the nature of case management, it is not surprising that there are no consensus- or empirically based standards of practice, although most reviews acknowledge the importance of a coordinated, multidisciplinary and multiagency approach (Committee on Educational Interventions for Children with Autism, 2001). Nonetheless, the state and federal regulations regarding the birth-to-3 transition and post-21 planning have no doubt increased continuity between services. Interest in post-21 planning has also helped spur the development of various models for the development of long-term plans, models that are more likely to recognize the person's rights to self-determination and quality of life.

Assessments of Cognitive and Adaptive Functioning

Formal assessments of overall functioning are conducted at some point—often at many points—in the life of a person with ASD, across school, hospital, and community settings. These can include assessments of overall cognitive or intellectual functioning (e.g., the Wechsler series of assessments), which are most often conducted by a licensed school or clinical psychologist. These can also include overall assessments of adaptive or daily living skills (e.g., the Vineland Adaptive Behavior Scales), which can be conducted by a variety of professionals. Virtually all of the instruments used to assess cognitive and adaptive functioning in people with ASD are also used in the assessment of other populations. Though many of the accommodations considered for people with ASD are also applicable to other populations, most would agree that specialized training and experience can greatly facilitate the assessment of people with ASD (Klin, Saulnier, Tsatsanis, & Volkmar, 2005).

✳ Case Studies

Overall assessment established Asif's eligibility for EI services.

These instruments serve primarily to establish overall eligibility and level of need for planning of services, as when access to developmental disabilities services requires that the person score below a specific cutoff. In research, these instruments are critical to precisely matching groups in an experimental design (e.g., treatment group versus a waiting-list control group). The reliability and validity of the majority of the most commonly used instruments are well established when used in the general population, although most agree that, for a variety of reasons, results obtained for people with ASD are more prone to error: Language deficits can lower estimates of other skills for tests that rely heavily on verbal instruction; markedly uneven skill profiles can make an overall IQ or other quotient less meaningful; estimates may also be lower for people with ASD who tend to be noncompliant or who are less motivated by interactions with an examiner. Although these tests remain the standard for establishing overall functioning levels, their utility in generating individualized intervention targets is limited. On the one hand, results may indicate general patterns of strength and weakness (e.g., strong abstract reasoning, weak social comprehension) that can sometimes help in broadly prioritizing needs, or may reveal areas of surprising strength that can inform instructional strategies. On the other hand, most instruments designed to reliably estimate overall functioning rarely provide the level of detail needed to set specific, measurable goals. Those seeking to identify a specific goal, and then track progress on a weekly or monthly basis, have increasingly turned to curriculum-based assessments (see the discussion later in the chapter).

HEALTH

People with ASD often require health care for many different reasons. I have grouped these under a number of categories (see Figure 2.3), primarily according to the level of specialization required, in anticipation of the kinds of professionals and settings involved. I recognize,

Primary care	Psychopharmacology
Specialized medical evaluation and outpatient treatment of co-occurring conditions	
Emergency medical care	Specialized inpatient behavioral stabilization[a]

Figure 2.3. Health services.
[a]Pivotal service

however, that the boundaries between the roles of generalists and specialists can sometimes be fluid, and so have also sought to capture that here.

Primary Care

Primary care refers here to the broad range of evaluation and treatment services provided by primary care physicians (PCPs) (e.g., pediatricians, family practitioners), nurse practitioners, and dentists. I also consider school nurses to function as PCPs in this context. All of these professionals play a critical role in the lives of people with ASD with respect to the following elements of health care. By definition, primary care is a basic service applicable to all people with disabilities.

- Preventative care and treatment of minor ailments (e.g., ear infections, cavities, minor gastrointestinal problems) is important because people with ASD cannot always communicate accurately regarding the source and extent of their pain and discomfort.

- Screening for conditions requiring more specialized care is important because of the opportunity for early detection of ASD (described earlier) and the higher risk for other medical conditions, especially when ASD is accompanied by significant intellectual disability (see the discussion later in the chapter). Screening for lead is especially important for those people with pica or persistent mouthing.

- Promotion of healthy behaviors is important because people with ASDs often have poor sleep, exercise, and diet (Myers, Johnson, & Council on Children with Disabilities, 2007).

- Overall case management allows the PCP to act as a gatekeeper for referrals to specialists and as a repository for the results and recommendations resulting from their work.

- When specialists are difficult to access (e.g., outside of urban areas and for traditionally underserved populations), PCPs may assume a greater role in long-term management of chronic physical conditions (e.g., allergies) and mental health conditions (e.g., anxiety, mood disorders).

Together, these roles can create a unique bond between PCPs and people with ASD and their caregivers. A PCP who fulfills these roles can become indispensable to the lifelong health and overall well-being of the person with ASD.

This potential is recognized in the concept of the "medical home," which aims to provide "primary medical care that is accessible, continuous, comprehensive, family-centered, coordinated, compassionate, and culturally effective" (Carbone, Behl, Azor, & Murphy, 2010, p. 317). Failure to fulfill one or more of these roles can have significant consequences: In my experience, acute conditions (e.g., ear infections, cavities, constipation) can lead to spikes that can render previously manageable behavior uncontrollable, while chronic conditions (e.g., reflux, sleep, allergies) that are not addressed can have a broad impact on the functioning of the person with ASD, if not their caregivers. Families face many different kinds of barriers to primary care, including the lack of experienced providers, transportation, insurance, and the child's behavior (Pennsylvania Bureau of Autism Services, 2011b). A review by Carbone and his colleagues (2010) concluded that caregivers of children with ASD are likely to report dissatisfaction with primary care, even relative to children with other special health care needs.

Case Studies

Asif's pediatrician helped to screen for possible seizures. Evan's practicing nurse practitioner (PNP) helped to resolve his sleep problems and ear infections. Sofia's physician and school nurse collaborated to better manage her constipation, but the failure of preventative dental care to detect Sofia's cavities likely resulted in unnecessary hospitalization.

Since 2000 there has been increasing recognition of the potential role of PCPs in overall health care. This has led to the development by the American Academy of Pediatrics of consensus-based guidelines for the identification and management of ASD (Johnson et al., 2007; Myers et al., 2007) and an accompanying resource toolkit (American Academy of Pediatrics Autism Expert Panel, 2007). The body of work on gastrointestinal (GI) disorders illustrates the potential convergence between research and practice. A number of reviews have failed to verify a causal link between GI disorders and ASD, but have suggested that specific problems such as selective feeding and constipation may be more prevalent among people with ASD (Ibrahim, Voigt, Katusic, Weaver, & Barbaresi, 2009). These sparked the development of consensus-based guidelines for the identification and treatment of GI disorders in people with ASD (Buie, Campell, et al., 2010; Buie, Fachs, et al., 2010). I believe that the kind of concrete recommendations and specific algorithms included in these guidelines will help PCPs feel confident in taking a more active role in the identification and management of GI problems, which are known to be of great concern to parents. As I discuss later, this has prompted other agencies to invest in the Autism Treatment Network to develop similar guidelines for sleep and other issues commonly addressed by PCPs.

Other Specialized Medical Evaluations and Treatments for Co-Occurring Conditions

There is increasing recognition that ASD is often accompanied by other medical conditions. Although specialized medical evaluations and treatments do not address the core symptoms of ASD, they nonetheless offer immediate opportunities to improve the quality of life for people with ASD. In my experience, PCPs may be more open to identifying and managing the more common of these co-occurring conditions than the diagnosis and management of ASD themselves.

Case Studies

Asif's family sought help from a neurologist for seizures and a gastroenterologist for reflux. Psychiatrists involved in Joshua's and Chloe's care sought to treat problems related to attention and anxiety.

Some of the co-occurring conditions described in Chapter 1 that impact physical and mental health may require more specialized evaluations than can be provided by PCPs. I believe that the effective use of specialists may also help PCPs assume a more active role as appropriate. For example, a neurologist can be a critical asset for the identification of seizures and the use of magnetic resonance imaging (MRI), computerized axial tomography (CAT), electroencephalogram (EEG), or other scans to search for structural or functional neurological anomalies. A psychiatrist can seek to disentangle ASD and other disorders such as attention deficit-hyperactivity disorder (ADHD), anxiety, depression, psychosis, bipolar disorder, and so forth. A geneticist can help determine if ASD is accompanied by other syndromes, and a gastroenterologist can rule out other disorders. A developmental pediatrician may play a role in each of these evaluations, undertaking these themselves, or referring to the previously named specialists. Although the aforementioned guidelines published for primary care practitioners (Johnson et al., 2007) should facilitate referrals to each of these specialists, significant shortages of these professionals represent a significant barrier to care, especially in rural regions. Families are on waiting lists for many months and sometimes must travel many miles for an evaluation. Specialists may compensate by broadening their area of practice; a developmental pediatrician may consult less frequently with a geneticist or psychiatrist, or a neurologist or psychiatrist primarily trained to work with adults may begin to see adolescents. Primary care physicians may compensate by undertaking the diagnosis of some of the more commonly co-occurring psychiatric conditions (e.g., ADHD, anxiety). These shortages, and the fact that many of these conditions are managed primarily through medication (see the discussion later in the chapter), increase the role of PCPs in treatment and evaluation. The identification of co-occurring neurological or genetic conditions may only offer insights into the possible etiology of ASD: With the exception of seizure disorder, they rarely suggest a course of treatment.

Psychopharmacology   A wide range of medications has been used to address the symptoms of ASD (e.g., repetitive behavior), other maladaptive behavior (e.g., aggression, self-injury), other co-occurring psychiatric conditions (e.g., ADHD, anxiety, depression, bipolar disorders), and sleep dysfunction. In their review, Myers, Johnson, and the Council on Children with Disabilities (2007) noted that "recent surveys indicate that approximately 45% of children and adolescents and up to 75% of adults with ASD are treated with psychotropic medication" (p. 1170). A study of national Medicaid claims data for children with ASD revealed that about 20% were prescribed three or more psychotropic medications, and that factors other than clinical presentation appear to be associated with prescription practices; for example, psychotropic use was relatively higher among those living in rural regions and among those counties with a greater proportion of white residents (Mandell et al., 2008).

✴ Case Studies

Medication helped Evan and Chloe with their anxiety. It was unclear whether Joshua or Sofia had ever benefited from medication for attention and self-injury, respectively.

Despite their widespread use, I know of no widely accepted consensus or evidence-based guidelines for psychopharmacology in ASD. A recent review of the medical treatments for ASD concluded that "although many children with ASDs are currently treated with medical interventions, strikingly little evidence exists to support benefit for most treatments. Risperidone and aripiprazole have shown benefit for challenging and repetitive behaviors, but associated adverse effects limit their use to patients with severe impairment or risk of injury" (McPheeters et al., 2011, p. E 1312). Other reviews have also concluded that the number of evidence-based pharmacological treatments for problem behaviors associated with ASD is limited (Myers et al., 2007; Scahill & Boorin, 2011). To date, only risperidone had received formal approval from the Food and Drug Administration for treatment of symptoms in individuals with ASD, and no consensus or evidence-based guidelines exist for the use of multiple medications.

Emergency Medical Care

In my experience, families of children with ASD, for a variety of reasons, turn to emergency rooms (ERs) more often than families of typical children. These families may hesitate to promptly address emerging medical concerns because of the behavior difficulties they present in the waiting room and with the physician. These same behavior difficulties may be exacerbated by the emerging medical problems, which creates a behavioral crisis and prompts an ER visit. People whose ASD is complicated by other specific genetic or neurological syndromes are at a higher risk of associated conditions (e.g., seizures), which may themselves precipitate an ER visit. Finally, parents may turn to the ER when behaviors such as aggression, self-injury, or suicidal thoughts or behaviors put the person with ASD at ready and immediate risk. For example, 3%–12% of Pennsylvania respondents reported ER use in the past year for behavioral or psychiatric reasons (Pennsylvania Bureau of Autism Services, 2011c). In my experience, general hospitals rarely have the specialized personnel or procedures necessary to easily accommodate people with ASD—especially those in behavioral crisis—and I know of no standards that have been widely adopted for emergency care of people with ASD. Faced with a behavioral or psychiatric crisis, most hospitals will seek placement in a psychiatric hospital or, when available, an inpatient program specializing in behavioral stabilization and short-term intensive treatment of people with ASD and related developmental disabilities (see the discussion later in the chapter).

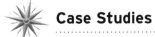 **Case Studies**

Evan's parents sometimes used the emergency room and an emergency clinic for basic care, and Sofia's parents turned to the emergency room to try to get help for her self-injury.

Specialized Inpatient Behavioral Stabilization

In my experience, parents will demonstrate incredible commitment and resourcefulness when their child demonstrates challenging behaviors. Similarly, I have encountered many schools, residential programs, and other service providers who take extraordinary measures to support people with ASD under these circumstances. Nonetheless, parents and providers are sometimes faced with aggression, self-injury, suicidal thoughts, or other behaviors that put the person with ASD or others at significant and immediate risk and that require a level of care that they can no longer provide. The options available at this point are usually very limited: Residential services rarely have either the available beds or the levels of specialized and intensive staffing support to respond in a crisis; community-based crisis centers and hospital emergency rooms may provide a safe place for a day or two while other options are explored; psychiatric hospitals do not always have expertise in developmental disabilities and may have already discovered that individuals with Asperger syndrome are a poor fit with the typical inpatient milieu. In my experience, such behavioral crises act as a pivotal point in the long-term outcomes for people with ASD: They often signal a breakdown not just in behavior planning but also in the coordination of services and supports across home, school, and community, and I have found that these crises often precede placement in a more restrictive setting—a placement that is too rarely reversed. The Pennsylvania 2011 Needs Assessment suggested that such crises are not a rare occurrence—3%–8% of caregivers of someone with ASD, or adults with ASD themselves, reported a hospitalization for behavioral or psychiatric reasons (Pennsylvania Bureau of Autism Services, 2011a).

In response to this need, a number of innovative programs have emerged to provide support during a behavioral crisis. Most of these are hospital-based, inpatient stabilization and short-term treatment programs specializing in people with ASD and related developmental disabilities. I know of a dozen such programs scattered across the United States, identified through the newly established Autism and Developmental Disorders Inpatient Research Collaborative (www.inpatientdevelopmental.com). A recently published survey of nine of these programs revealed many common characteristics across the sites (Siegel et al., 2012): small size (9–22 beds), each with short-term stays (mean of 30 days); a multi-disciplinary approach blending applied behavior analysis, pharmacotherapy, and other short-term treatments, with the goal of reintegrating the individual back into home and community settings as soon as possible; and inpatient services as part of a continuum of services. The limited number of total beds (137) and the concentration of the programs in the Northeast and Mid-Atlantic regions suggests that access will continue to be a significant problem for years to come. In Chapter 7, I describe another innovative approach within the Delaware public school system: A public school program offering part-time extended/residential programming, targeting children and adolescents with significant behavioral problems before behavioral crises necessitate a referral to hospital or residential services. All of these programs can draw on a range of evidence-based behavioral and pharmacological treatments for addressing challenging behaviors (National Autism Center, 2009; National Professional Development Center on Autism Spectrum Disorders, 2011; Powers et al., 2011; Scahill & Boorin, 2011).

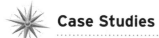 ## Case Studies

When Sofia presented in behavioral crisis at her local hospital's emergency room, the staff sought inpatient behavioral stabilization for her escalating self-injury.

EDUCATION

Education can take different forms (see Figure 2.4). In many respects, education is the foundation upon which many other interventions for children with ASD can—or should—be built. Education may well constitute the bulk of intervention received by children, when considered in terms of number of hours of services delivered directly by, or under the supervision of, a professional. It is the service most likely accessible to all children, regardless

Early intervention
Elementary/middle/high school
Higher education

Figure 2.4. Education services.

of where they live or what specific challenges they face and regardless of who their parents are or what they earn; it is a right guaranteed to all children, and which, at least in the United States, must be individualized to the needs of children with ASD and other disabilities. Education can be much more comprehensive than any specific therapy or intervention, and the benefits of education can extend beyond the walls of the school or university and throughout the lifetime of the individual.

Education of children and adolescents in the United States has been largely shaped by the predecessor to the Individuals with Disabilities Education Act (IDEA), originally passed in 1975. Key elements enshrined in IDEA which was and its amendments include a free appropriate public education (FAPE), or an individualized education plan designed to confer benefit and accord access to the regular curriculum; the least restrictive environment (LRE), ensuring that education must occur with nondisabled peers to the maximum extent appropriate; the individualized education program/individualized family service plan (IEP/IFSP), which sets standards for individualized goals and accommodations and the process around their development; protection from disciplinary action for behaviors attributable to the disability; and procedural safeguards or rules and regulations to protect these rights for children and caregivers (Mandlawitz, 2005). I expect that the vast majority of children with ASD benefit from IEPs/IFSPs, if not other formal mechanisms designed to accommodate their specific needs.

In the following sections, I attempt to highlight those elements of educational programs that are most likely to be adapted to meet the needs of people with ASD, that are most likely to be overlooked by those less familiar with education-based services, and that I feel can contribute most directly to positive outcomes. As discussed at the outset of this chapter, I also try to distinguish between those educational programs that are relatively more specialized from those that can be delivered in a broad range of settings. I do not address those elements of educational programming already discussed under cross-domain services (e.g., ASD identification, behavioral interventions, social skills training, other therapies, paraprofessional support, case management, and assessments of cognitive and adaptive functioning). Although some may be tempted to characterize education as simply a service through which these other, more specialized elements are provided, I argue that, even after these other services are carved out of educational programs, there still remains a tremendous range of skills to be addressed and learning opportunities upon which professionals can capitalize.

Early Intervention

Early intervention (EI; for purposes of discussion here, EI spans birth to 6 years of age, when many children enter kindergarten) begins once eligibility is established either because of a specific diagnosis of ASD or (as in the case studies presented here) after other evaluations had established the presence of significant developmental delays. Prior to age 3, EI programs are almost exclusively home-based, often delivered by an early childhood educator (or paraprofessional under his or her supervision) year-round with the consultation and support of other professionals (e.g., speech pathologists, occupational and/ or physical therapist), and usually part time (e.g., 10 hours per week or less). Early intervention is driven by an individualized family service plan (IFSP) and, as I discuss in Chapter 3, is funded and delivered by services based in the health and/or public welfare agencies. Publically funded services after age 3 are driven by an IEP and delivered by education agencies, usually offering part-time programs (e.g., from 3 to 5 half-days per week), sometimes based in specialized preschools rather than the home.

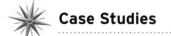 ## Case Studies

Asif and Evan had begun EI services even before being diagnosed with ASD.

By the early 1990s, the traditional methods and curricula used in most EI programs were challenged by the findings of Lovaas (1987) and his colleagues (described earlier in this chapter). These findings sparked lawsuits across the country by parents seeking similar programs for their preschoolers and school-age children with ASD. Although some school districts provided these services only in response to such lawsuits, and other school districts adapted their practices to include more ABA-based techniques and/or more intensive programming, I believe that most school districts have not fundamentally changed their approach to early intervention in response to these findings. As a result, some parents elected to pursue EIBI in place of, or as a supplement to, their other educational services, although the cost was prohibitive for most.

Since the publication of Lovaas's original findings, other comprehensive educational programs have become increasingly popular. For example, more developmental approaches place relatively greater emphasis on play-based interventions as a medium for developing social-emotional understanding (Gutstein & Sheely, 2002; Prizant et al., 2006). The Denver model emerged more recently as an attempt to bridge these gaps (Dawson et al., 2010), and is the first model since Lovaas to provide clear evidence of significant and positive outcomes, using a much more rigorous experimental design. Although I am skeptical that the EI programs offered by most school districts have fundamentally altered in response to Lovaas's findings or the programs that have since emerged, I do believe that some changes may still occur as the current generation of newly trained educators, better versed in these programs, begins to assume leadership positions (see Chapter 3).

One significant consequence of Lovaas's claims was the attempt to develop evidence-based standards for early education programs, beginning with the EI guidelines published by the New York State Department of Health (New York State Department of Health, 1999). This led to perhaps the most ambitious effort to date to develop national guidelines for educational programs, the *Educating Children with Autism* report by the National Research Center (Committee on Educational Interventions for Children with Autism, 2001). Although the report was a timely and comprehensive review of available evidence regarding a range of educational interventions, it is my opinion that the resulting recommendations were too broad and nonspecific to push early intervention programs toward important changes, with two exceptions: 1) as mentioned previously, the recommendation that programs do not attempt to differentiate within the autism spectrum when determining eligibility and 2) that children with ASD be eligible for 25 hours a week, year-round programs as soon as they are identified. The National Standards Project has since recommended EIBI as an evidenced-based program (National Autism Center, 2009), although a number of reviewers have emphasized that attempts to validate broad programs rather than specific methods may overlook the impact of nonspecific treatment variables (e.g., the intensity of programming, the quality of staff training, the reliance on data-based decision making) (Volkmar, Reichow, & Doehring, 2011).

The Role of Parent Training   Early intervention programs are particularly noteworthy for their unique emphasis on parent training and support, an emphasis that I believe should continue at least through childhood and adolescence. Whereas publicly funded EI programs explicitly include services provided to parents, publicly funded programs for older children define goals in relation to the child and deliver services to the child (albeit with the parent's input). Beginning with EIBI, most of the comprehensive EI approaches subjected to rigorous empirical review have included a significant parent training component. More than any other program, EIBI provided parents with all of the information (e.g., what research supports EIBI, how schools work) and practical tools (e.g., how to organize a home-based program, how to measure progress) they needed to become effective advocates (Maurice, Green, & Foxx, 2001; Maurice, Green, & Luce, 1996). The tremendous rise of EIBI programs illustrates how effective parents can be when they become engaged in their child's education and treatment and are optimistic about their progress. Although the potential for many children to recover, as originally claimed by Lovaas and his colleagues (Lovaas, 1987; McEachin & Lovaas, 1993), has since been disputed, I have little doubt that EIBI helped many parents become more ardent and effective advocates for their own children and helped to reshape services for the generation that followed. As I argue later in this chapter and in the final section of this book, this focus on parent training and advocacy should continue beyond the preschool years: A parent who is informed and supported can invigorate his or her child's program and ensure continuity of care across service systems that are often disconnected and at times dysfunctional.

Elementary/Middle/High School

For many children with ASD, a traditional public school education remains the primary mechanism through which they acquire the knowledge, understanding, and experience that prepares them to become full participants in society. Children with ASD attend public schools in the United States for 12–16 years (i.e., from age 5 or 6 until 18 or 21), for 1,000 to 1,200 or more hours per year (e.g., including summer programs), guaranteeing 12,000 to almost 18,000 hours of education. Any endeavor that seeks to scale up services and associated training, research, and policy at a regional, state, or national level must therefore consider how educational services are effectively adapted to the needs of children with ASD. I highlight some of the challenges to curriculum, methods, and the bundling of services in the next paragraphs, and continue this discussion by highlighting important elements of the IEP process, teacher training, and the complex educational infrastructure in Chapter 3.

Until recently, the array of legal and ethical "best practices" facing educators stands in stark contrast to the relative lack of evidence-based practices (Doehring & Winterling, 2011). As noted earlier, the work of the NRC (Committee on Educational Interventions for Children with Autism, 2001) resulted in little more than general recommendations. In this context, the work of both the National Professional Development Center (Chapter 13) and the National Standards Project (National Autism Center, 2009) to identify specific practices for teachers is a significant advance. These organizations and other authors (Doehring &

Winterling, 2011; Eren & Brucker, 2011) are also beginning to address the practical challenges of implementing these practices in public school settings. Other specific examples of public education programs seeking to implement best practices are also described in later chapters (see Chapters 5, 6, and 10).

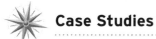 ## Case Studies

Evan and Liam attended a typical school with support, while Joshua attended a typical charter school. Sofia attended a specialized public school program.

The Impact of Intellectual Disability   Perhaps the most important variable determining the type and amount of educational services, as well as adaptations to curricula and methods, is the presence and extent of co-occurring ID. All school districts have at least a limited spectrum of more specialized services adapted to the needs of children with ID: separate classes for those who are least likely to benefit from a typical classroom, and which include substantially modified methods and curricula; and typical classes in which children with ID, ASD, and/or other disabilities can benefit from the support of teacher aides and/or other educational professionals. Other schools have a broad range of options in between, and creative ways of fully integrating children with even highly intense needs into regular educational programming. Although a program specialized in ASD will always develop expertise in ASD more quickly, I have found that a successful and well-structured program for children with at least moderate ID can often meet most of the needs of children whose ID is accompanied by ASD, if the program is led by a resourceful teacher who: 1) is versed in teaching techniques derived from applied behavior analysis (ABA); 2) is responsive to the individual needs of his or her students and their parents; 3) can readily gain access to behavior support to manage the unique challenges sometimes presented by children with ASD; and 4) has been given the flexibility and support by school leaders to adapt their schedule, methods, and curricula. When these children struggle to achieve their potential under these circumstances, this usually reflects the failure to provide teachers with the proper support, or the pressure to service a group of students that is either too large or too diverse in their needs; it does not necessarily reflect that the methods or curricula are inadequate. In this context, it is easy to understand how and why specialized private programs have emerged to fill these gaps.

I have found that schools are more likely to struggle to meet the needs of children with borderline or relatively mild ID, and those with ASD, especially as they approach the transition into adult services. Children with borderline or relatively mild ID accompanied by ASD may have unrealized potential because professionals relied on traditional assessments that underestimated the children's skills or failed to detect and fully exploit areas of exceptional interest or relatively intact skills (e.g., the ability to read). Children with ASD and with challenging behavior do not fit either in the typical classroom setting (especially if it lacks the additional resources to prevent or respond to a behavioral crisis) or in a classroom for children with conduct or other behavior problems (because they are vulnerable to bullying, and may find the academics understimulating). The kinds of individualized staffing, programming, and support require time, training, and other resources that schools may not have. Again, the emergence of specialized private programs is not surprising under these circumstances.

The Impact of Inclusion   The pressure to fully include children and to ensure their access to the regular curriculum has had both positive and negative impacts on the education of children with ASD. On the one hand, it has no doubt prevented children with ASD and not ID from being pushed out of regular classes. As a result, it has probably helped a generation of children realize their potential to graduate from high school if not attend college. It has also pushed teachers and other educators to find creative ways to integrate children with ID with their typical peers, helping the latter to fully appreciate and embrace the diversity of ability, and perhaps in adulthood making them likely to accept people with ID as colleagues in the workplace and citizens in the community.

On the other hand, the expectation central to more recent interpretations of IDEA and the general push to "highly effective teaching"—that all teachers become proficient in the implementation of the regular education curriculum—has come at the expense of adequate training in curricula and methods effective for children with ID, especially those based in ABA (see Chapter 3). Remarkably, the fact that this one-size-fits-all approach to curricula appears to contradict IDEA's prime directive—to ensure that education is adapted to the individual needs of the child—has not diminished this trend in any way. Teachers are neither provided with the training, the materials, nor the time to focus adequately on helping children with ID acquire the basic, functional, self-help, domestic, and community skills they need to become as independent as possible as adults. As a result, they expend their energies adapting complex language and math lessons that are part of the regular education curriculum to students with ID in their classroom, instead of teaching these students a functional curriculum that includes skills they can actually use in the real world, like ordering and paying for a meal in a restaurant. Inclusion's push to dissolve specialized classes and schools, and to educate children in their neighborhood school, has scattered teachers and children across districts, making it even more difficult to appreciate the need for—let alone develop—alternative programs for students with ASD and ID. I return to this issue in Chapter 14, to propose that a more coordinated regional and statewide approach to special education in the schools be implemented to counter the loss in quality that inevitably results under the circumstances described previously.

Vocational and Summer Programs   A related area important to future independence but often overlooked is vocational programming, or the training and support needed to transition into the workforce. Vocational programming already faces the challenges identified earlier: the failure of some schools to adopt a more functional curriculum, approach, and the challenges associated with developing more specialized programs with students with ID and ASD who are scattered across schools and districts. As described earlier, transition planning (of which vocational training is an integral part) can only work effectively when programs across different agencies serving children and adults can be actively coordinated at the level of the individual student, in some cases over a period to 5 or more years. I have also found that successful vocational programming requires that schools actively cultivate a network of vocational placements and experiences, a process that itself demands considerable time and experience. Without these efforts, students graduate with no prospect of employment, risk requiring programs that are more expensive and less likely to lead to greater independence, or simply languish at home in the care of parents too tired to undertake another battle, now for services that are neither mandated nor fully funded.

The impact of poor-quality summer programs on both the student and the family is also overlooked. In theory, individualized programming under IDEA should be constructed to prevent regression or to support the continued development of critical emerging skills during breaks in education, the longest of which occurs over the summertime. In practice, effective summer programs are as challenging to organize as those offered during the school year, but the resources needed to develop and deliver summer programs are the most vulnerable to cuts. As a result, many summer programs in nonspecialized public schools are part-time (e.g., no more than 4 mornings per week) and shortened to 5–6 weeks in length (e.g., leaving 2–3-week breaks at the beginning and the end of the program). When the quality of programming during the regular school year is poor, summer programs are abbreviated and underresourced, and the breaks before and after the summer program are long, summer school quickly devolves into little more than babysitting, and students begin the new school year 1–3 months behind where they had ended the previous school year. I expect that most children with ASD cannot be readily integrated into other summer programs (e.g., especially when their children are older, face more significant intellectual disabilities, present with challenging behaviors). Specialized summer programs for children with ASD are few and far between, and state funds available to defray their cost are often under pressure. As with after-school programming (see discussion later in the chapter), some families have no choice but to absorb considerable out-of-pocket costs for child care or have one spouse stay at home; for single-parent families or those struggling with poverty, even this option is unavailable.

Higher Education

Fifteen years ago, most parents and professionals would have concluded that the pursuit of higher education was an unrealistic goal for all but a handful of people with ASD. With the increasing recognition of the broader spectrum, and with a generation of children having benefited from advances in treatment, higher education has emerged as a viable option for a growing minority of young adults with ASD. A variety of supports have emerged as potentially important: accommodations for the completion of academic requirements; social skill training to navigate increasingly complex relationships; self-advocacy to help the person with ASD chart his or her course; and alternative housing to provide additional support for those not quite ready to live alone or in a regular college residence. These options can take advantage of more traditional mechanisms of support (e.g., college counseling services) and more innovative options (e.g., peer-led models) (see Chapter 4).

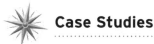 **Case Studies**

Peer and professional support for social and behavioral challenges helped Chloe at college.

COMMUNITY-BASED AND OTHER SUPPORT SERVICES

A variety of formal services and less formal—but nonetheless important—supports are delivered to people with ASD at every age and functioning level (see Figure 2.5).

Child and adult care[b]	Information, support, and advocacy for people living with autism spectrum disorder[a]
Vocational training	Residential program

Figure 2.5. Community services.
[a]Pivotal service.
[b]Babysitting, preschool, before/after-school care, respite, and summer camp.

Child and Adult Care

Regardless of which form it takes, most parents depend on some form of child care at some point in their life. Child care can become inaccessible to caregivers of people with ASD, however, because of the special challenges these people present.

- Parents employed outside of the home may rely upon day care or preschool until their children are old enough to attend school (e.g., day care or preschool).

- Once school has begun, parents employed outside of the home may relay on care at the beginning or end of the school day (e.g., before- or after-school care), and during the summer (e.g., summer camps).

- Parents of typical children may also use a couple of hours of "babysitting" to take care of tasks, or just reconnect. Parents of children with ASD are in even greater need of such support, especially when the behavior challenges prevent the child with ASD from accompanying parents on typical community outings: Child care arrangements at church may be unable to accommodate children with ASD; the one-to-one supervision required may preclude an evening at another family's house; other family outings (e.g., a movie, dinner, a sibling's soccer game) may provoke problem behavior.

- For parents of children with ASD and other disabilities, respite can provide a welcome or necessary break from the pressure of ongoing care. (Whereas the term *respite* is sometimes used for "babysitting," described previously, my use of the term is meant to emphasize the service more specific to people with disabilities.) For some caregivers, a 2- to 3-hour break to simply take care of chores such as shopping for food or gifts, without also supervising a person with ASD, itself provides the needed respite. For people with ASD who react poorly to changes in routines and environments, vacations can provoke a behavioral crisis: For these families, overnight respite may be the only way for them to ever take a break from care.

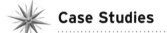 **Case Studies**

Various interventions helped to maintain Asif in his mosque's preschool, Joshua in summer camp, Evan in after-school care, and Sofia in respite with her grandmother.

In each of these contexts, child care is a loosely structured activity generally provided by nonprofessionals—for example, family members, child care assistants, and respite providers. This flexibility can allow the activity to be adjusted to the needs of the child, especially when the adult responsible is compassionate and responsive. Challenges arise when the person with ASD presents with specific behavioral problems: Child care providers rarely have the training or resources to provide more individualized support, and generally have little tolerance for aggression (especially directed to other children). Other challenges arise when the person with ASD begins to outgrow naturally available supports (e.g., there are no after-school programs for adolescents and adults). Caregivers of people with ASD who present with challenging behaviors or who have outgrown these natural supports may literally never get a break from their children. With some exceptions (see Chapter 6), I have found few programs that provide reliable and accessible respite or before- or after-school care after the early childhood years. Thus, it is not surprising that the majority of Pennsylvania care-givers (or their spouses) reported a significant change in their work situation because of their child's ASD (e.g., reducing work hours, losing a promotion, stopping work altogether) (Pennsylvania Bureau of Autism Services, 2011a).

Advocacy, Information, and Support for Caregivers and People with Autism Spectrum Disorder

People living with ASD—that is, both caregivers of and people with ASD—may seek in-formation about many topics important to them: What is ASD? What kinds of help might I need? Where might I find this help? Although this information can be obtained from a variety of written sources (books, the Internet, etc.), I focus here on local, community-based services that have emerged with a specific mission to help those living with ASD to take charge of their care. People living with ASD often play a major role in providing these services, if not leading the agency, though professionals may act in an advisory capacity. Services provided can include training (e.g., characteristics of ASD, effective interventions, systems of care, parental rights), general support (e.g., mentoring, ASD-friendly social activities), advocacy (e.g., help with negotiating the service system, understanding paren-tal rights, seeking to change local or regional policies). The focus on local, community-based services is not intended to discount the activities of national organizations (e.g., Autism Society of America, Autism Speaks), which are discussed in greater detail in the next chapter, but to emphasize the need for people living with ASD to gain to access infor-mation and support at the local level and that is immediately relevant to their individual circumstances.

 Case Studies

Asif's and Joshua's parents identified and advocated for services using information and support provided by various community-based groups. Self-advocacy helped Chloe to take steps to resolve sexual trauma.

I characterize advocacy, and the related services of information and support, as pivotal because, to a large extent, they complement those provided by other agencies by provid-ing critical information and support that people living with ASD might not otherwise get. Through the information and case studies provided in the previous chapter, I hope that readers can begin to appreciate just how hard it is for those living with ASD to know what to expect and what kinds of help to seek. Some may be surprised by the extent of even this most basic of needs: For example, the emerging results of the Pennsylvania Needs Assess-ment suggest that, even among the most recently diagnosed preschoolers, close to 30% were not referred to early intervention services (Pennsylvania Bureau of Autism Services, 2011a). In Chapter 4, I outline the bewildering array of service systems that people living with ASD must navigate to begin to get this help. In this chapter, I have tried to illustrate how case management and planning can be pivotal to coordinating care across disciplines and agencies in the short term, and assuring continuity of support in the long term. In the last section of this book, I propose that the central role of caregivers in the long-term coordina-tion of care be formally recognized, by providing caregivers with the training and support needed to accomplish this task, and providing other accommodations to facilitate this.

Vocational Training

Except for the minority of people with ASD who pursue higher education, all people with ASD should be prepared to perform some form of work as adults. I recognize that such work can ultimately take many forms, from more traditional options at the extremes (e.g., separate workshops for those with most intense and complex support needs, full employment for those with few or no specialized support needs), and less traditional options: community-based clusters of employees working in an enclave or a work crew with the full-time support of a professional; self-employment with the support of a caregiver and/or a professional; and individual job placement with part-time job coaching support provided formally with a job coach or informally (e.g., natural supports with co-workers). Regardless of which option is pursued, I have found that almost all people with ASD will require at least some preparation prior to leaving high school, and that most will require specific and intense preparation. This preparation can be provided by teachers and assistants in the school, but ideally should include community-based placements together with the support of someone with more specific vocational training and experience and whose responsibilities include the cultivation of a range of potential placements or in-house training opportunities. Once the person with ASD is no longer eligible for education-based services, he or she most often receives support through 1) community-based agencies that are either privately contracted to run separate centers, community-based programs, or, less often, individual job coaching and/or 2) publicly funded and administered vocational counselors who assist with placement and provide direct support. Statistics regarding the availability of this range of supports are not readily available, and I have found that options are very limited in most places: Although mandated transition planning obligates educators and caregivers to begin to consider vocational options, no such mandate guarantees support when education-based services cease.

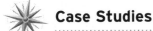 ## Case Studies

Liam benefited from vocational training and community placement organized by his teacher with support from other agencies.

Residential Services

Sometimes the deficits in critical skills of daily living are so pervasive and profound, the behavioral challenges are so intense, and/or the ability of the family to manage them so fragile, that caregivers cannot safely maintain the person with ASD in the family home. Under these circumstances, the most appropriate option in the short, medium, or long term might be some form of residential placement. In cases where the primary problem lies in the family's ability to provide care (e.g., as when the parent struggles with his or her own intellectual or psychiatric challenges, especially in a single-family household or one struggling economically), a specialized foster family placement might suffice. When the primary problems lie in deficits in independence, especially when combined with challenging behavior, the 24/7/365 support of a residential program is usually preferred. A recommendation for residential placement may also be sparked by a behavioral crisis, in some cases itself warranting hospitalization in an inpatient behavioral stabilization program (see earlier discussion). Some residential programs for children and adolescents include a day program, through which their educational needs can also be met. In any case, staff in such programs typically include nonprofessional direct care staff, professionals supervising day-to-day programming (usually with at least a bachelor's-level training from one of a variety of related fields), and a general clinical support team. In my experience, almost all requests signal a breakdown in services and supports within and/or across service systems, and a significant proportion can be prevented or at least forestalled by improvements to supports at school and/or at home. Nonetheless, at least a minority of such placements may be almost inevitable if the family does not have the resources to maintain extraordinary levels of support across the person's lifetime.

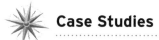 **Case Studies**

A residential program was suggested when Sofia's self-injury seemed too difficult to manage at home.

CONCLUSIONS

The Importance of Pivotal Services

Many services and supports shape the growth of people living with ASD at different points in their lifetime, but I believe that some of these merit the label of pivotal services. Just as Pivotal Response Training targets those skills and methods that prime the child to benefit from other interventions (Koegel et al., 2001), pivotal services help to integrate or to facilitate access to other services (see Figure 2.6). As illustrated by the case studies, pivotal services may also sometimes require relatively limited time or resources, and as such represent immediate opportunities for service, training, research, or policy initiatives. I return in the final chapter to discuss the most promising of these opportunities—that is, those informed by evidence-based practices—for new and more established programs.

- *ASD identification:* Though some people with ASD initially receive services through other diagnoses, screening and diagnosis is often essential to gaining to a wide range of services and supports more specific to ASD, as illustrated through Asif's story.

- *Case management:* As illustrated through Evan's story, case management can also facilitate eligibility and access, and can be essential to bridging gaps across agencies and professionals to solve specific problems.

- *Advocacy:* Joshua's caregivers were educated about his ASD and became more actively involved in advocating for him: This helped them to identify and pursue other services better tailored to their needs, and take a more active role in educating others about Joshua.

- *Behavioral support:* Evan and his parents needed support from many different professionals to address his behavior and related issues. Sofia's story reveals how a behavioral crisis can signal a breakdown in basic services and supports and potentially spur a significant change in placement. Liam's case illustrates how careful communication and collaboration can sometimes prevent a misunderstanding of sexual overtures, leading to more serious consequences.

A) Services facilitated by Asif's ASD identification

Service	Target	Professional (setting)
ASD identification	Screening/diagnosis ➔ referrals to:	Pediatrician (CLI)
Psychological assessment	Establish eligibility for other services	Psychologist (COM)
EI, other therapies	Address overall delays	PAR, TEA (spec. ed.), OT, SLP (HOM)
Specialized medical management	Evaluate for possible seizures	Neurologist (HO-S)
Resource utilization	Provide family with support	Advocate (PIC)

B) Services successfully obtained via Evan's case management

By his social worker

Service	Target	Professional (setting)
Information	Assist in accessing ID support for respite	Social worker (IDA)
Respite	Provide the parents with a break	PAR (COM)
Behavior support	Coordinate toilet-training at home & school	TEA, PAR, Behavior specialist (SC-R, HOM)

By his community-based pediatric nurse practitioner

ASD Identification	Screening led to ASD diagnosis in consultation with others, including evaluation for anxiety and support for interventions to improve sleep & toileting	Nurse (CLI)
Psychopharmacology		Nurse (CLI) in consultation with Developmental pediatrician (CLI)
Primary care		Nurse (CLI)

C) Services that Joshua's parents obtained through their advocacy

Specific service	Target	Professional (setting)
Social skills	Peer conflict	SLP (COM)
Baseball	General accommodations	Baseball coach (COM)
Summer camp		PAR–Camp counselor (COM)
Dentist, haircut, air travel		Behavior specialist, pediatrician (COM)

D) Outcomes of Evan's, Sofia's, and Liam's behavioral support

	Behavior	Professional (setting)	Impact of reductions in behavior
Evan	Anxiety	Nurse (CLI), developmental pediatrician (CLI) & behavior specialist (COM)	Improvements in other behaviors
	Sleep	Nurse (CLI) & developmental pediatrician (CLI)	Provides relief for parents, who are able to more effectively advocate for Evan
	Aggression	Behavior specialist (COM & SC-R)	Return to school
	Toileting	Behavior specialist & PAR (COM & SC-R); social worker (IDA)	Makes after-school care possible; father can return to work
Sofia	Self-injury	Behavior specialist & nurse (SC-S, CLI)	Improvements in other behaviors
		Dentist (COM) & ER team (HO-S)	Failure led to suspension, & referral to residential & inpatient treatment programs
Liam	Sexual overtures	Teacher (SC-R) / Public defender (COM)	Avoided suspension, and possibly incarceration

Figure 2.6. Outcomes associated with pivotal service. (*Key: professionals and settings*: ASD = autism spectrum disorder; CLI = clinic; COL = college; COM = community-based programs; HOM = home; HO = Hospital [-R, Regular; -S, Specialized]; IDA = country/state agency; OT = occupational therapist; PAR = paraprofessional; PIC = parent information center; RES = residential program; SC = school (-R, regular; -S, special); SLP = speech-language pathologist; TEA = teacher.)

Collaboration Between Disciplines, Agencies, and Caregivers/Professionals

The services and associated case studies summarized in this chapter—and especially the pivotal services described previously—illustrate the importance of collaboration across disciplines and agencies. Collaboration presumes that individual professionals understand and respect the other's expertise and role, and that agencies adjust the scope and/or methods of service delivery to that of other agencies. Sadly, this happens too rarely: I have found that professionals often misunderstand the role of other professionals and agencies, underestimate the barriers they face, and then are quick to scapegoat others when care fails. This ignorance and inflexibility, and territoriality that results, become exaggerated when resources are limited and pressure is increased, and hardens with each year and each failure. A similar pattern is noted in the caregiver/professional relationship: Each over- or underestimates the role they might play and the barriers they might face. Until professionals live with disability, either as a parent or as a professional responsible for comprehensive care, they will never fully appreciate the challenges faced by parents. For the cases presented here, most of the breakthroughs in care depended on this cross-discipline/agency and caregiver/professional collaboration. I return to discuss possible solutions to these problems in the next chapter, and in the final section of the book.

Basic Versus Specialized Services Throughout this chapter, I have repeated the distinction between needs that are more basic and those that are more specialized. This distinction captures the amount or training or level of specialization required by an individual, and has important implications in later chapters. Take, for example, important services that are needed by other populations (e.g., management of common gastrointestinal problems), those with important co-occurring conditions that sometimes overlap with ASD (e.g., those with ID but not ASD who need functional skills training), or those specific to ASD but that require minimal training (e.g., screening for ASD). In each of these cases, service professionals can potentially draw on a larger pool of less specialized providers who may require relatively little preparation to deliver an important service. Professionals who may have once hesitated to provide any services and supports, because they feared ASD is beyond their expertise, may become more open to providing other services as appropriate. For more specialized needs (e.g., disentangling ASD from other disorders such as severe intellectual disability, anxiety, psychosis), professionals should be helped to learn when and where such referrals might be needed, and then work with the appropriate agencies to assure the availability of specialists and appropriate training. This distinction also captures the fact that some needs are likely to be common to many people with ASD and others more rare. This information becomes important in later chapters when I seek to project service needs. For example, frequently needed services (e.g., behavior support, respite) should be available in all communities, whereas rarely needed services (e.g., inpatient behavioral stabilization) might only be available at the regional or state level.

Beyond Assessment to Intervention   My case studies underscore what many parents, policy makers, clinicians, and (increasingly) researchers now recognize: The challenge of ASD goes far beyond assessment and diagnosis. We recognize that ASD identification is critical to gaining more specialized services and supports. Research has been conducted to develop the tools to effectively diagnose most cases of ASD by 3 years of age, with some exceptions: For example, Asperger syndrome may continue to be diagnosed somewhat later, ASD may remain difficult to disentangle from severe intellectual disability or anxiety disorder. At this point, additional research on the characteristics of ASD or the finer points of diagnosis appears unlikely to improve access to high-quality service. The principal barriers to early identification now lie in implementation: ASD continues to be diagnosed later among traditionally underserved minorities, and the professions must identify how to help frontline professionals begin to comfortably and accurately diagnose children in their practice when appropriate. By acknowledging all that lies beyond assessment and diagnosis, I hope effort and resources can begin to shift to tackle the much more significant and complex challenges surrounding intervention and support.

REFERENCES

American Academy of Pediatrics. (1998). Auditory integration training and facilitated communication for autism. *Pediatrics, 102*(2), 431–433.

American Academy of Pediatrics Autism Expert Panel. (2007). *Autism: Caring for children with autism spectrum disorders: A resource toolkit for clinicians.* Elk Grove, IL: American Academy of Pediatrics.

Bambara, L.M., & Kern, L. (2005). *Individualized supports for children with problem behaviors: Designing positive behavior plans.* New York, NY: Guilford Press.

Baron-Cohen, S., Wheelwright, S., Cox, A., Baird, G., Charman, T., Swettenham, J., et al. (2000). Early identification of autism by the Checklist for Autism in Toddlers (CHAT). *Journal of the Royal Society of Medicine, 93*(10), 521–525.

Bondy, A., & Frost, L. (2001). The Picture Exchange Communication System. *Behavior Modification Special Autism, Part 1, 25*(5), 725–744.

Buie, T., Campbell, D.B., Fuchs III, G.J., Furuta, G.T., Levy, J., Vandewater, J., et al. (2010). Evaluation, diagnosis, and treatment of gastrointestinal disorders in individuals with ASDs:

A consensus report. *Pediatrics, 125*(Suppl. 1), S1–S18.

Buie, T., Fuchs III, G.J., Furuta, G.T., Kooros, K., Levy, J., Lewis, J.D., et al. (2010). Recommendations for evaluation and treatment of common gastrointestinal problems in children with ASDs. *Pediatrics, 125*(Suppl. 1), S19–S29.

Bureau of Autism Services, Pennsylvania Department of Public Welfare. (2011). *Pennsylvania Autism Needs Assessment: A survey of individuals and families living with autism: Unwanted outcomes-police contact & urgent hospital care.* Retrieved from http://www.paautism.org/asert/ASERT_Unwanted outcomes_August%202011.pdf

Carbone, P.S., Behl, D.D., Azor, V., & Murphy, N.A. (2010). The medical home for children with autism spectrum disorders: Parent and pediatrician perspectives. *Journal of Autism and Developmental Disorders, 40*(3), 317–324.

Carr, E.G., Dunlap, G., Horner, R.H., Koegel, R.L., Turnbull, A.P., Sailor, W., et al. (2002). Positive behavior support: Evolution of an applied science. *Journal of Positive Behavior Interventions, 4*(1), 4–16, 20.

Committee on Educational Interventions for Children with Autism. (2001). *Educating children with autism.* Washington, DC: National Academies Press.

Cooper, J., Heron, T., & Heward, W. (2007). *Applied behavior analysis* (2nd ed.). Upper Saddle River, NJ: Prentice-Hall.

Dawson, G., Rogers, S., Munson, J., Smith, M., Winter, J., Greenson, J., et al. (2010). Randomized, controlled trial of an intervention for toddlers with autism: The Early Start Denver Model. *Pediatrics, 125*, 17–23.

Doehring, P., & Winterling, V. (2011). The implementation of evidence-based practices in public schools. In B. Reichow, P. Doehring, D.V. Cicchetti, & F.R. Volkmar (Eds.), *Evidence-based practices and treatments for children with autism* (pp. 343–363). New York, NY: Springer.

Eren, R.B., & Brucker, P.O. (2011). Practicing evidence-based practices. In B. Reichow, P. Doehring, D.V. Cicchetti, & F.R. Volkmar (Eds.), *Evidence-based practices and treatments for children with autism* (pp. 309–341). New York, NY: Springer.

Ferraioli, S.J., & Harris, S.L. (2011). Treatments to increase social awareness and social skills. In B. Reichow, P. Doehring, D.V. Cicchetti, & F.R. Volkmar (Eds.), *Evidence-based practices and treatments for children with autism* (pp. 171–196). New York, NY: Springer.

Gutstein, S.E., & Sheely, R.K. (2002). *Relationship development intervention with children, adolescents, and adults: Social and emotional development activities for Asperger syndrome, Autism, PDD, and NLD.* Philadelphia, PA: Jessica Kingsley.

Hollon, S.D., & Ponniah, K. (2010). A review of empirically supported psychological therapies for mood disorders in adults. *Depression and Anxiety, 27*(10), 891–932.

Ibrahim, S.H., Voigt, R.G., Katusic, S.K., Weaver, A.L., & Barbaresi, W.J. (2009). Incidence of gastrointestinal symptoms in children with autism: A population-based study. *Pediatrics, 124*(2), 680–686.

Ingersoll, B., Lewis, E., & Kroman, E. (2007). Teaching the imitation and spontaneous use of descriptive gestures in young children with autism using a naturalistic behavioral intervention. *Journal of Autism and Developmental Disorders, 37*(8), 1446–1456.

Johnson, C.P., Myers, S.M., & and the Council on Children with Disabilities. (2007). Identification and evaluation of children with autism spectrum disorders. *Pediatrics, 120*(5), 1183–1215.

Kleinman, J.M., Robins, D.L., Ventola, P.E., Pandey, J., Boorstein, H.C., Esser, E.L., et al. (2008). The Modified Checklist for Autism in Toddlers: A follow-up study investigating the early detection of autism spectrum disorders. *Journal of Autism and Developmental Disorders, 38*(5), 827–839.

Klin, A., Saulnier, C., Tsatsanis, K., & Volkmar, F. (2005). Clinical evaluation in Autism Spectrum Disorders: Psychological assessment within a transdisciplinary framework. In F.R. Volkmar, R. Paul, A. Klin, & D. Cohen (Eds.), *Handbook of autism and pervasive developmental disorders: Assessment, interventions, and policy* (3rd ed., pp. 772–798). New York, NY: Wiley.

Koegel, R.L., Koegel, L.K., & McNerney, E.K. (2001). Pivotal areas in intervention for autism. *Journal of Clinical Child Psychology, 30*(1), 19–32.

Lord, C., Rutter, M., DiLavore, P.C., & Risi, S. (1999). *Autism Diagnostic Observation Schedule (ADOS).* Los Angeles, CA: Western Psychological Services.

Lord, C., Rutter, M., & Le Couteur, A. (1994). Autism Diagnostic Interview-Revised: A revised version of a diagnostic interview for caregivers of individuals with possible pervasive developmental disorders. *Journal of Autism and Developmental Disorders, 24*(5), 659–685.

Lovaas, O.I. (1987). Behavioral treatment and normal educational and intellectual functioning in young autistic children. *Journal of Consulting and Clinical Psychology, 55*(1), 3–9.

Mancil, G.R. (2006). Functional communication training: A review of the literature related to children with autism. *Education and Training in Developmental Disabilities, 41*(3), 213–224.

Mandell, D.S., Morales, K.H., Marcus, S.C., Stahmer, A.C., Doshi, J., & Polsky, D.E. (2008). Psychotropic medication use among Medicaid-enrolled children with autism spectrum disorders. *Pediatrics, 121*(3), e441–e448.

Mandlawitz, M. (2005). Educating children with autism: Current legal issues. In F.R. Volkmar, R. Paul, A. Klin, & D. Cohen (Eds.), *Handbook of autism and pervasive developmental disorders: Assessment, interventions, and policy* (3rd ed., pp. 1161–1174). New York, NY: Wiley.

Maurice, C., Green, G., & Foxx, R.M. (2001). *Making a difference: Behavioral intervention for autism.* Austin, TX: PRO-ED.

Maurice, C., Green, G., & Luce, S.C. (1996). *Behavioral intervention for young children with autism: A manual for parents and professionals.* Austin, TX: PRO-ED.

McEachin, J.J., & Lovaas, O.I. (1993). Long-term outcome for children with autism who received early intensive behavioral treatment. *American Journal on Mental Retardation, 97*(4), 359–372.

McPheeters, M.L., Warren, Z., Sathe, N., Bruzek, J.L., Krishnaswami, S., Jerome, R.N., et al. (2011). A systematic review of medical treatments for children with autism spectrum disorders. *Pediatrics, 127*(5), e1312–e1321.

Myers, S.M., Johnson, C.P., & the Council on Children with Disabilities. (2007). Management of children with autism spectrum disorders. *Pediatrics, 120*(5), 1162–1182.

National Autism Center. (2009). *The National Standards Project: Addressing the need for evidence based practice guidelines for autism spectrum disorders.* Randolph, MA: Author.

National Professional Development Center on Autism Spectrum Disorders. (2011). *Evidence-based practice briefs.* Chapel Hill: FPG Child Development Institute, University of North Carolina at Chapel Hill.

New York State Department of Health. (1999). *Clinical practice guideline: Report of the recommendations. Autism/pervasive developmental disorders, assessment and intervention for young children (0–3 years).* Albany: New York State Department of Health, Early Intervention Program.

O'Neill, R.E., Horner, R.H., Allard, A., Sproul, C.J., Storey, K., & Newton, J.S. (1997). *Functional assessment and program development for problem behavior: A practical handbook* (2nd ed.). Belmont, CA: Thomson Brooks/Cole.

Partington, J.W., & Sundberg, M.L. (1998). *The assessment of basic language and learning skills.* Pleasant Hill, CA: Behavior Analysts.

Pennsylvania Bureau of Autism Services. (2011a). *Pennsylvania Autism Needs Assessment. 1 (Statewide Summary).* Harrisburg: Pennsylvania Department of Public Welfare.

Pennsylvania Bureau of Autism Services. (2011b). *Pennsylvania Autism Needs Assessment: A Survey of Individuals and Families Living with Autism. 3: Barriers and limitations to accessing services.* Harrisburg: Pennsylvania Department of Public Welfare.

Pennsylvania Bureau of Autism Services. (2011c). *Pennsylvania Autism Needs Assessment: A Survey of Individuals and Families Living with Autism. 4: Unwanted outcomes—police contact and urgent hospital care.* Harrisburg: Pennsylvania Department of Public Welfare.

Powers, M.D., Palmieri, M.J., D'Eramo, K.S., & Powers, K.M. (2011). Evidence-based treatment of behavioral excesses and deficits for individuals with autism spectrum disorders. In B. Reichow, P. Doehring, D.V. Cicchetti, & F.R. Volkmar (Eds.), *Evidence-based practices and treatments for children with autism* (pp. 55–92). New York, NY: Springer.

Prelock, P.A., Paul, R., & Allen, E.M. (2011). Evidence-based treatments in communication for children with autism spectrum disorders. In B. Reichow, P. Doehring, D.V. Cicchetti, & F.R. Volkmar (Eds.), *Evidence-based practices and treatments for children with autism* (pp. 93–169). New York, NY: Springer.

Prizant, B.M., Wetherby, A.M., Rubin, E., Laurent, A.C., & Rydell, P.J. (2006). *The SCERTS® Model: A comprehensive educational approach for children with autism spectrum disorders: Program planning and intervention* (Vol. 2). Baltimore, MD: Paul H. Brookes Publishing.

Reichow, B., Doehring, P., Cicchetti, D.V., & Volkmar, F.R. (2011). *Evidence-based practices and treatments for children with autism.* New York, NY: Springer.

Rutter, M., Bailey, A., & Lord, C. (2003). *The Social Communication Questionnaire.* Los Angeles, CA: Western Psychological Services.

Scahill, L., & Boorin, S.G. (2011). Psychopharmacology in children with PDD: Review of current evidence. In B. Reichow, P. Doehring, D.V. Cicchetti, & F.R. Volkmar (Eds.), *Evidence-based practices and treatments for children with autism* (pp. 231–243). New York, NY: Springer.

Schaaf, R.C. (2011). Interventions that address sensory dysfunction for individuals with autism spectrum disorders: Preliminary evidence for the superiority of sensory integration compared to other sensory approaches. In B. Reichow, P. Doehring, D.V. Cicchetti, & F.R. Volkmar (Eds.), *Evidence-based practices and treatments for children with autism* (pp. 245–273). New York, NY: Springer.

Siegel, M., Doyle, K., Chemelski, B., Payne, D., Ellsworth, B., Harmon, J., et al. (2012). Specialized inpatient psychiatry units for children with autism and developmental disorders: A United States survey. *Journal of Autism and Developmental Disorders, 42*(9), 1–7.

Volkmar, F., Paul, R., Klin, A., & Cohen, D. (2005a). *Handbook of autism and pervasive developmental disorders: Assessment, interventions, and policy* (3rd ed.). New York, NY: Wiley.

Volkmar, F., Paul, R., Klin, A., & Cohen, D. (2005b). *Handbook of autism and pervasive developmental disorders: Diagnosis, development, neurobiology, and behavior* (3rd ed.). New York, NY: Wiley.

Volkmar, F.R., Reichow, B., & Doehring, P. (2011). Evidence-based practices in autism: Where we are now and where we need to go. In B. Reichow, P. Doehring, D.V. Cicchetti, &

F.R. Volkmar (Eds.), *Evidence-based practices and treatments for children with autism* (pp. 365–391). New York, NY: Springer.

Warren, Z., Stone, W., & Humberd, Q. (2009). A training model for the diagnosis of autism in community pediatric practice. *Journal of Developmental and Behavioral Pediatrics, 30*(5), 442–446.

Whalen, C., Schreibman, L., & Ingersoll, B. (2006). The collateral effects of joint attention training on social initiations, positive affect, imitation, and spontaneous speech for young children with autism. *Journal of Autism and Developmental Disorders, 36*(5), 655–664.

Wood, J.J., Fujii, C., & Renno, P. (2011). Cognitive behavioral therapy in high-functioning autism: Review and recommendations for treatment development. In B. Reichow, P. Doehring, D.V. Cicchetti, & F.R. Volkmar (Eds.), *Evidence-based practices and treatments for children with autism* (pp. 197–230). New York, NY: Springer.

World Health Organization. (2008). *ICD-10: International statistical classification of diseases and related health problems* (10th rev. ed.). New York, NY: Author

3

An Overview of the Training, Research, and Policy Supporting Systems of Services for People with Autism Spectrum Disorder

Peter Doehring

As outlined in the introduction, this chapter describes the training and research associated with the services listed in Chapter 2 provided to people with ASD, and the policy underlying all of these activities. Even though this infrastructure is described in reference to the subset of service introduced in the previous chapter, it illustrates the many mechanisms through which services can—or should—be identified, expanded, and sustained at the local, regional, state, and national levels. At various points throughout this chapter, I return to the cases introduced in Chapter 1 (and summarized in Table 3.1) to help imagine how training, research, and policy can translate into real and significant improvements in the lives of people living with ASD.

Table 3.1. Case studies—services and agencies

Name	Key Services Obtained or Sought[a]
Asif	Screening and diagnosis;[b] speech/occupational therapy; developmental assessment; primary care; specialized medical treatment for co-occurring conditions; early intervention; child care; advocacy[b]
Evan	Screening & diagnosis;[b] behavioral support;[b] case management;[b] primary care; psychopharmacology; emergency medical care; early intervention; regular school; child care/respite
Joshua	Social skills training; specialized medical treatment for co-occurring conditions; psychopharmacology; charter school; summer camp; advocacy[b]
Sophia	Behavioral support;[b] case management;[b] primary care; psychopharmacology; emergency medical care; inpatient stabilization; special school; respite; residential services
Liam	Case management; regular school; vocational training
Chloe	Social skills training; cognitive behavioral therapy; specialized medical treatment for co-occurring conditions; psychopharmacology; college; advocacy[b]

[a]All individuals benefited from paraprofessional support.
[b]Pivotal service.

TRAINING

Most comprehensive reviews of intervention for ASD have emphasized that one of the most significant barriers to scaling up high-quality services is the lack of training programs, generally, and trainers, specifically (Committee on Educational Interventions for Children with Autism, 2001). Although the amount of training has certainly increased significantly over the past two decades, the number and range of training opportunities has hardly kept pace with the increase in the number and range of people identified with ASD. As I argue next, many parents and practitioners value training, but few have recognized its full potential to fundamentally reshape services, and fewer still have exploited it. As a result, many rely on isolated training events around a relatively narrow range of topics, instead of committing time and resources to the kinds of coordinated, integrated, and comprehensive programs I describe next.

In this section, I provide examples of the kinds of training activities and programs that might prepare professionals and others to deliver the services listed in Chapter 2. Again, it is beyond the scope of this book to list all of the specific training activities involved for each type of service, discipline, and agency. My goal is to describe the range of activities and programs common to different types of providers, to help identify the best opportunities and the greatest barriers. These descriptions are derived from almost 20 years of experience across various settings leading the development of training programs, or contributing to implementation of other training programs for the full range of professionals and parents. This level of understanding is important because, as becomes evident further on in the chapter, opportunities for training specific to ASD during initial certification and licensure have been virtually nonexistent and may be difficult to create, although other opportunities may offer more promise.

The Content of Training Programs

Building on the characteristics of ASD listed in Chapter 1 and the types of services and themes listed in Chapter 2, I would argue that training for specific disciplines and professional groups should seek to develop breadth and depth in several areas of knowledge and expertise (see Figure 3.1). In sum, I believe that the multifaceted nature of ASD and their impact on people living with them demand a broad perspective that cuts across the life span. I have found that many professionals over time tend to specialize with respect to the range of interventions they use, the type of people they work with, and the types of agencies with which they are familiar: By at least ensuring a basic understanding of the full range of services, supports, and settings, I can help professionals be more open to collaboration. In a similar manner, awareness of the full impact of ASD may help professionals recognize that they are unlikely to meet all of a person's needs and provide greater impetus for collaboration. In general, I have also found that many professionals fail to grasp the full impact on people living with ASD, and are prone to overestimate the potential influence of their own profession or agency and underestimate the influence of others. Whether this is naturally corrected with experience appears to depend on the temperament of the professional: Those who are open-minded recognize the value of collaboration, whereas the more cynical become suspicious and entrenched in promoting their own contribution to the exclusion of others. The exception is professionals who either participate in a postgraduate training program or work in a setting that explicitly promotes community-focused, person-centered, and multidisciplinary treatment (see Chapter 14).

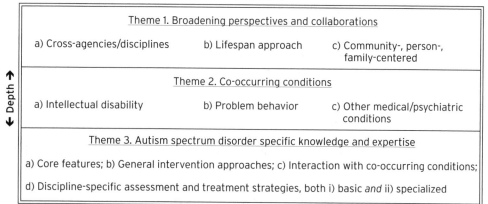

Figure 3.1. Content of ASD training programs.

As recommended in previous chapters, professionals should also be trained in the co-occurring conditions that are sometimes more prevalent or somewhat less complex than ASD (e.g., intellectual disability [ID], problem behaviors). Of the three content areas identified in Figure 3.1, I have found that professionals are more likely to have received a broad training in this area as part of their initial licensure, but may be unsure when and how these techniques should be adapted for people with ASD. The third broad content area is knowledge and expertise in ASD itself. In general, I have found that many practitioners became interested in ASD during their initial training and licensure, but that opportunities to acquire knowledge, let alone expertise, are very limited (see discussion later in the chapter). Specialization (e.g., provision of services specific to ASD, and/or especially rare or complex services) is generally acquired on the job and not as part of a structured training program.

This summary clearly does not begin to convey the challenge of developing a training program intended to create a new generation of specialists: That task is to be left to leaders in each of their respective fields. Nonetheless, this framework has helped me to focus my own training in ways that allow programs to be scaled up progressively. For example, I have found that even experienced professionals misunderstand the role of other professionals and agencies, and they have greatly appreciated my efforts to educate them about other disciplines and agencies. I also incorporate accounts of the experience of people with ASD—if not presentations from people with ASD itself—into most introductory trainings, and convey the impact of interventions on day-to-day functioning. Professionals have told me that these first-person accounts reinvigorate them, and people living with ASD making such presentations leave with a greater respect and understanding of the professionals with whom they work. Scaling up training programs by adopting a broader perspective is important given the much greater challenge of developing specific expertise in ASD, which I describe next.

The Structure of Training

Those seeking to develop specific expertise in ASD among professionals often turn first to existing, traditional training approaches. I begin by summarizing some of the strengths and limitations of existing programs with which I have worked, and then propose how existing programs can be reorganized and enhanced to build experts and leaders in ASD.

Programs Leading to Initial Licensure   Licensure itself, and the university-based programs that prepare individuals for licensure, seem to offer the best opportunities to increase the knowledge and expertise of practitioners because they must assure that critical content is covered, and critical supervised experience is provided. Almost all of the major professional groups listed in the last chapter (e.g., physicians, nurses, psychologists, teachers, speech pathologists, occupational therapists, social workers) are formally licensed at the state and/or national level, following completion of a degree program through a university. Other subspecialties may also be formally licensed (e.g., various medical specialists, pediatric nurse practitioners, special education teachers). Licensing bodies also verify that the university-based program has met certain criteria that typically include types of courses and/or course content, plus one or more practicum placements that may add up to more than 1,000 hours of fieldwork. Professions such as medicine and psychology that require a doctorate and postgraduate fieldwork of several years provide even greater opportunities for specialization. Psychology doctorates (PhD or PsyD) requiring a thesis based on a literature review and/or empirical research provide other opportunities to develop additional expertise, albeit usually more academic than clinical.

Supplementary Licensure

Initial training and licensure is often ill-suited to develop autism spectrum disorder expertise. Supplementary licensure or endorsement (e.g., specialized post-graduate training in ASD) is more realistic (see Chapter 7 for an example).

My experience has led me to conclude, however, that programs leading to initial licensure rarely ensure that the individual graduates have enough specific knowledge regarding ASD to immediately become more specialized, though specific courses and practicum opportunities can provide valuable exposure to people with disabilities. For example, I have found very few formal training programs leading to a universally recognized initial license that require a specific course in ASD. Although their discipline-specific training in disabilities or psychiatric conditions may well include ASD, I have found that the competing pressures to prepare the professional to potentially work with a range of populations often preclude any requirement for such specialization. Moreover, the coursework and curricula are hotly debated by academics, and the effort required to inject significant content specific to ASD above and beyond the core features of ASD (Theme 3a) is difficult to justify given the difficulty students have integrating all of this information, especially in the absence of relevant fieldwork. Training programs that rely primarily on one field or practicum placement usually structure these placements not to specialize but to ensure exposure to a range of populations. For these reasons, I feel that it is perhaps easier to promote the first two themes (i.e., a broad approach and knowledge of co-occurring conditions). I would advocate that clinical programs support practicum placements wherever possible, to build collaborations with specific training programs, and entice trainees to consider pursuing additional training or at least sensitize them to the issues involved in the treatment of ASD.

These programs also provide relatively few opportunities for those who want to embark on a path to specialization during this initial phase of their training. Programs that include multiple field placements with a significant time commitment (e.g., 500 hours or more) may allow one of these placements to be more narrowly focused (e.g., serving primarily those with ASD). Though this rarely provides the trainee with enough experience to immediately specialize upon graduation, it can stoke his or her interest to seek employment in an agency serving primarily people with ASD, or to seek additional, more specialized, postgraduate training. Postgraduate practica (e.g., medical residency or postdoctoral psychology internships) are designed to support greater specialization. Doctoral research of a clinical nature can also provide experience that can help the professional more quickly specialize in ASD. Of course, focusing on programs leading to initial licensure does little to help professionals already in the field, and who are more likely to be in positions of program leadership.

For other professional groups that are not formally licensed, there are no guarantees that certain training requirements have been met. Although national standards have been defined for Board Certified Behavior Analysts (BCBAs), many states have yet to formally recognize BCBAs as a separate professional group. As a result, professionals in those states may use other titles (e.g., behavior consultant/therapist). Consistency nationwide in the state licensing of BCBAs offers great promise: I have found that behavior analyst training programs offer the highest concentration of coursework more directly related to clinical intervention specific to ASD, as well as practicum placements focused on people with ASD. Some other kinds of titles commonly used (e.g., therapist, case manager, residential advisor, job coach) are often not associated with a specific credentialing body. In each of these cases, the agency if not the state has broadly defined criteria that often include completion of an undergraduate or graduate degree in a related field, but without the rigor or detail of a formal licensing body. As a group, those acting in a paraprofessional capacity are very rarely credentialed. Though some agencies may require completion of an undergraduate degree in a related field, many will not have done so.

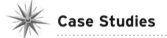

Case Studies

Relatively few cases benefited from professionals who received training in ASD during initial licensure, with the exception of the Board Certified Behavior Analysts (BCBAs), who all received coursework and practica experience in ASD. Other exceptions included the work-study program for Joshua's camp counselors and the specialized program in developmental disabilities completed by his speech pathologist.

Other Training Channels   Given the limited opportunities to develop knowledge and expertise specific to ASD during initial training and licensure, I next turn to other kinds of training opportunities. *Postgraduate university programs* specializing in ASD and/or severe disabilities are increasingly popular, especially in fields such as special education. Such programs are not constrained by licensure requirements, and so can target specific areas. Sometimes these programs are structured as a specialized certificate, and other times are structured as an area of specialization within a specialized degree (e.g., a master's in special education with a concentration in ASD); the latter are more likely be formally recognized by employers (e.g., in establishing seniority, pay grade). Although I am skeptical about the benefits of an isolated course, I believe that a well-designed program that includes at least three courses specific to ASD can help build specialization for professionals who are also working predominantly with people with ASD.

✳ Case Studies

All of the cases benefited from professionals who received training via other channels. *Specialized postgraduate training* programs helped Evan's teacher (teaching certification in ASD). *Agency-specific training* helped Sofia's aide know how to accommodate her needs in the emergency room. *Specialized workshops* helped Asif's pediatrician (screening for ASD) and family (advocacy), Evan's nurse (diagnosis of ASD), and Joshua's teacher. *Case consultation* helped Liam's teacher anticipate needs related to his sexuality.

The most immediate opportunity to develop expertise specific to ASD often lies in *agency-specific professional development activities.* For example, mandatory trainings conducted as part of initial orientation can potentially reach all employees, and ensure that critical content is covered. When core principles of assessment and intervention are described with reference to agency-specific expectations and activities (e.g., a specific assessment protocol, how results are reported and used), the information is more relevant and meaningful to practice, and more likely to be consolidated than the more abstract principles too often covered in these training programs. Agency-specific continuing education activities offer an opportunity to bring in specific experts to provide specific training and consultation. Training provided in a timely manner in response to an expressed staff need can lead to immediate implementation. With the right supervision, development and implementation of an in-house training program can help to groom promising staff to become trainers and program leaders. The effort needed to develop an in-house program may be difficult to justify, however, for a small- or medium-size agency, but is certainly worthwhile for larger agencies or for a consortium of small- to medium-size agencies.

Many people pursue ongoing professional development through *presentations, workshops, and professional conferences.* Although such activities can certainly increase awareness and perhaps generally shape the practice of an experienced professional, I doubt that these activities in isolation will contribute significantly and reliably to the development of expertise in ASD in a less experienced professional, with some exceptions. Intensive workshops that focus on the use of a specific technique, that describe clear parameters for when and with whom the technique should be used, that include opportunities for practice and feedback, and that provide supporting materials (e.g., a manual, kit, data sheets) can help the professional adopt a new practice as long as there are plenty of opportunities and no significant barriers to its immediate implementation. Too often, I have participated in less intensive and specialized workshops that focus too much on theory and too little on real-world applications, assuming that all participating professionals can translate general principles into practice. I have had the privilege of participating in and organizing formal workshops on the use of the Autism Diagnostic Observation Schedule (Lord, Rutter, DiLavore, & Risi, 1999) and Autism Diagnostic Interview–Revised (Lord, Rutter, & Le Couteur, 1994), and have observed how these workshops have evolved to include all of the ingredients listed earlier: They provide detailed manuals and scoring protocols, workshops include observation of live and videotaped assessments, and participants can often pursue opportunities to have a videotape of their practice testing reviewed by an experienced administrator. It is clear when these instruments should be used, and many participants have enough opportunities to apply the skill.

Finally, I have also found that *enhanced case consultation* can be one of the most powerful training tools, but only when it is strategically employed. Case consultation often begins when a parent, school, or other provider is seeking guidance regarding a specific skill or school, usually for a specific person living with ASD. If the consultation is limited to this specific situation, little opportunity might exist to expand the training goals: The consultation might be very narrowly focused, and responding to a crisis situation may produce too much stress to promote a more thoughtful approach to learning. When the case consultation is provided proactively to address known areas of weakness, and to increase a broader range of skills, it can become much more powerful: Professionals invest in the training, and gain immediate opportunities to practice. Pairing this case consultation with on-site coaching is perhaps the best way to promote fidelity of intervention. I elaborate on such a model later in this section, but mention here that this training emerges naturally when a program leader recognizes an emerging need, can find a local expert experienced not just in intervention but also in staff training, and can secure the resources to support a program that extends beyond crisis-oriented case consultation. Case consultation is particularly useful in helping to compensate for the lack of specialized programming in smaller organizations in rural regions.

One other factor influencing the ease with which professionals can acquire knowledge and expertise bears mention here: experience either as a family member or working in a

---

Helping Paraprofessionals Become Teachers

The state of Delaware, school districts, and University of Delaware collaborated to create a program whereby working paraprofessionals can complete teacher training quickly and at low cost, while maintaining their employment. Autism Delaware and other related groups have offered scholarships to paraprofessionals who completed their teacher training.

---

paraprofessional role. The former can help to ensure that the professional is committed and understands the challenges of living with ASD every day. A careful reading reveals that almost all of the cases here benefited from a professional who was himself or herself a family member of someone with ASD. For that reason, I have actively sought to recruit trainees with this background. The latter can also help to convey the complexity of providing care (especially the challenges facing frontline staff), and can help in the acquisition of specific skills when the experience is acquired in a high-quality program. The only potential drawback is when this professional has adopted a rigid set of practices based on this experience, and is unwilling to consider other practices. I have therefore learned to weigh this experience appropriately when considering prospective students or employees, and carefully evaluating the person's capacity to be self-critical. I have also actively promoted programs that help subsidize paraprofessionals who are interested in pursuing higher education (see the "Helping Paraprofessionals Become Teachers" sidebar).

Where Do We Go From Here?
A Comprehensive and Integrated Approach to Training

Individual Training Activities Evolve Over Time into a Broad Training Program   As described earlier, individual expertise will rarely be conferred by attending a single course or workshop. As described in the following paragraphs, isolated training activities will rarely bring about systemic change. A coordinated program of training (e.g., a series of workshops, a course, a certificate program) can increase the total training time by stretching it across multiple days to accommodate other valuable activities—demonstrations, practice, self-assessments, group discussion, case consultation, development of supporting materials, and so forth (see Table 3.2). Breaking training into chunks makes it more manageable (e.g., easier for the trainer to prepare), more efficient (e.g., trainees are easier to keep engaged for 90 minutes than for 6 hours), and perhaps more easily scheduled (e.g., a 60–90 minute session can be scheduled at the beginning or the end of the workday). Stretching training over time gives trainees opportunities to practice skills, share successes and failures, and connect with other trainees in similar roles at other participating sites or agencies. Periodic updates can help to realign training to new research findings, reenergize practitioners who may have little chance to share successes and failures because they are the only expert in their program.

This evolution extends to the development of the program itself. A comprehensive training program cannot be developed overnight; hence the need for sustained support and a designated leader. In the beginning, a program may strive to develop a curriculum through the initial training presentation, with opportunities for practice and coaching, a preliminary literature review to ensure it is consistent with best practice, and opportunities to draw feedback from participants. In a second phase, the training can seek to develop additional supporting materials (e.g., annotated bibliographies, written guidelines), expand the use of practice and coaching (e.g., with case consultation, fidelity checks), and enhance the initial presentation (e.g., with video clips of the practice in action, pre- and/or posttests).

Identify and Support a Leader and/or Lead Agency   The kinds of training programs needed to build and maintain effective, evidenced-based services require careful planning, coordination, and follow-up if awareness and expertise is to grow and a common vision is to be established. Too often, I have watched as agencies advance a training initiative under the direction of an ambitious professional: Both underestimate the time and resources required to prepare and provide even an isolated workshop, and the training

Table 3.2. Comprehensive Training Programs

Include these **Components**	Draw upon these **Strategies:** To ...	Seek these **Goals:** To ...
a) **Individual training: Activities** are combined into a **broad training program** b) with the guidance and support of a designated **Leader**	c) ... Carefully assess **resources** and **barriers** to sustaining implementation d) ... Develop collaboration and a shared vision across the entire **network** of services e) ... Be **data-driven**	f) ... Establish **Best Practice Guidelines** aligned with empirical research and legal standards g) ... Build and sustain both **knowledge** and **expertise**

program flounders. In my experience, 2–5 hours are needed to prepare materials for every hour of training when first designing an isolated course or workshop, and sustained effort and support is needed to develop a more integrated program as described next. Without a significant time commitment (e.g., at least 2 days per week over an 18- to 24-month period), I have found that it is difficult to develop and run a training program in the manner described next. Sharing the responsibilities among multiple individuals is rarely a solution, unless the individuals share a clearly articulated vision. Ad-hoc committees can be important to developing consensus among professionals and independent experts, and commitment at state and local levels, but there are often too many details for such a committee to efficiently implement the training itself. Moreover, expertise in the subject area of the training program (e.g., ASD identification) is necessary but insufficient in a trainer: The person must become a model presenter and consultant, build bridges with other professionals and agencies, understand all of the components of the program, and adapt the program to the needs of the participating professional and agency.

Assess Resources and Barriers to Implementation
Training programs may fall short of long-term goals not because of lack of proficiency in the specific assessment / intervention method itself, but because of the many potential barriers to implementation. Before training begins, it is important to identify all of these potential barriers, and to secure commitments for any significant reallocations of time and/or resources.

• *Adequate personnel:* Agencies may be unwilling to hire new staff, adjust caseloads for existing staff, or otherwise commit the time needed to implement new interventions.

• *Identified clients:* There may not be enough clients to justify the ongoing expense of delivering the service, or the clients themselves may not be able to attend because of other barriers (e.g., transportation, time).

• *Supporting materials:* The newly trained staff may struggle if they do not have all of the materials, data forms, and examples of lesson or treatment plans ideally bundled into a package that includes detailed guidelines that answer most questions likely to come up. An annotated bibliography of relevant research and regulations, together with a directory of service providers or other resources, can support follow-up.

• *Coaching and consultation:* Even after an intensive training workshop that includes opportunities for practice, questions inevitably emerge once professionals begin to implement the intervention on their own. Opportunities for case consultation can help to answer these questions, and coaching (on-site or via video review) can increase treatment fidelity. By building these services and costs into the contract of an external expert, the expert can commit to tweak the training based on areas of difficulty identified via coaching.

Build Consensus and Collaboration Across the Entire Network of Services
As demonstrated in Chapters 1 and 2, different professionals and agencies can play complementary roles—if not actively collaborate—in the delivery of services. The development and implementation of a training initiative supporting a new program, or improving or expanding an existing one, is an ideal opportunity to strengthen this collaboration and build consensus regarding shared goals. In each case, the information presented to different professionals and agencies should be tailored to their role: For a training program in ASD identification, a presentation to potential referral sources can emphasize the importance of early intervention rather than a discussion about the causes of ASD.

Similarly, these same participants could be involved in the design of the program, which may increase their investment to change. Sometimes elements of a training initiative can build a shared vision and energy across all stakeholders; for example, presentations to professionals and parents regarding the importance of early identification together with an awareness campaign using alternative media (e.g., newspaper, website) can generate enthusiasm among the broader community. I have found that such presentations can also help to dispel common myths, or help everyone to use the same vocabulary (e.g., to recognize that they must focus on the broader autism spectrum).

Data-Driven Training   An evolving training program must be shaped by data of various types. Trainees are also consumers and customers, and so training must not just inform them but also engage and motivate them. Pre- and posttests are invaluable, especially when the questions tap critical knowledge. Opportunities to practice the skill during and after training can also reveal areas where training needs to be improved, especially when combined with fidelity checklists. When providing training to more experienced professionals, especially as part of an ongoing program, asking professionals what they want to learn can help to tailor the training to their needs.

Establish Best-Practice Guidelines Aligned with Scientific, Legal, and Regulatory Standards   As described later in this chapter, professionals are now beginning to identify evidence-based practices (EBP) by systematically evaluating and summarizing outcome research. Most professionals, and publicly funded and regulated agencies, are also bound by legal and regulatory standards. At the very least, training programs must be explicitly aligned with these standards. Annotated bibliographies that include references to scientific research, professional standards, and state/federal regulations help the trainers ensure that the necessary ground is covered and provide the trainee with additional information should the person wish to read further. Over time, a training program can seek to develop very specific guidelines that integrate scientific and regulatory standards and express these as core principles and practices. When properly designed, core principles and practices can guide the day-to-day work of professionals and feed directly into assessments of program integrity and treatment fidelity.

Build and Sustain Expertise   The lack of autism experts has been universally acknowledged as a barrier to the improvement of services (Committee on Educational Interventions for Children with Autism, 2001). I believe that expertise can be developed and demonstrated in stages in coordination with the design and delivery of an integrated training program. The leader of a training program can become more expert as he or she integrates the feedback of consultants into the program. Training activities themselves, especially those that include opportunities to practice and receive feedback, can help a trainer to initially identify individuals with the knowledge and other skills needed to become leaders and experts within their agencies. I also believe that active participation in the development and use of materials to assess fidelity of implementation can help to shape expertise. A train-the-trainer model that includes regular refreshers can help maintain expertise. Independent experts external to the program are often a critical part of developing internal expertise, as well as the design and delivery of an integrated training program, if there is an opportunity for their input to be shaped by trainees: No matter what their background, independent experts almost always need the eyes and ears of frontline professionals to tailor the training program to local needs and conditions.

What Might a More Integrated and Comprehensive Program of Training Look Like?

In Figure 3.2 I describe the elements of training programs for ASD diagnosis and behavior support consistent with the principles identified earlier. This description is a conglomeration of programs I have developed for hospital-, school-, and community-based programs.

FOR BOTH DOMAINS

- Program evolves over 2–5 years,[a,b] with some grant support for lead trainer, research assistant, and consultant.
- Training activities include annotated bibliographies, sample data sheets/reports, and provider directory.[c,d]
- Training includes opportunities for on-site, follow-up consultation with designated leaders.[c,g]
- Training is organized around written protocol that integrates scientific findings and recommendations from professional organizations[f]; involves trainees in shaping standards and expanding protocol;[e,g] and includes tools for agencies to conduct self-evaluations to evaluate compliance.[e]
- Funding pays for tools for agencies to participate via webconferencing.[c]
  Before training begins, meetings are held with each agency to assure support for increased time needed for training program, and enhanced diagnostic evaluation[c] and to gather information about waiting lists, and so forth.[e]

ASD Identification

- As the lead agency, a research clinic establishes itself as an expert resource in the center of a regional network including the participating agencies, bringing in research participants.[d]
- Program draws on data demonstrating delays in diagnosis for traditionally underserved populations.[e]
- Phase I: i) Consultant provides initial Autism Diagnostic Observation Schedule and Autism Diagnostic Interview–Revised workshops for diagnosticians[g]; ii) workshops for referral sources on autism spectrum disorder screening[d]; iii) workshops for general public on importance of early identification.[d]
- Phase II: Workshops by consultant and lead trainer[b,g] for diagnosticians on differential diagnosis and co-occurring conditions, research update on instruments, and case presentations by diagnosticians.[c,g]

Behavior Support

- Lead agency has clinical oversight for a multisite program that includes specialized programming for children with intensive behavior needs and that acts as a hub for affiliated regional partners.[d]
- Phase I: i) Initial standards established for functional behavioral assessment (FBA) and model emphasizing evidence-based behavior support strategies positive behavior support (PBS), ii) mechanism for independent consultant review of plans for more intense behaviors, iii) initial training program in crisis response.
- Phase II: Continue and elaborate on Phase I, plus i) core training in FBA and PBS strategies for all behavior support consultants (BSCs) in program, and inviting other partner agencies and ii) other trainings for parents and other professionals in the program promoting positive, proactive behavior support strategies,
- Phase III: Continue previous phases, plus i) other training topics for BSCs (e.g., data collection and analysis, specific intervention strategies) with program partners,[d] ii) more senior BSCs selected for multiday training in advanced assessment techniques with experts[g] that includes case presentations, iii) teams participate in conference presentations on related topics.[g]

Figure 3.2.   Imagining comprehensive training programs.

[a]Combine individual activities into a program.
[b]Identify a leader.
[c]Assess barriers to implementation.
[d]Build consensus and collaboration across a network.
[e]Use data.
[f]Establish Practice Standards.
[g]Build expertise.

ASD Identification: Refer to Chapter 6 for more details regarding elements of a program for training public school personnel in ASD identification. Other training programs described in this book also include some or most of these elements. For example, the Learn the Signs. Act Early. program (Chapter 12) promotes a wide range of activities to build consensus regarding the need for early identification, explicitly addresses barriers to implementation, gathers data to identify primary areas of need, and so forth.

Behavior Support: Refer to Chapter 6 for more details regarding elements of a program for training public school personnel in behavior support. Some of the elements are also consistent with well-designed programs for positive behavior support. Other chapters in Parts II and III also embody many of these principles.

RESEARCH

What role can research play in services, training, and policy? I believe that several different kinds of research questions can help direct services, to design relevant training programs to improve these services, and to drive the policy needed to support these service, training, and research activities. Many of these questions are relevant to service, training, and policy regarding ASD as a whole, and to specific service needs.

1. Can professionals assure the early and accurate *identification* of ASD and critical characteristics? This helps to provide the right education and treatment to those who need it most.

2. What is the *prevalence* of ASD? This helps to know how many programs must be created and professionals trained to meet the growing need.

3. What are the *evidence-based interventions* for ASD? This helps to prioritize program development, by focusing initial effects on those interventions demonstrated to be effective.

4. What are the *costs* associated with the identification and treatment of ASD (or the failure to do so)? This helps to project the resources needed.

5. What are the *barriers* to the identification and treatment of ASD? This helps to make attempts to improve identification and treatment as efficient as possible.

In the following sections, I describe examples of research that addresses each of these questions, to illustrate how they can help direct services, design training, and drive policy. In Chapter 14, I describe some specific principles for improving the integration of research with services, training, and policy at the local, regional, and national level. In Chapter 15, I propose specific research strategies as part of specific networks and programs.

Before describing examples of research, it may be helpful to distinguish between different research approaches (see Figure 3.3). I would expect that the vast majority (perhaps more than 80%) of research funded, conducted, and published would fall in a category of *basic research.* This kind of research seeks to discover immutable facts or "truths" about ASD related to its causes and characteristics, its relationship to other conditions, its prevalence, its assessment and diagnosis, and how it changes over time. Basic research would therefore address Questions 1 (identification), 2 (prevalence), and part of 4 (aspects of cost related to general outcomes not reflecting the impact of a specific program or intervention). *Intervention research* directly and specifically addresses Question 3, or the effect of broad programs and specific interventions, as well as the development and validation of formal assessment

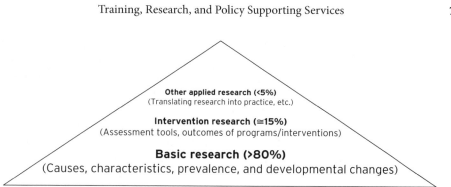

Figure 3.3. Types of research and examples of research questions.

tools used in practice. I would estimate that that may constitute no more than 14% of peer-reviewed research publications (Volkmar, Reichow, & Doehring, 2011). I might describe the very small proportion addressing remaining issues related to the costs and barriers as *other applied research;* for example, *translational research* describes how to take methods developed in the laboratory and implement them in the community, whereas *other research* describes the access to and utilization of services and supports in the community. By making these distinctions, I hope to educate those readers less familiar with the many different kinds of questions that research can answer. These distinctions will also help to begin to identify what kinds of research will become most important in scaling services and training up at the regional and national level, as I shall discuss at the end of this section.

The Identification of Autism Spectrum Disorder

ASD identification is often essential to establishing eligibility for specialized services and supports, and early identification is universally recognized as important to maximizing the benefits of such interventions (Levy, Mandell, & Schultz, 2009; Johnson, Myers, & and the Council on Children with Disabilities, 2007). As described in Chapter 2, considerable research has helped to establish the validity and reliability of instruments used in screening for ASD and diagnosis, and researchers focusing on the early symptoms of ASD are able to reliably identify ASD in children 24 months of age and younger (Zwaigenbaum et al., 2009). The development of instruments for early screening and diagnosis has grown directly from a large body of basic research undertaken to distinguish ASD across ages and developmental levels.

The understanding of the essential characteristics of ASD appears to have far outstripped, however, our ability to translate this knowledge into early and accurate identification in the community. Screening for ASD is particularly relevant because screening instruments are by definition designed to be quick and easy to administer, and to specifically facilitate early and accurate identification (Baron-Cohen et al., 2000). Considerable research was conducted to help the original Checklist with Autism in Toddlers (CHAT; Baron-Cohen et al., 2000) develop into the Modified Checklist with Autism in Toddlers (M-CHAT; Robins, 2008) capable of reliably signaling most children at risk for ASD prior to 24 or 30 months of age (Kleinman et al., 2008). Recent reports from the Autism and Developmental Disabilities Monitoring (ADDM) network suggest that 70%–95% of parents had noted developmental concerns prior to 3 years of age (Autism and Developmental Disabilities Monitoring Network Surveillance Year 2006 Principal Investigators & Centers for Disease Control and Prevention [CDC], 2009), and so may be expected to bring these concerns quickly to a professional's attention. Nevertheless, the ADDM network has reported that the mean age of first diagnosis for its 2006 cohort was 50 to 60 months: Although this represented a reduction of 5 months in the mean age of diagnosis relative to the 2002 cohort, diagnosis appears to still occur at least 12 to 24 months after many parents first noted concerns (Autism and Developmental Disabilities Monitoring Network Surveillance Year 2006 Principal Investigators & CDC, 2009). This suggests that, despite our understanding of the early manifestations of ASD, and the availability of reliable and valid tools, professionals lack cost-effective models translating this understanding into community practice.

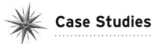 ## Case Studies

The screening for ASD that helped Asif and Evan more quickly gain access to specialized supports and the diagnostic evaluation that helped to disentangle Joshua's and Chloe's ASD from their other psychiatric conditions, was made possible by basic research into the characteristics of ASD and the validation of assessment protocols.

The Prevalence of Autism Spectrum Disorder

Accurate estimates regarding the prevalence of ASD are important if professionals are to project the resources needed to ensure adequate services and supports. Since the 1990s, new research findings on the overall prevalence of ASD have generated considerable professional and public debate, especially regarding the causes of ASD. Changes in the estimated prevalence from 1 in 2,500 to current estimates of 1 in 110 (Autism and Developmental Disabilities Monitoring Network Surveillance Year 2006 Principal Investigators & CDC, 2009) have led many advocates to characterize ASD as an "epidemic," and is probably the fact most often cited in proposals to increase services, training, and research. Efforts to establish the prevalence of ASD have also been undertaken in countries such as Finland (Mattila et al., 2007), Great Britain (Baird et al., 2006), China (Charman et al., 2009; Wong & Hui, 2008), Sweden (Nygren et al., 2011), and elsewhere.

To the extent that overall estimates of the prevalence of ASD will continue to drive policy discussions, some methodological questions surrounding changes and variations in these estimates must be addressed. The potential for confusion is exemplified by discussions surrounding changes in the rates of identification of ASD in schools in the United States. Dramatic increases in rates of identification of ASD in special education data compiled by states had been frequently cited as evidence of an ASD epidemic. Reanalyses of rates in California suggested that at least 25% of the increase in rates of identification of ASD is the result of diagnostic change in ASD relative to mental retardation classification, such as changes to diagnostic practices (e.g., changes to the medical or state regulatory criteria), diagnostic substitution (e.g., substitution of an autism diagnosis for a diagnosis of mental retardation), or diagnostic accretion (e.g., the addition of an autism diagnosis to a diagnosis of mental retardation) (King & Bearman, 2009). Reanalyses of other population-based data by Baird and her colleagues found that application of the least demanding diagnostic criteria increased the estimated rates by 4.5 times, as compared to the rate achieved when the most demanding criteria were applied (Baird et al., 2006). Prevalence estimates, therefore, can be expected to continue to fluctuate with the impending changes under the *Diagnostic and Statistical*

Manual of Mental Disorders, Fifth Edition (DSM-5; American Psychiatric Association, in press). Many other factors are also likely to significantly affect the rate and rapidity of diagnosis among different groups, as described later in this section as barriers to identification and intervention. Going forward, fluctuations in estimates of the prevalence of ASD seem more likely to reflect changes in how ASD are defined or identified and less likely to reflect changes in its true prevalence. In this context, "true" prevalence may never be established, as long as professionals continue to change the threshold at which a diagnosis is assigned.

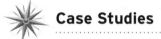 **Case Studies**

Increasing prevalence estimates generated via basic research sparked a focus on early screening and diagnosis to the benefit of Asif and Evan. Although co-occurring neurological, behavioral, psychiatric, and other medical problems complicated the treatment of Asif, Evan, Joshua, Sofia, Liam, and Chloe, basic research has yet, in most cases, to reliably establish their prevalence.

For the purposes of planning treatment, the prevalence of conditions associated with ASD should also be considered. As described earlier, researchers and practitioners who are concerned about mitigating the impact of ASD have increasingly recognized the contribution of common, co-occurring or comorbid conditions such as behavioral problems (e.g., aggression, self-injury), neurological functioning (e.g., intellectual disability, seizures), other psychiatric diagnoses (e.g., anxiety, depression, attention problems), and physical health (e.g., gastrointestinal problems, sleep disorders). Accurate estimates of the prevalence of these co-occurring conditions are important to establishing priorities for services and training, but in most cases are not widely available or have fluctuated greatly. In this context, the range of estimates in recent reviews is informative: 5%–49% will have a seizure disorder; 30%–80% will have a co-occurring ID; 9%–90% will have a gastrointestinal disorder; 8%–32% will have a behavioral disorder; 43%–84% will have anxiety; 2%–30% will have depression; and 52%–73% will have a sleep disorder (Johnson et al., 2007; Levy et al., 2009; Myers, Johnson, & the Council on Children with Disabilities, 2007). It is therefore not surprising that parents and professionals may not be confident when identifying and treating these comorbid and co-occurring conditions.

The Treatment of Autism Spectrum Disorder

Research on the effectiveness of interventions is critical to professionals and policy makers seeking to prioritize services and training. As discussed briefly in Chapter 2, a number of reviews have sought to identify evidence-based practices (EBP) by systematically applying rigorous standards to studies evaluating specific treatment outcomes. This includes the reviews of the National Autism Center (2009), the National Professional Development Center on Autism Spectrum Disorders (2011), and those that my colleagues and I have undertaken (Reichow, Doehring, Cicchetti, & Volkmar, 2011). There is considerable overlap in the criteria adopted by these reviewers, and most notably the recognition of two factors: 1) the validity of single-case designs used often in research derived from applied behavior analysis (ABA); and 2) that the traditional standards established in medical research (i.e., a randomized, double-blind, placebo control design) was unnecessary; unrealistic; and, at least in most community-based treatment contexts, perhaps unethical. By recognizing the potential contribution of studies that do not necessarily achieve these standards, more researchers might be prepared to contribute to the body of EBP.

The application of these new standards to the growing body of high-quality outcome research has already revealed certain methods more likely to be effective. For example, all of these reviews agree that a broad range of interventions based in ABA, that emphasize proactive and preventative strategies, and that build on a functional approach to understanding problem behavior, all help to decrease problem behavior. All of these reviews also identified a variety of interventions that help to develop social and communication skills, and an increasing number of interventions specifically benefiting individuals with Asperger syndrome. These new approaches all offer policy makers a way to look beyond individual studies more confidently. Some of the areas of improvement noted by reviewers will also help in the design of future intervention programs (Volkmar et al., 2011). For example, the drive toward manualized interventions and the emphasis on treatment fidelity will help transfer these advances into community settings, especially when incorporated into the comprehensive training programs described earlier.

Despite the growing availability of EBPs, important gaps persist. Many practices in common use are not evidence based: Although this does not preclude their application, especially in areas of significant need, this makes it more difficult to design programs to maximize their cost-effectiveness. This gap becomes wider when you consider how the implementation of EBPs by community-based practitioners is likely to vary from standards established in the laboratory because of lack of training. One of the most striking examples illustrating both the challenge and the potential lies in approaches to managing problem behavior. On the one hand, a wide range of interventions have been identified as effective in reducing problem behavior, interventions drawn from behavior analysis and other educational and therapeutic approaches. On the other hand, only a handful of medications commonly used in behavior management are evidence based (McPheeters et al., 2011; Scahill & Boorin, 2011), even though recent surveys indicate 35%–55% of children with ASD are on at least one psychotropic medication (Logan et al., 2012; Mandell et al., 2008; Rosenberg et al., 2010). Again, the available evidence in no way precludes the potential benefits of medication in managing behavior in an individual with ASD. Nonetheless, I have found that the lack of training in the effective application of evidence-based interventions for behavior management, the ease with which medications can be prescribed, and the failure of most professionals to engage in data-based decision making (see discussion later in the chapter) together results in the relative overreliance on psychopharmacological approaches and underutilization of EBPs for behavior management. This example illustrates that professionals may know what to do but lack the knowledge and resources to disseminate and apply this knowledge in community settings.

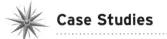

Case Studies

Although all of the cases responded positively to most of the interventions described in Chapter 2, relatively few of these are clearly evidence based. The relative lack of treatment research makes it difficult for individual clinicians to confidently determine methods and goals and for programs to confidently set broad priorities for services and training.

One of the most important, controversial, and often overlooked dimensions of treatment is treatment intensity. Treatment intensity came to prominence when Lovaas and his colleagues (Lovaas, 1987; McEachin & Lovaas, 1993), describing the results of their early intensive behavioral intervention (EIBI) program, reported that almost one half of participants in the EIBI group made significant gains following 2 years of intensive intervention (including one-to-one teaching for 40 hours per week for at least 2 years) in comparison to the minimal gains made by a control group receiving "treatment as usual" at a much less intensive rate. Others at the time questioned whether the positive effects reflected the specific impact of Lovaas's methods or the benefits of intensive one-to-one support regardless of the techniques used (Schopler, Short, & Mesibov, 1987). Nonetheless, countless successful lawsuits brought by parents seeking to implement EIBI specifically cited the level of treatment intensity desired. With the exception of attempts to replicate Lovaas's findings, I know of no studies outside of psychopharmacology that have examined treatment intensity per se, and the failure to establish the optimal dose response represents a major limitation to applying EBP (Volkmar et al., 2011). From a practical standpoint, I have found that treatment intensity (e.g., number of hours of intervention per week, and the staff-to-child ratio) is one of the most important determinants of the cost of treatment, and in my experience can be one of the most important factors in positive outcomes.

Other practical but important barriers to the application of EBP persist. For example, most clinicians need to identify specific treatment goals for an individual with specific characteristics (e.g., an intervention to teach requesting skills in a child with autism with no independent verbal or nonverbal means of communication), but most reviewers are limited to drawing conclusions about the impact of an intervention on a broadly defined target for a broadly defined population (e.g., Picture Exchange Communication System is an EBP for communication skills). This may begin to change as researchers evaluate how people with different skill profiles respond differentially to different treatments (Yoder & Stone, 2006) and as other approaches are developed to reanalyze outcome data to identify more individualized goals and practices (Doehring & Winterling, 2011). It is also surprising to note that the increased interest in autism research has not resulted in a concomitant increase in outcome research specifically: Whereas more than 28% of studies published in 2000 addressed treatment, this proportion dropped to 14% in 2008 (Volkmar et al., 2011). Continued efforts to improve treatment fidelity will positively impact both the quality of the research, and the ability of practitioners to quickly and faithfully replicate the practice in the community. Finally, it is important to recognize that professionals in the community cannot easily—or simply do not—gain access to information about EBP (Volkmar et al., 2011), although some of the strategies described in the section on training (e.g., development of EBP guidelines, annotated bibliographies) may help to address this.

Costs Associated with Identification and Treatment

Although the cost of services is usually far from the minds of those conducting basic research, it is of primary concern to those conducting other applied research more directly relevant to policy surrounding ASD, and to caregivers who pay for services directly. This is because the costs of identification and treatment for people with ASD are from 3 to 10 times higher than for people without ASD (Liptak, Stuart, & Auinger, 2006; Mandell, Cao, Ittenbach, & Pinto-Martin, 2006) and have been rising as much as 10% per year (Wang & Leslie, 2010). One of the arguments made in support of EIBI is that its increased costs are more than recouped by the savings that result from improved outcomes (Jacobson &

Mulick, 2000). These efforts have been criticized because projections depended entirely on difficult-to-calculate estimates of the potential benefit, ignored the possibility that children may make some (albeit perhaps modest) gains even with "teaching as usual," and could shift significantly based on projected costs of long-term care (Marcus, Rubin, & Rubin, 2000). Nevertheless, even with the most conservative estimates, many will agree that the cumulative lifetime cost of ASD is likely to be very significant. The efforts to account for all costs also reveal the scope of the challenge and the potential. Thus, Jacobson and Mulick's (2000) analysis suggests that costs associated with care of adults accounted for the majority of total lifetime costs, especially in residential support. This fact is important because services for children in the United States are more likely to be protected (if not guaranteed) in fiscally conservative times, whereas services for adults with developmental disabilities are traditionally more vulnerable to cuts. These authors also included in their calculations the potential contributions that individuals with the most optimal outcomes may make to society, at least in terms of income generated.

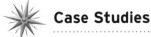 ## Case Studies

Each case required significant medical, educational, behavioral, and additional support to assure independence and a reasonable quality of life. The failure to manage Sofia's problem behavior led to the consideration of very expensive treatment options. Evan's, Joshua's, and Sofia's parents also incurred significant direct and indirect financial costs.

Other efforts to calculate costs have also been informative. Jabrink's (2007) efforts to estimate the total cost of caring for a child with ASD across home and school environments revealed that 75% of the total costs for education were accounted for by the residential school or treatment home required for 7% of the sample. This suggests that, from a cost-benefit perspective, policy makers might focus on the minority of people with ASD who incur the majority of costs. The hidden costs to families were also significant: The annual loss of income to families through sick leave, early retirement, and the choice to work part-time was very high (more than $6,000); most (41%) of the 977 hours of additional unpaid time that families spent annually on caring for their child's ASD could have been used for salaried activities, and together these accounted for 15% of the total societal costs estimated at more than $70,000 annually. More recently, Bouder, Spielman, and Mandell (2009) sought to precisely calculate the increase in insurance premiums resulting from the enactment of insurance legislation for ASD. By taking into account many factors more unique to privately funded services, and by focusing on "treated prevalence" (or the actual proportion of people seeking treatment for a given condition), they found that enacting such insurance would increase premiums by about 1%.

Barriers to Identification and Treatment

Gaining Access to Services   A fundamental barrier to ASD treatment is the variability in their identification, and some of the discussion regarding this variability illustrates the different priorities set by those focused on questions of basic research and those driven to quickly improve the lives of people living with ASD. On the one hand, those interested in establishing the most accurate prevalence estimates may be less interested by changes in rates of identification within administrative systems (e.g., such as rates of identification in special education or developmental disability services), having concluded that these rates are confounded by too many factors to be meaningful. These people may advocate increased investment in more rigorously controlled approaches such as the ADDM network (Rice et al., 2010). Given the efforts invested in the ADDM network and in similar projects undertaken in other countries, I expect that researchers in 2013 are now much closer to the most accurate estimate possible than they were in the 1990s, and that new findings regarding ASD's true prevalence are unlikely to have the same dramatic effect on perception and policy.

On the other hand, those interested in determining how close service professionals are to meeting the needs of all people living with ASD may be shocked by the gap between current estimates of the prevalence of ASD, and rates of identification within administrative systems. The Pennsylvania Autism Census revealed that the number of people receiving services through publicly funded administrative systems is likely to be dramatically less than the total number of potentially eligible individuals, and seems more likely to reflect the impact of factors such as the availability of qualified diagnosticians than true differences in prevalence (Lawer & Mandel, 2009). This gap is illustrated by contrasting the proportion of people receiving services in Pennsylvania, in the most and the least prevalent counties, with the most recent national estimates of true prevalence (see Table 3.3). Even within Pennsylvania, rates of identification in some counties were up to three times greater than in other counties, and suggest that most people with ASD in Pennsylvania (e.g., between 64% and 90%) do not appear to be receiving publicly funded ASD services in health or education. This gap is surprising given that Pennsylvania has a relatively well-developed system of services and supports. Although a small proportion of people with ASD may not in fact need such services, or may seek services privately, I would expect that most people with ASD would have sought out such services. The gap is also the accumulated result of years of underidentification. More than one half of those identified were between 5 and 12 years of age, suggesting that a much higher proportion of children with ASD are receiving health or education services under this label. This makes the gaps in identification among adults even more striking, however: Even at current (albeit inadequate) rates of identification (as of 2012), the number of adults seeking services is projected to increase by 621% between 2005 and 2015.

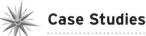

Case Studies

Asif and Evan benefited from programs designed in response to research demonstrating disparities in access to services for traditionally underrepresented groups.

The magnitude of this variability is consistent with rates reported in other states (Bryson, Corrigan, McDonald, & Holmes, 2008), and variations in rates of identification reported from state to state (Autism and Developmental Disabilities Monitoring Network Surveillance Year 2006 Principal Investigators & CDC, 2009). These variations are not ascribed to differences in true prevalence but to factors such as variations in policies from one region to another (King & Bearman, 2009; Mandell et al., 2010). Most analyses have also revealed underidentification among racial and ethnic minorities and those living in poverty (Autism and Developmental Disabilities Monitoring Network Surveillance Year 2006 Principal Investigators & CDC, 2009; Fountain, King, & Bearman, 2011; Liptak

Table 3.3. Pennsylvanians with Autism Spectrum Disorder Not Receiving Publicly Funded Services

Source	Rates	
ADDM (CDC, 2009)	0.9%, or 9 per 1,000	
Pennsylvania Autism Census (Lawer & Mandell, 2009)		Percentage not receiving publicly funded services
Most prevalent county	0.32%, or 3.2 per 1,000	64%
Least prevalent county	0.09%, or 0.9 per 1,000	90%

et al., 2008; Mandell, Listerud, Levy, & Pinto-Martin, 2002; Mandell et al., 2010), and these disparities extend to the ability of these populations to gain access to services (Lawer, Brusilovskiy, Salzer, & Mandell, 2009; Liptak et al., 2008). Current administrative systems for identifying people with ASD in need of services are clearly broken, and it seems clear that far greater progress in closing these gaps could be made by addressing differences in policy or increasing access to traditionally underserved populations rather than investing resources in research likely to yield marginal improvements in the best estimate of ASD's "true" prevalence.

Translating Research Into Practice   Transferring knowledge gleaned in the laboratory into day-to-day practice in the community remains a significant barrier to improving services. In contrast to the wealth of basic research on the potential causes, characteristics, and trajectory of ASD, there is almost no research to address this challenge, except perhaps in the area of ASD identification. One example of such research describes the practical, organizational changes needed to assure that most young children within a practice are cost-effectively screened for ASD (Allen, Berry, Brewster, Chalasani, & Mack, 2010; Gura, Champagne, & Blood-Siegfried, 2011), including the need to potentially screen outside of well-child checkups (Miller et al., 2011). Even more significant is the lack of research demonstrating the widespread application of a specific, cost-effective, and reliable protocol by community-based practitioners for ASD diagnosis. On the one hand, the considerable effort invested in the development of tools reliable enough for research purposes, such as the Autism Diagnostic Observation Schedule (ADOS; Lord et al., 1999) and the Autism Diagnostic Interview–Revised (ADI-R; Lord et al., 1994), has been critical to the success of basic research in ASD. On the other hand, I have found that tools such as the ADOS and ADI-R are simply too cumbersome and complex for day-to-day use by community-based practitioners, and I have explored a two-stage evaluation process consistent with the recommendations of other panels (Levy et al., 2009), whereby community-based practitioners refer to more specialized teams when the results are contradictory, or when initial screening suggests the presence of complicating, comorbid conditions. Efforts to date to demonstrate a reliable protocol for training community-based practitioners in diagnosis suggest that ASD can be accurately identified in many cases, though overidentification remains a significant problem (Warren, Stone, & Humberd, 2009). I would expect that this overidentification, together with instability in diagnoses of pervasive developmental disorder-not otherwise specified (PDD-NOS) and Asperger syndrome among community-based practitioners (Daniels et al., 2011), will perpetuate the delays in identification already rampant across the United States. Research on ASD diagnosis in Denmark (where most children must receive an ASD diagnosis by a hospital-based team prior to receiving special education services) suggests that hospital-based clinical teams can become highly reliable (Lauritsen et al., 2010), though application of this solution requires a considerable investment in training and services.

Where Do We Go From Here? Research Opportunities and Priorities

Changing Research Priorities to Help People with Autism Spectrum Disorder Now I must repeat here my belief that the ultimate goal of research is to discover how to improve the lives of people living with ASD. Research that identifies EBPs and research that helps specify the costs and overcomes barriers to identification and treatment clearly helps us progress immediately toward this goal. Several decades of intense investment in basic research have provided us with a number of important insights that ultimately improved practice: Detailed descriptions of the characteristics of ASD led directly to improvements in screening and diagnostic tools; other detailed descriptions of the developmental course and trajectory of ASD reaffirmed the need for individualized treatment and the potential for progress; painstaking efforts to establish the prevalence of ASD helped to establish the extent of the need. Nonetheless, I must question whether the continued emphasis on basic research to the exclusion of other kinds of research will assure reasonable progress toward a goal of helping to improve the lives of all those living with ASD. Given the complexity of ASD and the amount of basic research already conducted, such basic research appears increasingly unlikely to quickly and significantly help those living with ASD.

Given the diminishing returns offered by basic research, why is it continuing to be funded to the exclusion of other kinds of research? I believe that this reflects the prevailing, implicit model of science that pursues simple and dramatic causes and theories, underestimates the complex relationships between people and environments, and undervalues the cumulative impact of technological advances. Throughout the 19th and 20th centuries, researchers have successfully derived effective treatments for countless disorders by first understanding their causes. In the case of ASD, the available research would lead us to frankly conclude that this strategy seems unlikely to help us make significant progress toward this goal, at least in the short- and medium-term. To date, no single "cause" for ASD has been discovered: In fact, recent research findings suggest that perhaps 25% of ASD is associated with specific combinations of rare and common genetic variants (Glessner et al., 2009; Wang et al., 2009). Countless studies have also sought to identify functional or structural neurological characteristics distinct to ASD, yet no such anomaly has been found to reliably explain ASD in a majority of cases. Moreover, the research is hard pressed to identify any one assessment or treatment approach recognized as a "best practice" in recent reviews (National Autism Center, 2009; Reichow et al., 2011) that has been primarily—or even substantially—informed by research findings related to the cause(s) or neurological substrate(s) of ASD. I would argue that knowledge about the cause(s) or neurological substrate of ASDs is neither sufficient nor even necessary to developing effective interventions, as demonstrated by the impact of interventions based in applied behavioral analysis that have been derived with little reference to a presumed genetic or biological substrate. Why have those in the field continued to invest in basic research that has failed to contribute to the identification and treatment of ASD? Like a number of other authors (Doehring, 2002), I believe that much research and clinical work continues to be rooted in a 19th- and 20th-century positivistic, premodern model of science that seeks to discover objective truths and trace complex phenomena back to simple, immutable causes. A postmodern, postpositivistic 21st-century model of science acknowledges that behavior and pathology may sometimes have multiple explanations, with solutions that are dependent on context.

The failure of research on the genetic and neurological substrates of ASD to contribute meaningfully to treatment is in stark contrast to the needs and to opportunities that exist today in other areas of research. Thus, research has helped to identify ways to reliably diagnose ASD and ways to cost-effectively screen for ASD in very young children, but research suggests that many people are diagnosed much later in childhood if at all. By broadening the range of designs considered valid for outcome research, and identifying approaches to deriving clear conclusions from outcome research, professionals could usher in a new era of scientifically driven practice, yet the proportion of studies on treatment outcomes is shrinking. Researchers can develop tools for mapping neurological substrates with extraordinary precision, with no reasonable guarantee this understanding will ever actually help anyone now living with ASD, but they somehow cannot assure that traditionally underserved populations will have reasonable access to the most basic of diagnostic services. I hope professionals and others can find the will and the vision to invest in the development of practical tools and technologies that build on what is already known about ASD, and that offer help now and not just hope for the future.

The understanding of ASD is beginning to far outstrip the ability to apply this knowledge to the betterment of people living with ASD, and continued investment in basic research will only widen—never close—this gap. Although researchers might imagine how basic research may eventually lead to an improved quality of life, program leaders are accountable for helping Asif, Evan, Joshua, Sofia, Liam, and Chloe, and others now. To begin to use the knowledge already available to face autism nationally, and to prepare to use the knowledge that will be gleaned from future research efforts, researchers need to reverse the current research priorities. They must emphasize the development and validation of EBP and must better understand how to translate these EBP into practice, while continuing to devote some limited resources to exploring questions of causes and characteristics of ASD (see Figure 3.4). At the end of this section, I describe how research on screening for ASD may come the closest to supporting the logical transfer of knowledge from the laboratory to the community. In the next section on policy, I discuss how agencies can play a role by mandating the research programs to address the questions of treatment outcomes, and to demonstrate how to overcome barriers to implementation. In Chapter 14, I offer suggestions for how these new priorities can fuel new and more meaningful collaborations between researchers, and practitioners and policy makers.

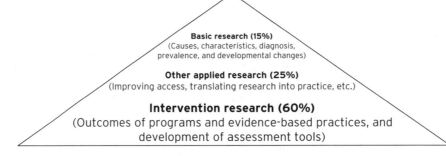

Figure 3.4. Research categories, questions, and priorities—revised.

Creating a Culture of Data-Based Decision Making   Research can shape practice and policy not just through the results it yields, but also through the methods it employs, by helping to create a culture of data-based decision making. This is especially true when seeking to face autism nationally, because of the challenge of scaling up services and training in a cost-effective manner. When done well, research provides professionals with the template to find the best possible answers to even complex questions: they become more focused and transparent by establishing measurable goals to a clearly defined population; they become more accountable by carefully measuring progress toward outcomes; they replicate successful programs by applying rigorous methods and procedures; and they adapt by making decisions based on the data they have gathered and the results they have obtained, and not on convention and tradition. Although few disagree with the benefits of data-based decision making in theory, far fewer seem to truly employ this practice.

Data-based decision making can help at all levels of service delivery, training, program development, and policy. Data-based decision making derived from the principles of single-case design provides a powerful template to help the professional working with the individual with an ASD to quickly assess the impact of interventions. When these data are gathered across patients, an organization can identify nodes of success or failure that can be targeted by training and support. Looking at the outcomes for one individual over time, or across groups of individuals, can inoculate professionals and program leaders from placing too much weight on the success or the failure of isolated cases, and is essential to tracking the slow but steady progress programs may make in meeting the needs of a broadly targeted population. In Chapter 14, I further expand upon the potential of data-based decision making by proposing that organizations supplement more traditional, narrowly defined skill-based outcomes by also considering broader goals related to quality of life.

Bridging the Gap Between Research and Practice   A need implicit to the recommendations offered earlier—changing research priorities to help people with ASD now, and creating cultures of data-based decision making—is the need to close the gap between research and practice. One of the most important factors contributing to this gap is the increasing specialization of the individual professionals in either research or practice. Part of this problem lies in their initial training. At present, there are relatively few training programs that can assure that graduates are ready to practice independently as a clinician *and* able to initiate an independent program of research worthy of grant support within 3 years of graduation. As a group, the scientist practitioner model in psychology may come the closest, if the individual's postdoctoral training includes clinical research, but even then many programs tend to emphasize the scientist or the practitioner role to the detriment of the other.

The problem worsens as professionals advance in their career. As the number of researchers and practitioners entering the field grows, there is increasing pressure for them to specialize as either researchers or practitioners if they are to remain competitive. For example, academic advancement in a research setting is almost always largely dependent on productivity defined with respect to research grants and publications: Those who devote significant effort to clinical activities are almost always at a disadvantage when they are competing for tenure with nonclinical counterparts. The pressure to specialize may be even greater for those aspiring to leadership positions, for which some degree of expertise is usually required.

I believe that one consequence of this gap is the lack of productive debate between researchers and practitioners regarding their respective roles and responsibilities in improving care for people living with ASD. Without ongoing and meaningful dialogue about treatment outcomes, I have watched practitioners fall back on untested traditions instead of embracing new EBPs, because researchers never developed the understanding of treatment needed to make a credible counterargument. Likewise, I have seen researchers proclaim the effectiveness of a new treatment approach and then blame practitioners for failing to implement it properly when results do not replicate in the community, instead of considering barriers to implementation. At the same time, practitioners are too intimidated by pronouncements of new research "breakthroughs," lack the knowledge of research to glimpse behind the curtain, and then fail to hold researchers accountable for a plan to ensure the research findings will be clinically relevant. In each case, researchers and practitioners tend to shield themselves behind the language and concepts of their trade and the self-serving belief that their work is too complex for the other to understand. And in the competition for limited resources or in reaction to their own insecurity, researchers and practitioners may minimize the potential contributions of the other.

Researchers and practitioners must learn to share the stage, and recognize that both are indispensable to the challenge of improving the lives of those with ASD. Researchers and practitioners should also recognize that collaboration does not develop overnight, and usually requires that each be prepared to adjust goals and expectations in response. Researchers and practitioners may not recognize the extent to which they speak a different language and have different priorities. For those who have invested significantly in a career and an identity as a researcher or a practitioner, this kind of collaboration can be surprisingly humbling; they appreciate the true extent of the challenge for the first time, or become uncomfortable or even angry when this debate throws the fundamental tenets and value of their life's work into question. This collaboration is ultimately enriching for both: The practitioner will learn that he or she is not fumbling in the dark and will discover new areas of research from which he or she can draw inspiration, while researchers can begin to see the true potential of their work on the lives of people with ASD.

Similar conditions and dynamics characterize the relationship between agencies focused on research, and agencies delivering services and training. Agencies and organizations are themselves becoming increasingly specialized in the competition for limited resources: Whether they are seeking increased internal funding, support from community leaders or donors, or competing for state and federal grants, agencies are more likely to stand out when they acquire national recognition for a very specific area of work. Yet agencies have other means at their disposal to begin to close this gap. Whereas it is difficult for one individual to quickly acquire research and clinical expertise, an agency can create expertise across a team by engaging individuals with complementary backgrounds, and promoting interdisciplinary collaboration. Funding agencies can also help close the gap by setting specific expectations for the integration of research and practice when designing policy or developing a grant program.

In the short term, other strategies may help to close this gap. Programs for training researchers and practitioners can include an introductory course, or offer credit for practical experience. Academic researchers can make greater efforts to translate findings into language comprehensible to nonresearchers by offering presentations to local groups of parents and clinicians, and inviting active discussion and debate regarding the findings. Participating in the board of an agency offers many opportunities: Researchers and practitioners can go beyond just presenting their respective points of view, but engage actively in shaping policy; practitioners can help to reenergize interest of the public in research by providing concrete examples of the benefits of research; researchers can help build the culture of data-based decision making described earlier. Some of the training strategies described earlier also help to bridge this gap—for example, EBP guidelines that systematically evaluate and summarize outcome research, or annotated bibliographies that save practitioners the trouble of sifting through the dizzying array of journals and studies.

What Might a More Integrated and Comprehensive Program of Research Look Like?: Screening for Autism Spectrum Disorder One other way to close the gap between research and practice is to illustrate how research might progress in a deliberate and logical way from laboratory to the community, and result in the development and widespread application of an evidence-based standard of practice with demonstrable fidelity. Given the amount of research conducted to date, it is remarkable that few interventions can be described as having demonstrated this optimal trajectory from research to practice, to become a widely and reliably applied standard. As suggested earlier, there might be few examples because of the relative lack of other applied research addressing critical issues of access and implementation, and because of the lack of an efficient training infrastructure.

One of the few examples approaching this optimal trajectory from research to practice to standard, and conveying both its potential and its challenges, is the development and implementation of tools used in screening for ASD (see also Figure 3.5). The original CHAT (Baron-Cohen, Allen, & Gillberg, 1992) drew from two sets of basic research findings: 1) evidence that the siblings of children already identified with ASD are at significantly increased risk for the disorder; and 2) increasing evidence that young children with ASD demonstrated specific deficits in joint attention, play, imitation, and other skills that not only offered insight into the core characteristics of ASD, but that also suggested specific markers of emerging ASD in very young children (Baron-Cohen et al., 1992). Based on these findings, Baron-Cohen and his colleagues piloted a simple screening procedure (CHAT) with the high-risk 18-month-old siblings of children already identified with ASD and a control

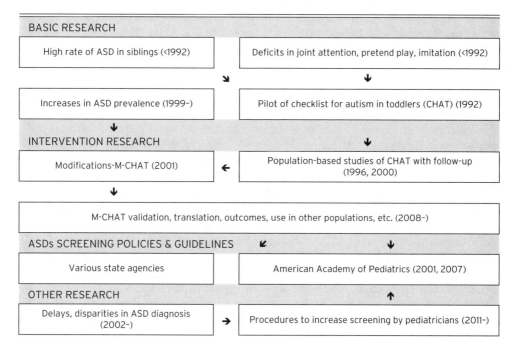

Figure 3.5. Interrelationship of research types and findings: Screening for autism spectrum disorder (ASD).

group of typical toddlers. The CHAT was relatively easy to administer, consisting of 9 questions asked of parents, and 5 observations made by the practitioner. Whereas none of the typical toddlers failed the CHAT, 4 of the 12 high-risk toddlers failed the CHAT, and were subsequently diagnosed with autism.

The next study of the CHAT signaled a shift from basic to intervention research. Baron-Cohen and his colleagues administered the CHAT as part of routine developmental screening in southeast England to more than 16,000 18-month-olds (Baron-Cohen et al., 1996) to validate its more widespread use. Almost all of those who failed the CHAT at 18 months in the high-risk group went on to receive a provisional ASD diagnosis at 20 months, whereas many of those in the moderate-risk group were identified with other significant language and developmental delays. A reevaluation of this same group of children 2 years later (Baird et al., 2000) yielded mixed findings: 1) those in the moderate- to high-risk group generally maintained their ASD diagnoses or shifted from another developmental disorder to ASD; 2) for every child who failed the CHAT at 18 months and went on to receive a diagnosis of ASD at 42 months, 2–3 children passed the CHAT at 18 months yet went on to develop ASD by 42 months. This illustrates how critical shortcomings may only become evident when a practice developed in the laboratory is tested in the field.

The potential for instruments such as the CHAT was heightened by findings emerging from another area of basic research—the prevalence of ASD. A reexamination of epidemiological research suggested that ASD was in fact "not an extremely rare disorder" (Gillberg & Wing, 1999). A detailed investigation of a potential spike in ASD in Brick Township, New Jersey (Bertrand et al., 2001), fueled speculation that the prevalence of ASD may be increasing, and was an important factor in the creation of the ADDM network.

The increased interest in screening for ASD, and the recognition of the CHAT's shortcomings, led to other intervention research seeking to identify alternative screening instruments. Perhaps the most successful of these is the M-CHAT. By eliminating the observations, transforming the interview into a questionnaire, adding other questions, and expanding the target population to children between 16 and 30 months of age, Robins and her colleagues (Robins, Fein, Barton, & Green, 2001) were able to simplify screening for ASD. A subsequent series of studies indicate that the M-CHAT was a very promising instrument when risk status was verified by a follow-up readministration of critical items (Kleinman et al., 2008), and suggested the potential use in other communities (Canal-Bedia et al., 2011; Eldin et al., 2008; Perera, Wijewardena, & Aluthwelage, 2009).

Even prior to the publication of other intervention studies seeking to validate ASD-specific screening instruments, agencies began to publish guidelines for screening for ASD and diagnosis. The American Academy of Pediatrics first described approaches to screening for ASD and diagnosis in a series of papers in 2001 (American Academy of Pediatrics, 2001; American Academy of Pediatrics, Committee on Children with Disabilities, 2001), but listed a wide range of instruments without endorsing a specific protocol. Updated guidelines published 6 years later (Johnson et al., 2007) included a detailed screening algorithm that recommended the use of ASD-specific screening instruments for all children at 18- and 24-month well-child checkups. A number of states have also set standards for screening for ASD and diagnosis (California Department of Developmental Services, 2002; Frant, 2005; Pennsylvania Autism Assessment and Diagnosis Expert Work Group, 2007).

Notwithstanding advances in screening for ASD instruments and the endorsement of detailed guidelines by prominent agencies, remarkably little research has sought to identify and address barriers to screening for ASD. Some of the research cited earlier in this chapter regarding delays and disparities to the diagnosis of ASD indirectly revealed barriers to screening. Informal descriptions of approaches to training and supporting community-based practices in the implementation of screening for ASD suggested some general strategies (Gura et al., 2011). Other studies suggest that simple but important adjustments to screening practices (e.g., not restricting screening to well-child checkups) may increase the likelihood of detection (Miller et al., 2011). Other studies demonstrated that the majority of children at risk for ASD may go undetected if pediatricians rely solely on screening instruments not specific to ASD (Pinto-Martin et al., 2008).

The shifts from research to practice to standard should logically evolve over time, through the contribution of different types of research (basic, intervention, and other applied research), and their progressive integration into training and policy. This logical evolution is not evident in the case of screening for ASD, and is likely to characterize almost all other critical areas of assessment and intervention for which professionals and advocates have eagerly sought to set standards. Unable to draw on supporting intervention and other applied research, professionals and advocates have often found themselves limited to setting very general standards that lack the research support needed to convince service providers of the need to change their practice and to convince policy makers to provide the necessary infrastructure and funding.

There are also many reasons why standards for screening for ASD should be relatively easy to develop and implement, and so the failure of research to inform and help engender the widespread adoption of screening for ASD is particularly telling. The benefits of screening for ASD are almost universal: All children are eligible for screening for ASD, many children ultimately identified with ASD would be identified earlier with screening for ASD, and early intervention is universally recognized as one of the most important contributors to positive treatment outcomes. Screening itself takes little time, has minimal costs, and can be implemented with relatively little training. The outcomes of screening (e.g., does it result in the efficient and accurate identification of children at high risk for ASD and who merit a diagnostic evaluation) are much easier to evaluate than the outcomes of other interventions. As I discuss later, this failure may also reveal the limits of examining practices in isolation, and the need to consider these practices within a broader network. I have found, for example, that community-based practitioners are much less likely to identify children at risk of ASD when waiting lists for diagnostic evaluation are long or the practitioner lacks awareness of or confidence in the services and supports subsequently available to those diagnosed with ASD. I elaborate more on the importance of an integrated network in the final section of this book.

The remarkable failure of research to inform practice even in the case of screening for ASD may also reveal a fundamental flaw in our model of science: that basic research findings will naturally trickle down to shape practice. In fact, few interventions can clearly trace their unique focus and methodology back to a specific cause, characteristic, or treatment strategy revealed primarily through basic research. For example, most interventions for ASD are designed to address characteristics already accepted as important to overall functioning (e.g., language deficits, social skill deficits) using methods similar to those in use elsewhere. This is not to diminish the importance of interventions that propose very specific methodologies (e.g., cognitive-behavioral therapy, Social Stories, Pictures Exchange Communication System), especially practices based in ABA; nonetheless, it is difficult to argue that these interventions depended significantly on methodological breakthroughs derived from basic research. Similarly, I do not intend to diminish the many insights into the characteristics and developmental trajectory of ASD revealed through decades of basic research: Nonetheless, it appears to me that the characteristics now addressed by cutting-edge treatments have been generally recognized for some years. In each of these cases, many of the methods and targets of intervention research emerging within the last decade appear to have been inspired by the insights of practitioners, or informed by the results of intervention research, and not primarily by basic research.

POLICY RELATED TO SERVICES, TRAINING, AND RESEARCH FOR AUTISM SPECTRUM DISORDER

Policy decisions occur at all levels of an organizational entity. Within the education system, for example, decisions can be made at the level of the school (e.g., a principal designates staff to specifically support students with ASD during recess), the school district (e.g., a special education director decides to contract out speech and language services instead of hiring a school district speech pathologist), the county level (e.g., several neighboring school districts agree to funnel resources to develop a highly specialized vocational program into one single school district), the state level (e.g., the state department of education realigns educational classification criteria for autism to better capture the spectrum), and the federal level (e.g., a federal agency creates a grand program to support pilot programs for the identification of ASD). From these examples, it is also clear that policy potentially affects all aspects of the infrastructure of services, training, and research, from providing funding and other resources, to defining mandates and setting standards.

Policy surrounding the ASD is therefore a very broad umbrella under which many potential issues might be addressed at many different levels. One of the most immediate effects of policy is to create or shape the infrastructure of services, training, and research, and identify funding sources. I address this in the next chapter, by providing a broad overview of funding and infrastructure at different levels (i.e., local, regional, state, and federal) including examples of agencies. In the following section, I focus discussion on a subset of proposed policy principles (see Figure 3.6). In each case, I illustrate these principles

	Screening	Registry	Specialist
i) A good first step to building awareness and taking action			
• Increases awareness about ASD and a specific concern	✓✓	✓	✓
• First step in a long-term plan for change	✓	?	X
• Low cost	✓✓	X	✓
• Addresses a need easily recognized as important	✓	X	✓
• Can be readily attained	✓	?	✓
ii) Builds on ongoing assessment of understanding and resources			
• Takes advantage of new research findings	✓✓	?	✓
• Draws upon reviews or policies developed by others	✓	✓	?
• Begins by creating inventory of current resources	?	✓	✓
• Generates data about needs and capacity	?	✓	?
iii) Develops standards and oversight to drive services and training			
• Promotes evidence-based practice guidelines	✓✓	?	✓
• Includes regulations that establish minimum standards	?	?	?
• Oversight enforces compliance *and* builds on strengths	?	?	?

Figure 3.6. Policy principles and examples of autism spectrum disorder (ASD) initiatives. (*Key:* ✓✓, Very Successful; ✓, Successful; ?, May or May Not Be Successful; X, Not Successful)

by describing examples of recent or common policy initiatives at the state level that have helped to build capacity or have fallen short of expectations: Relatively small examples (e.g., screening for ASD, registries for ASD, and specialized positions for ASD) as described within these sections, and two larger examples (insurance for ASD and the Combating Autism Act) are described separately at the end. Although I focus on policy decisions at the state and national level, I believe that the principles and examples can be applied to other types of public agencies and private organizations. In the final chapter in this volume, I return to some of these examples to recommend which policy initiatives might be undertaken by regions just beginning to build coordinated systems of services, training, research, and policy, and which initiatives may be within the reach of more established agencies.

Policy Principles

The First Policy Steps Build Awareness and Momentum for Other Changes
A policy decision is ultimately a call to action, in both the policy itself and the process by which policies are developed. As a call to action, a policy decision places an issue into the political and public consciousness. Whereas advocates may have a deep and rich understanding as to why early identification of ASD, services for adults, and other issues are important, policy makers and the general public may lack this understanding and the resulting commitment to change. To the extent that any policy decision affirms that an issue is worthy of attention and action, it can set an important precedent and constitute the first step in a broader program. For this reason, a first goal for any new policy initiative may be to implicitly or explicitly raise awareness about a specific issue.

A policy decision is also a test of the process by which policies are developed and implemented, and therefore serves as a means to a more complex and distant end. Who are the champions among the leaders and decision makers, what kinds of issues are personally important to them, and what kinds of information and interactions influence their decisions? The best advocates seek to understand what informs and drives leaders and policy makers, not with the goal of manipulating them, but to develop a true partnership for change. What are the avenues for change in a given organization? As entities grow in size and influence, they acquire more and more layers and avenues: Whereas special education policy in a school district may be led largely by a special education director and an ardent school board member, special education policy at the state level involves multiple committees within the state department of education and within the state legislature.

A policy decision may be but a single step on a longer road to change. Few single policy decisions bring about all of the changes sought by advocates. For this reason, advocates seeking improvements across a broad set of related but complex issues (say, the appropriate treatment of people with ASD within the legal system) may begin by selecting a specific goal that increases awareness about the core issue and represents a first step in a broader plan. Ideally, this specific goal is also relatively low cost, is not controversial, is readily attainable, and that gathers more information about the extent of the issue.

Screening for Autism Spectrum Disorder
Proposed goal: We will ensure timely access to early diagnosis and intervention by increasing screening for ASD in preschoolers.
Initiatives to promote screening for ASD in a state with limited services are one example of a specific strategy to begin to address the broader and more complex challenge of developing an integrated and intensive program of early intervention. Screening for ASD is a relatively low-cost service, as is its associated training. Through its emphasis on the signs

of ASD observed by parents and professionals, screening automatically promotes greater awareness of ASD. Screening for ASD is a necessary important part of any program of early intervention, and can provide the specific information needed to project the capacity needed to complete subsequent diagnostic assessments. Once fully implemented, however, a program of screening for ASD will quickly flood a poorly organized early intervention system, and so initiatives to improve diagnosis and intervention should follow quickly. Otherwise, the goodwill generated by a first promising step can turn quickly into bitterness and disillusionment for advocates and professionals alike.

Public Registries for Autism Spectrum Disorder   *Proposed goal: To improve statewide planning and delivery of services, we will create a state registry for children identified with ASD.*[1]

A number of states have implemented registries for ASD in which practitioners are invited or required to provide basic information about ASD cases under their care to a central repository. In my experience, the development and implementation of a registry for ASD will likely raise awareness of ASD, at least among the professionals responsible for enrolling registrants. The place of a registry for ASD in a longer-term program of change may not be clear, however: It may be redundant to the extent that it gathers information available elsewhere (e.g., the prevalence of ASD—see discussion later in the chapter), and examples in which state-based registries further participation in research are still relatively rare (Goin-Kochel & Cohen, 2008). The full cost of registries is often underestimated; centralized data repositories that allow practitioners to quickly and securely input sensitive information can be difficult to set up cheaply, and the time for practitioners to enroll a patient or client is not reimbursed, which inevitably creates resistance. I describe in the final chapter some other (albeit more costly) strategies to gather information for planning purposes.

Autism Spectrum Disorder Specialist   *Proposed goal: To improve the coordination of ASD information and policy, we will create the position of an ASD specialist.*

There are many examples of public and private agencies that begin by designating one person to respond to issues related to ASD. In my experience, this strategy can have an immediate and positive impact on awareness of ASD; by serving as the agency's representative on key committees, the person relieves others from this burden, provides a perspective specific to ASD, and can begin to build bridges across committees and initiatives. It is a low-cost solution that can quickly and easily draw on the growing body of committed advocates. The benefits of improved awareness and coordination of initiatives is short lived, however, unless the person gains additional personnel support or budgetary oversight (e.g., if the position develops into a specialized agency, as in the example of the Pennsylvania Bureau of Autism Services described in Chapters 4 and 6).

Policy Should Build on a Careful and Ongoing Assessment of Current Understanding and Resources   Even though the Internet has created many ways to quickly search for information about practices and policies surrounding ASD, a surprising number of policies fail to build on what is already known and what has already been done.

---

1. I consider a public registry to be somewhat different from a research registry, the primary goal of which is to identify a pool of people interested in participating in ASD research. Though a population registry may help to efficiently create a research registry (e.g., by providing a means to solicit potential participants for research), the reverse is unlikely to occur, because the pool of research participants is unlikely to be large enough or representative enough to provide any reasonable estimates of the characteristics of the general population.

For example, the explosion of autism research continues to suggest new needs and opportunities for intervention. In fact, increased estimates of ASD prevalence may be the greatest force driving new policy at the state and national level. Whenever possible, policy proponents should consider forging a partnership with researchers so that they can recognize which scientific advances might provide a general impetus for new policy, if not suggest specific objectives. Proponents advocating for a new line of policy (e.g., services for adults) may consider tethering their proposal to new research findings as these emerge (e.g., proposing tax deductions for the cost of adult care when new findings about the dearth of adult services emerge). This partnership may also help to reshape the work of researchers by helping them to appreciate the potential contribution of their findings.

I am also somewhat disappointed by the number of white papers, bills, and other policy initiatives at the state and the local level that fail to reference, let alone capitalize on, specific legislation or recommendations made by others. For example, many different agencies and organizations have developed white papers, strategic plans, and/or actual policies around issues such as identification, EBP, and so forth. I recognize that the process of assembling information, and drawing conclusions from it, can help a group of proponents discover shared values and special relevance to their organization. These potential benefits are far outweighed, however, by the amount of effort required to complete such reviews, the potential for misinterpretation, and the overall delays in implementation that result. Since the mid-1990s, for example, a number of different state and national agencies and organizations have dedicated considerable resources to conducting their own reviews, developing their own position papers, and making their own recommendations surrounding ASD identification and intervention. Most do not appear to have drawn significantly from authoritative reviews already conducted by groups such as the National Research Council and American Academy of Pediatrics. As a result, most of these reviews, papers, and recommendations simply repeated what these more authoritative groups had already concluded, missing the opportunity of using specific recommendations arising from these more authoritative reviews as a springboard for substantial policy changes. Thus, more than a decade after their publication, few states have implemented the universal screening for ASD recommended by the American Academy of Pediatrics (2001), or provided the 25 hours a week of year-long educational programming recommended by the National Research Council (Committee on Educational Interventions for Children with Autism, 2001).

At a more practical level, some policy initiatives fall short of expectations because they do not include a careful inventory of existing resources. Such resources can include specific services, training, or research programs or other related initiatives in development. By conducting an inventory, proponents may help identify a specific program that can serve as a foundation for new efforts or offer lessons on how to avoid potential pitfalls. Too often, proponents are quick to propose entirely new programs and fail to evaluate the potential for existing programs to be improved or expanded.

Finally, policy proponents should seriously consider how to gather and use data to bolster their case when proposing new initiatives and better target initiatives through their development and implementation phases. When a policy debate driven solely by opinions becomes rancorous, a proposal to gather additional data may help cooler heads break a stalemate. Policy makers dubious of the impact or concerned about the cost of a new program may be more supportive of a proposal to evaluate existing needs. Similarly, policy makers may value the opportunity to make ongoing funding contingent upon the results of data gathered and formally analyzed after an interim period, instead of committing to longer-term funding. This is especially important in developing new services because of the cost, the investment in associated training, and the challenge of ensuring that these services are accessible to those most in need. In general, I have found that new programs are most likely to fall short of expectations when they underestimate need and overestimate capacity. I return in Chapter 14 to discuss specific strategies for taking all of these factors into account.

- *Screening for ASD:* As described earlier in this chapter, screening for ASD initiatives have been able to draw on a wide range of research, from the early characteristics of ASD to its growing prevalence. Nonetheless, it is only since the mid-2000s and the implementation of the initiatives such as First Signs that new screening for ASD programs have begun to build on the experience of others. Only with the advent of the Combating Autism Act have new initiatives included systematic efforts to inventory current resources and generate data (see Chapter 13).

- *ASD public registries:* Some ASD registries appear to have been motivated by concerns over the growing prevalence of ASD: Although these are in response to research, I know of no registries able to gather data rigorously enough to contribute to estimates of prevalence. Enough registries have been created, however, to allow some more recent initiatives to be able to draw lessons from previous efforts. Registries have the natural potential to inventory current resources related to assessment (e.g., by tracking the number and type of diagnosticians who contribute registrants) and to crudely estimate need (e.g., by tracking the age and location of registrants). The effectiveness of registries in meeting these goals decreases rapidly, however, as the proportion of people with ASD actually enrolled drops.

- *Specialist in ASD:* A specialist in ASD is well suited to centralize information about ASD resources and initiatives inside and outside of the organization. In my experience, proponents invariably overestimate a specialist's ability to provide significant services, training, or research beyond this role, without an infusion of other resources. Even the task of gathering more objective and systematic data about needs and capacity may be challenging for a single specialist unless the person has specific experience or other resources to draw upon. Similarly, it is unclear how such a specialist can do more to promote new research advances other than to communicate the latest research findings to others, unless the specialist can also serve as a go-between for researchers and initiatives in the organization.

Policy Can Promote the Convergence of Scientific, Ethical, and Legal Standards and Oversight to Drive Programs of Services and Training

When a group of leaders seek to create new programs or fundamentally reshape existing ones, they usually begin by defining laws and public policies that convey the broad ethical and other principles guiding practice. When these are clear and well-crafted, these principles can be translated in a second phase in specific standards that redefine practice, as in the case of the principles of free appropriate public education in the least restrictive environment in the Individuals with Disabilities Education Act (IDEA) and its amendments. It is very difficult to undertake more ambitious change without a two-step process in which a second, larger group laboriously crafts these standards. Here I focus on two types of standards: 1) specific, research-based practice guidelines for professionals and 2) regulations, licensing standards, policy/procedures manuals, and requests for proposals that govern the implementation of programs. At the very least, all of these should set the minimum standards for specific elements of service, training, and/or research programs: defining the scope of the program, the individuals or organizations that can provide the program, the population of people with ASD who are eligible for the program, and so forth.

By specific practice guidelines, I mean the research-based standards set by a group or body of professionals for a specific practice—for example, screening for ASD or diagnosis. Thus, I am distinguishing these from the general practice standard that a licensing agency might set (e.g., the regulations surrounding the practice of medicine or psychology set by a state or national board), because these govern many different actions taken with many different populations. The position papers outlining the pediatrician's role in the identification and management of ASD (Johnson et al., 2007; Myers et al., 2007) are perhaps the only ones beginning to illustrate this potential: These are based on summary reviews of the relevant scientific literature, the specific algorithm recommended for screening for ASD represents a significant incremental step forward in ASD identification, and they carry the weight of a respected professional body, though they ultimately fall short of providing specific guidelines surrounding practices other than initial identification. The development of more prescriptive standards is, however, challenging; as described earlier in this chapter, outcome research that supports more individualized recommendations is rare; professional bodies err toward granting professionals the opportunity to exercise their judgment; and discussions that should be guided by research are equally influenced by individual opinions and professional politics. In the final chapters, I return to propose areas where the development of such guidelines is perhaps more realistic.

The regulations accompanying state and federal laws, and other related elements (e.g., the requests for proposals soliciting applicants for grants and policy and procedure manuals adopted by other organizations), are other important means for translating policy principles into practice. Regulations and other related elements can include components that are nonnegotiable (e.g., the need for an assessment to occur within a specific time period) and those that present some flexibility (e.g., the ability to choose an assessment instrument, perhaps given a range of options). Through such regulations and other elements, a policy principle can be invigorated and extended, or it can be effectively dismembered and quietly crushed. Consider the example of regulations seeking to improve behavior support by requiring that people who provide in-home services meet new training requirements: Loose regulations sanction less-qualified practitioners and dilute the intended impact; overly restrictive regulations create barriers for practitioners seeking to enter the field, limiting the number of such practitioners and ultimately limiting access to this service; requirements that strike the right balance improve the training received by practitioners, and by extension the services they provide. Regulations are more likely to strike the right balance when practitioners familiar with the challenges of day-to-day implementation *and* stakeholders who helped to craft the original principles contribute equally to the development of the regulations. In the ideal world, development of these regulations and other elements is informed by, if not coordinated with, EBP guidelines; in the final chapters of this book, I suggest some ways this might be done.

Whether standards for services, training, and research are defined by a professional body or via regulations and related elements, they will have an even greater impact when they are paired with formal mechanisms of oversight. Although I hope that most individuals and organizations are inherently motivated to aspire to such standards, intelligent oversight can greatly increase this motivation. As with standards, oversight must achieve a balanced mix of sticks (compliance) and carrots (performance improvement) to be most effective. Oversight should have the potential to formally sanction—if not actually shut down—an inadequate program, even though it usually would focus on areas of improvement and strengths. Oversight must be provided by people and agencies that are independent of those reviewed, but who ultimately come from similar backgrounds and areas of expertise, and who can act as partners in a common goal of program improvement. Some form of objective rating must ultimately underlie any system with the potential to shut an ineffective program down, but these ratings must be accompanied by concrete examples and recommendations if they are to build on strengths. The burden of meaningfully documenting compliance with the standard should draw on data that programs are already gathering to set internal performance improvement goals. The independent peer review of behavior support plans described in Chapter 8 exemplifies some of these principles.

- *Screening for ASD:* For the past decade, screening for ASD initiatives have been able to take advantage of increasingly specific, research-based practice guidelines. I have yet to see examples of regulations that establish minimum standards, let alone mechanisms of oversight.

- *Public registries for ASD:* Although public registries could be one mechanism for promoting evidence-based practices for diagnosis, are often accompanied by formal regulations, and sometimes mandate the reporting of ASD, I know of no public registry that formally enforces such standards.

- *Specialist in ASD:* Such specialists are well placed to promote evidence-based practice guidelines and to better advocate for regulations that establish minimum standards, but in my experience often act in an advisory role and so have little opportunity to enforce compliance.

Other Principles for More Ambitious Initiatives   The examples described earlier are intended to convey the opportunities and barriers for policies that are more targeted, and therefore readily attainable for a smaller organization. I next describe examples of two more ambitious initiatives to illustrate other opportunities and barriers.

Combating Autism Act   The Combating Autism Act (CAA) was passed by the U.S. House of Representatives in December 2006 and represented perhaps the single most coordinated and comprehensive piece of legislation targeting a specific condition to that date. CAA originally included a more than $600-million investment in autism research, treatment, and services and $700 million more when reauthorized in September 2011. Given the amount of energy and resources invested into CAA, it will likely remain the most important federal legislation addressing ASD for decades to come.

An initiative as large and complex as CAA requires a clearly articulated strategic plan; for CAA, this was developed through an expansion of an existing committee, the Interagency Autism Coordinating Committee (IACC). The primary goals of the IACC are to

> provide advice to the Secretary of Health and Human Services regarding Federal activities related to autism spectrum disorder; facilitate the exchange of information on and coordination of ASD activities among the member agencies and organizations; and increase public understanding of the member agencies' activities, programs, policies, and research by providing a public forum for discussions related to ASD research and services. (http://iacc.hhs.gov/)

The IACC seeks to balance representation from both government and nongovernment sources—including those living with ASD—and this may have contributed to the inclusion of research topics of particular concern to parents (e.g., the association between the measles, mumps, and rubella vaccine; gastrointestinal tract disorders; and autism). I believe that the alignment of priorities via a strategic plan helped to ensure the inclusion of training and implementation programs, such as the funding of the Autism Intervention Research Networks on Physical Health and Behavioral Health (AIR-P and AIR-B Networks).

CAA also illustrates the pressure for major initiatives to reinforce existing approaches, rather than promote radically new approaches. In part, this is perhaps the natural consequence of a process whereby major stakeholders (e.g., other government agencies, major research institutions) help to shape the legislation. This is evident in the distribution of funding, which continues to reflect the belief that the most significant progress will be made by understanding causes and characteristics. More than 60% of funding was allotted to the National Institutes of Health alone, with more themes related to basic research (e.g., identifying biomarkers, establishing ASD registries, understanding genetic and environmental risk factors, evaluating interactions between the immune and central nervous systems), as opposed to assessment research (e.g., improving screening for ASD) and intervention research. CAA also reinforced the traditional distinctions between health and education; remarkably, CAA is almost entirely driven by health services and priorities, even though the majority of services to people under 21 years of age is provided through educational systems.

CAA also illustrates the pressure for major initiatives to bundle new programs and existing programs, rather than focus largely on creating new programs. The strategy of bundling existing programs under the umbrella of a "new" act can be interpreted in different ways: The cynic might conclude that it simply serves to inflate the estimate of the increase represented by the act; the optimist might believe that it results in a perfect alignment of programs; the pragmatist recognizes that ambitious acts must generate enthusiasm to be passed, accepts that it is more expedient to revitalize established programs than to create new ones, and is encouraged that any increase in the coordination of programs helps us to move incrementally forward toward a more integrated network of services, training, and research. For example, the Leadership Education in Neurodevelopmental and Related Disabilities (LEND) Programs referenced earlier in this chapter were expanded and bundled into CAA: CAA funded new components that help LEND programs provide training more specific to ASD to the next generation of clinical leaders; the entire budget of the preexisting LEND program was subsumed under CAA, even though LEND provides training related to a broad range of disabilities.

Autism Insurance   Since the early 2000s, perhaps the most significant effort to broaden and increase funding for services has come through autism insurance legislation. Until recently, most private health insurers excluded autism-specific interventions. Autism insurance legislation typically compels private health insurance providers to cover those costs for screening for ASD, diagnosis, and treatment that are not already covered elsewhere, to a level comparable to the coverage of physical illness (e.g., to achieve parity). Such legislation often covers the costs of some treatments otherwise often excluded, including applied behavior analysis. As of April 2013, 32 states had passed such legislation, although 10 more had endorsed or were activity pursuing such legislation (Autism Speaks, 2013). In the following examples, I cite some examples of Pennsylvania's experience since the passage of autism insurance legislation (Act 62) in 2008.

The efforts to pass autism insurance legislation reveal the tremendous potential impact when advocacy is coordinated. Autism Speaks has assumed a leading role in promoting such legislation in states such as Pennsylvania, using its growing number of chapters and members to build interest and momentum. This is also the first time that information about major ASD state legislation in negotiation or enacted in one state is made easily accessible to advocates in other states. As a result, states are less likely to repeat earlier missteps, and Autism Speaks has now developed and disseminated model legislation. The precedent established because of the number of states that have passed autism insurance legislation is probably a significant factor in the decision to include behavioral health treatments in the Essential Health Benefits package of the Affordable Care Act of 2010. Thus, every health plan offered through the state exchange system is required to incorporate behavioral health treatments—including applied behavior analysis for autism—in these benefits by 2014.

These efforts have also drawn explicitly and strategically on available data sources. Previously, those advocating for increased early intervention often focused on applied behavior analysis, citing Lovaas's original 1987 findings and more recent analyses suggesting potential lifetime savings of at least $1 million for each child who received intensive early intervention (Jacobson & Mulick, 2000). Advocates for autism insurance have managed to overcome the questions that have dogged the acceptance of these claims of recovery and dramatic cost-savings by referencing broader reviews that recognize the general impact of early and intensive intervention, the general evidence supporting behavioral and other approaches, and the cascading effect of early intervention on later functioning. Proponents have also considered more carefully the specific costs associated with such legislation, concluding that these would increase insurance costs by 1% (Bouder et al., 2009). For Pennsylvania, all of this information is clearly articulated in a position paper commissioned by the Pennsylvania Health Care Cost Containment Council (Ganz et al., 2012).

Efforts to enact autism insurance legislation have already run headlong into a first line of significant barriers, with a second line of barriers laying still beyond these. As described earlier, major initiatives naturally reinforce existing institutions, approaches, and distinctions, unless new ones are specifically promoted. For example, autism insurance legislation was driven by the promise of increased skill acquisition through early and intensive behavioral intervention, yet such legislation has sought to leverage behavioral health services that traditionally focus on rehabilitation (e.g., preventing or redressing the loss of previously acquired skills) and specifically exclude education and habilitation (e.g., the acquisition of new skills). Some of the language included in Pennsylvania legislation (e.g., "to produce socially significant improvement in human behavior or to prevent loss of attained skill or function") may help to break through the traditional limitations arising from a reliance on "rehabilitative" services and broaden the range of goals addressed.

The development, implementation, and enforcement of the rules and regulations that actually guide the implementation of law can be an immediate opportunity or a barrier, as also evident by the experience of Pennsylvania. Although the passage of significant legislation to create a new and costly program will always be an arduous task, and the signing of bill into law will always represent a watershed in the development of new programs, this may sometimes only represent the end of the beginning, especially for ambitious and/or complex legislation. Yet the development of regulations is also challenging because the negotiations can be just as political and pressurized as those involved in the initial passage of the law, but may not be as transparent. Thus, entities originally opposed to a bill can use the regulatory process to effectively emasculate it, and the full impact may not be evident until the regulations are fully implemented and proponents become confused because the expected benefits have failed to materialize. For example, autism insurance was signed into law with much fanfare in Pennsylvania in 2008, but it was only after the passage of regulations that the administrative burden for health providers became apparent, with the result that many potential providers have thus far not elected to offer services funded through Act 62. Well-crafted regulations can also improve services by clarifying which procedures should be applied, when, by whom, and with what mechanisms of accountability and oversight. Thus Pennsylvania's law mandated the Department of Public Welfare to promulgate regulations to license autism "behavior specialists" responsible for delivering behavioral treatment. Regulations published in June 2012 expanded on this opportunity by clearly outlining additional, more specialized training that includes topics that are not addressed in many traditional behavioral training programs for ASD, such as addressing co-occurring conditions, working with families, and so forth.

Some of the other elements in the second line of barriers to improving services have already been described: ensuring access to timely and accurate diagnosis for all, the recognition of co-occurring conditions, the identification of EBPs, and so forth. One such element immediately relevant to autism insurance legislation in Pennsylvania and elsewhere is the lack of specialized training capacity. Earlier in this chapter, I outlined how training capacity is likely to develop through the interaction of various factors; now it is possible to project why it might be at least 5 years from the passage of legislation in Pennsylvania before the new autism behavior specialists envisioned in this legislation are beginning to provide services, and at least 7 years before enough specialists are available to begin to meet the needs of traditionally underserved populations.

- Act 62 was passed in July 2008.

- Regulations guiding the certification of autism behavior specialists must be promulgated; in Pennsylvania, these were published in June 2012 (i.e., 4 years after the passage of the original act).

- The necessary training program must be developed through colleges and universities, unless this training is delivered by the service providers themselves or available through some other mechanism. College and universities must be convinced that the opportunity justifies the investment of resources needed, and then must create the necessary programs. A first wave of trainees may be created relatively quickly through well-established behavioral training programs, which need only to create new course(s) or adapt existing ones. Nonetheless, these modifications are unlikely to be online until at least 6–12 months after the publication of the regulations, and will only result in a first cohort of new specialists 6–12 months after that (e.g., 5–6 years after the passage of the original act). Given the large number of autism behavior specialists needed and the relatively limited number of established training programs, this first wave is unlikely to generate the capacity needed across the Commonwealth to ensure access to traditionally underserved regions and populations.

- To generate full capacity, other college or university programs will require a more extensive investment; the designation of specialized faculty, the creation of a new certificate program or specialized master's degree program, and so forth. Given this investment, these new training programs for ASD may not be online until at least 12–24 months after the publication of the regulations, and will only result in a first cohort of new specialists 6–12 months after that (e.g., 6–7 years after the passage of the original act).

REFERENCES

Allen, S.G., Berry, A.D., Brewster, J.A., Chalasani, R.K., & Mack, P.K. (2010). Enhancing developmentally oriented primary care: An Illinois initiative to increase developmental screening in medical homes. *Pediatrics, 126*(Suppl. 3), S160–S164.

American Academy of Pediatrics. (2001). Technical report: The pediatrician's role in the diagnosis and management of autistic spectrum disorder in children. *Pediatrics, 107*(5), 1–18.

American Academy of Pediatrics (Committee on Children with Disabilities). (2001). Developmental surveillance and screening of infants and young children (RE0062). *Pediatrics, 108*(1), 192–196.

Autism and Developmental Disabilities Monitoring Network Surveillance Year 2006 Principal Investigators & Centers for Disease Control and Prevention (CDC). (2009). Prevalence of autism spectrum disorders—Autism and Developmental Disabilities Monitoring Network. *MMWR Surveillance Summary, 58*(10), 1–20.

Autism Speaks. (2013, April 8). *State initiatives.* Autism Speaks. Retrieved from http://www.autismspeaks.org/sites/default/files/docs/gr/states_4.8.2013.pdf

Baird, G., Charman, T., Baron-Cohen, S., Cox, A., Swettenham, J., Wheelwright, S., et al. (2000). A screening instrument for autism at 18 month age: A six-year follow-up study. *Journal of the American Academy of Child and Adolescent Psychiatry, 39,* 694–702.

Baird, G., Simonoff, E., Pickles, A., Chandler, S., Loucas, T., Meldrum, D., et al. (2006). Prevalence of disorders of the autism spectrum in a population cohort of children in South Thames: The Special Needs and Autism Project (SNAP). *Lancet, 368*(9531), 210–215.

Baron-Cohen, S., Allen, J., & Gillberg, C. (1992). Can autism be detected at 18 months? The needle, the haystack, and the CHAT. *British Journal of Psychiatry, 161,* 839–843.

Baron-Cohen, S., Cox, A., Baird, G., Swettenham, J., Nightingale, N., Morgan, K., et al. (1996). Psychological markers in the detection of autism in infancy in a large population. *British Journal of Psychiatry, 168,* 1–6.

Baron-Cohen, S., Wheelwright, S., Cox, A., Baird, G., Charman, T., Swettenham, J., et al. (2000). Early identification of autism by the Checklist for Autism in Toddlers (CHAT). *Journal of the Royal Society of Medicine, 93*(10), 521–525.

Bertrand, J., Mars, A., Boyle, C., Bove, F., Yeargin-Allsopp, M., & Decoufle, P. (2001). Prevalence of autism in a United States population: The Brick Township, New Jersey, investigation. *Pediatrics, 108*(5), 1155–1161.

Bouder, J.N., Spielman, S., & Mandell, D.S. (2009). Brief report: Quantifying the impact of autism coverage on private insurance premiums. *Journal of Autism and Developmental Disorders, 39*(6), 953–957.

Bryson, S.A., Corrigan, S.K., McDonald, T.P., & Holmes, C. (2008). Characteristics of children with autism spectrum disorders who received services through community mental health centers. *Autism, 12*(1), 65–82.

California Department of Developmental Services. (2002). *Autistic spectrum disorders: Best practice guidelines for screening, diagnosis, and assessment.* Sacramento, CA: Author.

Canal-Bedia, R., Garcia-Primo, P., Martin-Cilleros, M.V., Santos-Borbujo, J., Guisuraga-Fernandez, Z., Herraez-Garcia, L., et al. (2011). Modified checklist for autism in toddlers: Cross-cultural adaptation and validation in Spain. *Journal of Autism and Developmental Disorders, 41*(10), 1342–1351.

Charman, T., Pickles, A., Chandler, S., Wing, L., Bryson, S., Simonoff, E., et al. (2009). Commentary: Effects of diagnostic thresholds and research vs. service and administrative diagnosis on autism prevalence. *International Journal of Epidemiology, 38*(5), 1234–1238.

Committee on Educational Interventions for Children with Autism. (2001). *Educating children with autism.* Washington, DC: National Academies Press.

Daniels, A.M., Rosenberg, R.E., Law, J.K., Lord, C., Kaufmann, W.E., & Law, P.A. (2011). Stability of initial autism spectrum disorder diagnoses in community settings. *Journal of Autism and Developmental Disorders, 41*(1), 110–121.

Doehring, P. (2002). *Research strategies in human communication disorders* (3rd ed.). Austin, TX: PRO-ED.

Doehring, P., & Winterling, V. (2011). The implementation of evidence-based practices in public schools. In B. Reichow, P. Doehring, D.V. Cicchetti, & F.R. Volkmar (Eds.), *Evidence-based practices and treatments for children with autism* (pp. 343–363). New York, NY: Springer.

Eldin, A.S., Habib, D., Noufal, A., Farrag, S., Bazaid, K., Al-Sharbati, M., et al. (2008). Use of M-CHAT for a multinational screening of young children with autism in the Arab countries. [Special Issue: A global perspective on child and adolescent mental health]. *International Review of Psychiatry, 20*(3), 281–289.

Fountain, C., King, M.D., & Bearman, P.S. (2011). Age of diagnosis for autism: Individual and community factors across 10 birth cohorts. *Journal of Epidemiology and Community Health, 65*(6), 503–510.

Frant, Roger. (2005). *Guidelines for identification and education of children and youth with autism.* New Haven: Connecticut State Department of Education.

Ganz, M., Lavange, L., Mauch, D., Morrissey, J.P.C., Schlenger, W., & Sikich, L. (2012). *Autism spectrum disorders mandated benefits review panel report: Evidence submitted concerning Pennsylvania HB 1150.* Durham, NC: Abt Associates.

Gillberg, C., & Wing, L. (1999). Autism: Not an extremely rare disorder. *Acta Psychiatrica Scandinavica, 99*(6), 399–406.

Glessner, J.T., Wang, K., Cai, G.Q., Korvatska, O., Kim, C.E., Wood, S., et al. (2009). Autism genome-wide copy number variation reveals ubiquitin and neuronal genes. *Nature, 459*(7246), 569–573.

Goin-Kochel, R.P. & Cohen, R. (2008). Screening cases within a statewide autism registry: A comparison of parental reports using DSM-IV-TR criteria versus the SCQ. *Focus on Autism and Other Developmental Disabilities, 23,* 148–154.

Gura, G.F., Champagne, M.T., & Blood-Siegfried, J.E. (2011). Autism spectrum disorder screening in primary care. *Journal of Developmental and Behavioral Pediatrics, 32*(1), 48–51.

Jabrink, K. (2007). The economic consequences of autistic spectrum disorder among children in a Swedish municipality. *Autism, 11*(5), 453–463.

Jacobson, J.W., & Mulick, J.A. (2000). System and cost research issues in treatments for people with autistic disorders. *Journal of Autism and Developmental Disorders, 30*(6), 585–593.

Johnson, C.P., Myers, S.M., & the Council on Children with Disabilities. (2007). Identification and evaluation of children with autism spectrum disorders. *Pediatrics, 120*(5), 1183–1215.

King, M., & Bearman, P. (2009). Diagnostic change and the increased prevalence of autism. *International Journal of Epidemiology, 38*(5), 1224–1234.

Kleinman, J.M., Robins, D.L., Ventola, P.E., Pandey, J., Boorstein, H.C., Esser, E.L., et al. (2008). The Modified Checklist for Autism in Toddlers: A follow-up study investigating the early detection of autism spectrum disorders. *Journal of Autism and Developmental Disorders, 38*(5), 827–839.

Lauritsen, M.B., Jorgensen, M., Madsen, K.M., Lemcke, S., Toft, S., Grove, J., et al. (2010). Validity of childhood autism in the Danish Psychiatric Central Register: Findings from a cohort sample born 1990–1999. *Journal of Autism and Developmental Disorders, 40*(2), 139–148.

Lawer, L., Brusilovskiy, E., Salzer, M.S., & Mandell, D.S. (2009). Use of vocational rehabilitative services among adults with autism. *Journal of Autism and Developmental Disorders, 39*(3), 487–494.

Lawer, L., & Mandel, D.S. (2009). *Pennsylvania Autism Census Project: Final report.* Harrisburg: Bureau of Autism Services, Pennsylvania Department of Public Welfare.

Levy, S.E., Mandell, D.S., & Schultz, R.T. (2009). Autism. *Lancet, 374*(9701), 1627–1638.

Liptak, G.S., Benzoni, L.B., Mruzek, D.W., Nolan, K.W., Thingvoll, M.A., Wade, C.M., et al. (2008). Disparities in diagnosis and access to health services for children with autism: Data from the National Survey of Children's Health. *Journal of Developmental and Behavioral Pediatrics, 29*(3), 152–160.

Liptak, G.S., Stuart, T., & Auinger, P. (2006). Health care utilization and expenditures for children with autism: Data from U.S. national samples. *Journal of Autism and Developmental Disorders, 36*(7), 871–879.

Logan, S.L., Nicholas, J.S., Carpenter, L.A., King, L.B., Garrett-Mayer, E., & Charles, J.M. (2012). High prescription drug use and associated costs among Medicaid-eligible children with autism spectrum disorders identified by a population-based surveillance network. *Annals of Epidemiology, 22*(1), 1–8.

Lord, C., Rutter, M., DiLavore, P.C., & Risi, S. (1999). *Autism Diagnostic Observation Schedule (ADOS).* Los Angeles, CA: Western Psychological Services.

Lord, C., Rutter, M., & Le Couteur, A. (1994). Autism Diagnostic Interview-Revised: A revised version of a diagnostic interview for caregivers of individuals with possible pervasive developmental disorders. *Journal of Autism and Developmental Disorders, 24*(5), 659–685.

Lovaas, O.I. (1987). Behavioral treatment and normal educational and intellectual functioning in young autistic children. *Journal of Consulting and Clinical Psychology, 55*(1), 3–9.

Mandell, D.S., Cao, J., Ittenbach, R., & Pinto-Martin, J. (2006). Medicaid expenditures for children with autistic spectrum disorders: 1994 to 1999. *Journal of Autism and Developmental Disorders, 36*(4), 475–485.

Mandell, D.S., Listerud, J., Levy, S.E., & Pinto-Martin, J.A. (2002). Race differences in the age at diagnosis among Medicaid-eligible children with autism. *Journal of the American Academy of Child and Adolescent Psychiatry, 41*(12), 1447–1453.

Mandell, D.S., Morales, K.H., Marcus, S.C., Stahmer, A.C., Doshi, J., & Polsky, D.E. (2008). Psychotropic medication use among Medicaid-enrolled children with autism spectrum disorders. *Pediatrics, 121*(3), e441–e448.

Mandell, D.S., Morales, K.H., Xie, M., Polsky, D., Stahmer, A., & Marcus, S.C. (2010). County-level variation in the prevalence of Medicaid enrolled children with autism spectrum disorders. *Journal of Autism and Developmental Disorders, 40*(10), 1241–1246.

Marcus, L.M., Rubin, J.S., & Rubin, M.A. (2000). Benefit-cost analysis and autism services: A response to Jacobson and Mulick. *Journal of Autism and Developmental Disorders, 30*(6), 595–598.

Mattila, M.L., Kielinen, M., Jussila, K., Linna, S.L., Bloigu, R., Ebeling, H. et al. (2007). An epidemiological and diagnostic study of Asperger Syndrome according to four sets of diagnostic criteria. *Journal of the American Academy of Child & Adolescent Psychiatry, 46*(5), 636–646.

McEachin, J.J., & Lovaas, O.I. (1993). Long-term outcome for children with autism who received early intensive behavioral treatment. *American Journal on Mental Retardation, 97*(4), 359–372.

McPheeters, M.L., Warren, Z., Sathe, N., Bruzek, J.L., Krishnaswami, S., Jerome, R.N., et al. (2011). A systematic review of medical treatments for children with autism spectrum disorders. *Pediatrics, 127*(5), e1312–e1321.

Miller, J.S., Gabrielsen, T., Villalobos, M., Alleman, R., Wahmhoff, N., Carbone, P.S., et al. (2011). The Each Child Study: Systematic screening for autism spectrum disorders in a pediatric setting. *Pediatrics, 127*(5), 866–871.

Myers, S.M., Johnson, C.P., & the Council on Children with Disabilities. (2007). Management of children with autism spectrum disorders. *Pediatrics, 120*(5), 1162–1182.

National Autism Center. (2009). *The National Standards Project: Addressing the need for evidence based practice guidelines for autism spectrum disorders.* Randolph, MA: Author.

National Professional Development Center on Autism Spectrum Disorders. (2011). *Evidence-based practice briefs.* Chapel Hill: FPG Child Development Institute, University of North Carolina at Chapel Hill.

Nygren, G., Cederlund, M., Sandberg, E., Gillstedt, F., Arvidsson, T., Carina-Gillber, I., et al. (2011). The prevalence of autism spectrum disorders in toddlers: A population study of 2-year-old Swedish children. *Journal of Autism and Developmental Disorders, 42*(7), 1491–1497.

Pennsylvania Autism Assessment and Diagnosis Expert Work Group. (2007). *Supporting quality diagnostic practices for persons with suspected autism spectrum disorder.* Harrisburg: Pennsylvania Department of Public Welfare.

Perera, H., Wijewardena, K., & Aluthwelage, R. (2009). Screening of 18–24-month-old children for autism in a semi-urban community in Sri Lanka. *Journal of Tropical Pediatrics, 55*(6), 402–405.

Pinto-Martin, J.A., Young, L.M., Mandell, D.S., Poghosyan, L., Giarelli, E., & Levy, S.E. (2008). Screening strategies for autism spectrum disorders in pediatric primary care. *Journal of Developmental and Behavioral Pediatrics, 29*(5), 345–350.

Reichow, B., Doehring, P., Cicchetti, D.V., & Volkmar, F.R. (2011). *Evidence-based practices and treatments for children with autism.* New York, NY: Springer.

Rice, C., Nicholas, J., Baio, J., Pettygrove, S., Lee, L.C., Van Naarden, B.K., et al. (2010). Changes in autism spectrum disorder prevalence in 4 areas of the United States. *Disability and Health Journal, 3*(3), 186–201.

Robins, D.L. (2008). Screening for autism spectrum disorders in primary care settings. [Special Issue: Early detection]. *Autism, 12*(5), 537–556.

Robins, D.L., Fein, D., Barton, M.L., & Green, J.A. (2001). The modified checklist for autism in toddlers: An initial study investigating the early detection of autism and pervasive developmental disorders. *Journal of Autism and Developmental Disorders, 31*(2), 131–144.

Rosenberg, R.E., Mandell, D.S., Farmer, J.E., Law, J.K., Marvin, A.R., & Law, P.A. (2010). Psychotropic medication use among children with autism spectrum disorders enrolled in a national registry, 2007–2008. *Journal of Autism and Developmental Disorders, 40*(3), 342–351.

Scahill, L., & Boorin, S.G. (2011). Psychopharmacology in children with PDD: Review of current evidence. In B. Reichow, P. Doehring, D.V. Cicchetti, & F.R. Volkmar (Eds.), *Evidence-based practices and treatments for children with autism* (pp. 231–243). New York, NY: Springer.

Schopler, E., Short, A., & Mesibov, G. (1987). Relation of behavioral treatment to "normal function": Comment on Lovaas. *Journal of Consulting and Clinical Psychology, 57*(1), 162–164.

Volkmar, F.R., Reichow, B., & Doehring, P. (2011). Evidence-based practices in autism: Where we are now and where we need to go. In B. Reichow, P. Doehring, D.V. Cicchetti, & F.R. Volkmar (Eds.), *Evidence-based practices and treatments for children with autism* (pp. 365–391). New York, NY: Springer.

Wang, K., Zhang, H.T., Ma, D.Q., Bucan, M., Glessner, J.T., Abrahams, B.S., et al. (2009). Common genetic variants on 5p14.1 associate with autism spectrum disorders. *Nature, 459*(7246), 528–533.

Wang, L., & Leslie, D.L. (2010). Health care expenditures for children with autism spectrum disorders in Medicaid. *Journal of the American Academy of Child and Adolescent Psychiatry, 49*(11), 1165–1171.

Warren, Z., Stone, W., & Humberd, Q. (2009). A training model for the diagnosis of autism in community pediatric practice. *Journal of Developmental and Behavioral Pediatrics, 30*(5), 442–446.

Wong, V.C., & Hui, S.L. (2008). Epidemiological study of autism spectrum disorder in China. *Journal of Child Neurology, 23*(1), 67–72.

Yoder, P., & Stone, W.L. (2006). Randomized comparison of two communication interventions for preschoolers with autism spectrum disorders. *Journal of Consulting and Clinical Psychology, 74*(3), 426–435.

Zwaigenbaum, L., Bryson, S., Lord, C., Rogers, S., Carter, A., Carver, L., et al. (2009). Clinical assessment and management of toddlers with suspected autism spectrum disorder: Insights from studies of high-risk infants. *Pediatrics, 123*(5), 1383–1391.

4

How It Works

The Infrastructure of Agencies and Organizations That Support Services, Training, Research, and Policy

Peter Doehring

Anyone seeking to develop programs addressing training, research, and policy described in Chapter 3 needs some understanding of the array of agencies and organizations that support these activities. This understanding is even more essential to those programs intended to create ongoing services such as those described in Chapter 2. On the one hand, significant policy changes can be made without any commitment regarding funding, and many research projects and training events are themselves time limited and thus well suited to grant funding or other nonrenewable sources. On the other hand, the commitment to develop a service often requires a long-term investment that includes staff training and support, the identification of a need and a clientele, and a stable source of funding. Too often, the best new services cannot be implemented, or the most promising pilot projects continued, because the funding streams and infrastructure needed to sustain services have not been identified.

I focus much of the discussion on two critical dimensions—the sector (public versus private) and the level (local, regional, state, and national)—but begin with an overview of other important and distinguishing elements (funding, mandate, oversight, and domain). I conclude by illustrating the intersection of all of these elements in agencies and programs such as those referenced elsewhere in this book. At several points, I refer to the cases introduced in Chapter 1 to try to capture the important roles played by many different agencies in the lives of people living with autism spectrum disorder (ASD). As this discussion illustrates, many of the most important and challenging needs of people living with ASD will never be met by a single agency acting alone, no matter how large, influential, or well funded. The continued evolution of programs will therefore depend on improvements in the understanding of and collaborations between programs, improvements that themselves depend on an understanding of their infrastructure.

In the concluding section of this book, I propose some general principles that describe the complex interrelationship of local, state, and national agencies and private organizations in the United States in providing services, conducting research or training, or helping to shape policy in ASD. At no time do I seek to provide an exhaustive review of the available agencies, organizations, or funding sources, or pretend to offer expertise in government policy: Instead, I draw on examples specific to ASD to capture the range of roles played by these agencies. I found almost no peer-reviewed publications that provide data documenting the range and sources of variability in service delivery, and so have relied on my own experiences supplemented by comments from colleagues familiar with these issues. Although I normally hesitate to offer suggestions based on the quality of evidence available, I felt that the need was too great. My hope is that this description encourages those advocating for change to undertake a more thorough review of the infrastructure related to the programs of interest to them, guided by the framework and the examples provided here.

COMMON ELEMENTS

Funding

At least in the short term, the most important variable determining the development of new service, training, and research initiatives across all types of agencies may be neither the documented existence of a need nor the scientific demonstration of an effective outcome, but the nature of the funding source: No new initiative can be developed, and no successful initiative will be sustained, without a clearly identified and viable funding source. New initiatives can be supported via a new funding source or the reallocation of existing funding. For small or new projects, the need to identify new funding can be delayed: Most parent-volunteers and providers are willing to stretch their resources to accommodate a short-term and exploratory project. Once the project appears viable, a delay in the identification of additional funding can stall the momentum and then dampen the enthusiasm for a new project: Even the most promising project will invariably overstretch the energy of the parent-volunteer or discretionary resources of a provider. The identification of a new funding source is relatively straightforward, because the range of funding options is relatively discrete: 1) a grant or other time-limited source may be sufficient for a pilot project, 2) ongoing public funds can be raised through increased taxes, 3) ongoing public or private funds might be raised by increased fees, or 4) ongoing public or private funds may be created by reallocating funding from elsewhere.

By necessity, every organization has professionals with intimate knowledge about the organization's funding, although these professionals are rarely as knowledgeable about the full extent of the needs of people living with ASD. The challenge when developing new initiatives is to ensure that these professionals can participate fully and frankly in discussions regarding funding. I have been gratified by an emerging cultural shift in most agencies, at least in the United States, that has allowed these discussions to occur with program leaders and people living with ASD without the smoke and mirrors that had so often obfuscated such discussions in the past. Sometimes the identification of a funding source is still the elephant in the room: The element that must be discussed at some point, but that proponents fear might doom any commitment or dampen enthusiasm for a new program. Other times, the identification of a funding source is almost irrelevant to the overall challenge of a more ambitious project. The protracted debates risk polarizing stakeholders into groups perceived as those with imagination unfettered by such petty things as funding versus those who cannot see beyond the bottom line. Although the identification of a funding source is necessary, it may distract from discussion of other, more significant threats to the project. Here are some of the other lessons I have learned.

1. *Always consider whether new funding can be offset with efficiencies elsewhere.* There is almost always competition for resources, and so discussions regarding funding should

always begin by considering whether the proposed program has the potential to decrease costs elsewhere or justify reallocation of resources. Too often, the reallocation of existing funds is overlooked because it can require difficult cuts elsewhere, but it should always be seriously considered by program leaders.

2. *Long-term salary commitments often outweigh short-term construction and technology costs.* It is difficult to work in cramped conditions with outdated equipment, and everyone is excited by new technology and new facilities. Although these costs can represent a significant proportion of the initial investment in any new program, salaries often represent from 75% to 85% of ongoing program costs (especially when the full costs, including taxes and benefits, are considered). This is why funders are more excited by construction, because over the 10-year span of a program it may well constitute less than 10% of the total operational costs.

3. *Increases in funding will usually not result in changes overnight.* Funding is best understood as a link in a complex chain of events leading to a true increase in capacity. Funding will not increase services and training if the clients do not recognize the need for the service, if professionals and providers are not convinced that the opportunity is worth the investment of time and resources, if there is no one to provide training, and if there are no standards on which training can be based. Almost all new projects will depend to some degree on new personnel; the greater the specialization required, the more difficult it will be to find such personnel, and almost every leader with whom I have worked has underestimated the difficulty of finding trained and/or experienced personnel. This problem is magnified when there are significant changes either in the type or the number of personnel or providers needed.

The slow pace of change following the passage of autism insurance legislation, as discussed in the previous chapter, illustrates this chain of events. First, a new cohort of professionals must be trained and hired and new providers may need to be identified, but professionals and providers are unlikely to reinvest their time and resources to take advantage of these new opportunities until they are confident that the investment is worthwhile. Autism insurance legislation also introduces two other sources of delay: the need to pass state regulations and the need for individual families to establish their eligibility and petition for services.

Mandate

The mandate of an agency or program is critical to defining its mission and infrastructure. Well-crafted mandates can help ensure that there are no gaps; overly rigid mandates can create service silos that prevent agencies from collaborating to address complex problems.

Domain   What is the scope of the services or training provided, or the research and policy addressed? Traditional distinctions between service domains described in Chapter 3 (e.g., health, education, community) are reflected in the allocation of disciplines and agencies (e.g., doctors deliver services in hospitals, teachers in schools) and the fact that services are largely clustered around the service need (e.g., medical centers serving many different types of people) rather than the disability (e.g., a stand-alone multidisciplinary center focused on ASD). These distinctions are also reflected in the funding source (e.g., funding from education, health). As emphasized earlier, these distinctions do not meaningfully demarcate the needs of people with ASD—indeed, examples throughout this book emphasize the need for cross-discipline and cross-agency collaboration to meet the complex needs of people with ASD—but simply acknowledge the reality that this infrastructure is too entrenched to change quickly. These distinctions can be nonetheless useful in promoting: 1) the specialization needed to identify new, specific approaches (e.g., a specialist is more likely to make advances than a generalist); 2) the sharing of ideas across disabilities but with in domains (e.g., advances made with other disabilities are more likely to cross-pollinate in domain-specific institutions rather than a multidisciplinary center focused solely on ASD); and 3) accountability (e.g., multidisciplinary and multi-agency approaches can dilute and diffuse responsibility and accountability).

Eligibility   Who is eligible for services or training? Eligibility can be defined in terms of:

- *Age:* For example, people are typically ineligible for education-based services at the end of their 22nd year.

- *Diagnosis:* For example, recent insurance legislation provides support to people with ASD but not intellectual disability (ID), even though the latter can benefit from many of the same interventions.

- *ID:* For example, state developmental disabilities agencies often provide services only to those with significant impairment in intellectual functioning, excluding those with Asperger syndrome.

Setting   Where can the services be provided? Agencies are typically reluctant to provide services outside of specific settings. Schools hesitate to provide services outside of the school setting or beyond the school day or school year, unless there is a clearly documented need to do so. Community-based behavioral rehabilitation services may not interface with schools. To some extent, this may reflect a reasonable desire to avoid interfering with the work of another agency, but is more likely to reflect an attempt to limit their responsibility for—and ultimately the cost of—services. This can create unforeseen gaps: For example, no support for in-home toilet training may result when the school staff feels they lack the mandate to address toilet-training needs beyond the school day and when a behavioral rehabilitation agency views toilet training as falling outside of the scope of rehabilitation.

Other Examples   Sometimes the mandate also specifies the time frame within which a service must be provided: For example, the requirement that an evaluation be completed with a specified number of days since referral. Sometimes mandated collaboration can prevent gaps from occurring between agencies. For example, mandated transition planning into and out of education-based services (e.g., prior to age 3 and after age 21) is critical to assuring at least that caregivers, people with ASD, and providers meet to lay out a course of action.

Standards and Oversight

Laws, regulations, and licensing can dictate the type and amount of services and associated training with extraordinary detail, but can offer no assurance of quality unless standards of practice and mechanisms for oversight are clearly defined. Even though regulations rarely incorporate evidence-based practices in more than name only, they nonetheless can set useful, minimal standards of practice and define a process of periodic review for verifying that these standards are being met. When mechanisms of oversight are well designed and carefully implemented, they can contribute significantly to program consistency and quality.

Well-crafted mandates and regulatory standards can help reinstate some of the control a public agency otherwise relinquishes by contracting out to a private agency. When mechanisms of oversight are poorly crafted and/or arbitrarily implemented, they can introduce additional administrative inefficiencies that ultimately detract from the quality of services provided. Following are a few lessons I have learned.

1. *Seek to operationalize intelligent, practical, and observable if not measurable standards.* Whether drawing from agency-specific guidelines, the interpretation of state or federal regulations, or the regulations themselves, oversight functions most effectively when it is based on clear and relevant standards. How long should it take to meet a standard? What are the final products(s)? How is compliance evaluated? The development of such standards ideally evolves through negotiations between those who implement the practice and those who oversee it.

2. *Provide independent oversight with teeth.* Many of those providing services, training, and research have the best of intentions, and many organizations have internal standards and mechanisms of oversight. Nonetheless it is easy for practices to drift over time, for new organizations to be confused about standards, or for agencies to consider cutting corners under pressure. In these cases, it can be very helpful for knowledgeable professionals, independent of the agency, to audit compliance with the practice, and to compel providers who fall short of the standards to improve. For many health and mental health agencies, this function is accomplished through the process of licensure: Periodic site visits can ensure that providers comply with defined standards of practice, or face censure through loss of their license. Without periodic visits and the specter of censure, compliance is less consistent.

3. *Create a culture of shared accountability.* Agencies that implement the steps described earlier can create tremendous pressure for reviewers and for those reviewed, especially when the viability of a program or an agency hangs in the balance. This pressure can create a culture of "us versus them," splitting reviewers and those reviewed into their respective corners where they lose sight of a broader, shared goal: to improve the quality and availability of services. Those subjected to oversight must accept that accurate documentation of compliance is essential to the system of services. Those providing oversight must recognize that a heavy hand can destroy the very services, training, and research they are promoting. I believe that both the reviewers and those reviewed must engage in a responsible dialogue to shape these standards to achieve these broader, shared goals.

THE PUBLIC AND PRIVATE SECTORS

Many people will naturally categorize programs into those that are public (i.e., city, county, state, and federal agencies) and those that are private. Until recently, publicly administered and/or funded agencies provided the stable infrastructure and source of funding needed to build capacity over a period of multiple years. To some extent, this is hardly surprising, given that many of these focused on services for the public good, intended to reach a large and diverse clientele, for which there is little room or incentive for profit. Yet such agencies are often territorial, slow to develop and change, constrained by rules and regulations, and increasingly subject to the whims of the party in power. In contrast, private agencies can develop quickly to address changing needs and exploit emerging opportunities, but may lack the stable funding and infrastructure needed to develop an initiative over a longer period of time. The distinction between public- and private-sector agencies is not, however, always simple or clear, because one must consider the organization's role in providing the program, the funding of the program, the source and amount of regulatory oversight, and the scope and mandate of the program. These elements can be intertwined in complex ways that vary from program to program and from agency to agency.

Public- versus Private-Sector Agencies: Structure, Funding, and Mandate

Single-Sector Programs   Sometimes the organization essentially runs the program of services, training, research, and/or policy independently: It provides programming through its own personnel, it obtains most or all of its funding from a single sector (e.g., either public or private), and it determines the mandate (e.g., what the program consists of, how the program is delivered, who is eligible for the program). Many public agencies largely operate in this manner at each of the levels of government. For example, a public school provides education through personnel that it hires, and it receives its funding and is regulated by other public agencies. Note that this model is rarely as simple as it seems when multiple levels of funding and oversight are involved: The levels of funding and oversight provided by local, state, or federal programs can each vary greatly, and gaps in programs emerge with surprising frequency. Some private agencies may also fit this description: They may receive little or no public funding and may perform activities that are loosely regulated by public entities. For example, an advocacy group for ASD may operate entirely through fund-raising, and the scope of its advocacy efforts may not be subject to oversight by any specific public agency. In many cases, however, private agencies may benefit from grants or tax incentives provided through public agencies.

Public-Private Hybrids   Many readers will be surprised to learn that most programs function as hybrids: Many involve a mix of public and private funding, and programs that offer services are all subjected to some degree of public oversight. Public agencies can also fund privately run programs, with varying degrees and mechanisms of oversight. One example of this kind of hybrid is a traditional publicly grant-funded program for services, research, training, and policy: The program is funded largely or exclusively through a single grant; the original request soliciting applicants for the grant program defines the mandate; and the level of oversight can vary greatly from the expectation that a final report will be delivered, to ongoing monitoring via site visits. In my experience, many research, training, and policy programs are funded in this way, as well as some newly emerging programs focused on service delivery. These same grant-funding mechanisms have been used with great success by private agencies, even for very large and complex programs (see discussion later in the chapter). Grants can be an excellent way to help to develop a new sector, to inspire an innovative approach, and encourage an agency to become involved in programming. On the one hand, many grants operate on a short cycle (e.g., 1–5 years), and thus provide the opportunity for the funding agency to rework the program as needs change. On the other hand, this cycle creates instability in the funded program, making it hard to depend on grants to craft a long-term strategy.

Another example of a publicly funded but privately run hybrid program increasingly common in the United States is the public agency that no longer runs the program itself but contracts out to a private agency. The original request soliciting applicants for the contract (e.g., a request for proposal) may define the mandate of the program in a manner similar to a grant. Otherwise, the scope and mandate of the contract and the mechanisms of oversight may be much more variable. For example, a county early intervention agency may contract its early intervention services program out to one or more private agencies. This can save the public agency from the challenge of developing and overseeing the entire service, including obligations for health and pension benefits. Sometimes these services are contracted out on a per-head basis: For example, a charter school may receive funding from the local school district on a per-student basis to provide education. Sometimes only specific services are contracted: A public school may contract out for an entire department (e.g., speech-language therapy) or for a specific student (e.g., a one-to-one assistant provided by a private agency). This may save a public agency from developing a specific capacity or program for a service that is infrequently needed: For example, a private agency may be able to provide better and cheaper speech-language therapy via contracts to several school districts than had the individual school districts each developed their own departments. I have observed each of these kinds of relationships across different agencies within health, education, and rehabilitation contexts. I have found that the efficiency of these arrangements depends on the prevalence of the need (e.g., how many people are likely to benefit from the program) and the specialization of the program (e.g., how much training is required of the person delivering the program), factors that I discuss in the final section of this book.

Another commonly used mechanism by which public agencies fund a private professional or program is a simple fee-for-service arrangement. This can work well for discrete, time-limited, and/or specialized services. For example, a program might pay a trainer to provide a workshop, or may pay the registration fee for a staff member to attend a conference (please refer to the "Training" section in Chapter 3 for a discussion of the limitations of this approach). A school may pay an independent professional to conduct an educational evaluation more specialized than can be delivered by its own staff (e.g., a neuropsychological evaluation) when that is deemed essential to that student's programming. Unless the public agency monitors the frequency with which the service or training is needed, it may fail to recognize when it is more efficient to replace a fee-for-service arrangement with a contractual arrangement or by developing that capacity in-house. I believe that agencies should not underestimate the potential for increased accountability, commitment, and collaboration that a contractual arrangement can offer relative to a fee-for-service arrangement: A conscientious trainer who returns to coach trainees after an initial workshop, as part of an ongoing contract, can recognize and potentially rectify the shortcomings of the original training. The provider and the recipient of the training both benefit from increased understanding of the challenges that each faces, and the trust that can emerge from this understanding can support more active collaboration.

Other important variations are domain specific. For example, service-delivery organizations are sometimes divided between public, private for-profit, and private not-for-profit entities. A private for-profit institution is subjected to the full range of taxes, can disperse profits to shareholders, and has wide discretion in the range of services it provides and to whom. A private not-for-profit organization benefits from certain tax exemptions at multiple levels (e.g., reduced property tax, taxes on incomes), but is expected to make certain services more accessible to all potential clients.

Advantages and Limitations of Public- versus Private-Sector Agencies

As is the case throughout this volume, professionals and agencies working in one area often misunderstand the strengths and limitations of those working in other areas. In my role as a leader of programs in the public and the private sectors, I have found that professionals in each sector tend to overestimate the contribution of their own sector and undervalue the contribution of the other. When resources clearly fall short of meeting a specified need, this misunderstanding breeds competition, further clouds what are already complex relationships between the public and private sector, and undercuts collaboration for the common good. To begin to close this gap of understanding, I briefly describe here what I believe to be some of the broad characteristics and culture of public- and private-sector programs, and link this to some of the needs of people living with ASD.

Programs in the Public Sector   I believe that public-sector programs, especially those focused on service delivery, have a distinct role and culture.

- Many public agencies are institutions with a specific role to be easily accessible to all those in need. Given the high prevalence of ASD and disparities in access noted earlier, this appears to be an important characteristic.

- As institutions, many public agencies can offer a stable service that, under the right circumstances, can evolve over many years to provide quality services adapted to the needs of the community. The many layers (local, state, federal) of funding and oversight also help to assure some consistency and continuity in services across regions, while also allowing for some region-to-region variation. This stability and consistency is important given that ASD is, for many, a lifelong need, and because the field continues to evolve.

- I believe that the role of public-sector agencies in promoting equal opportunity for all, regardless of the family's income or background, instills a sense of pride among professionals providing services through these agencies. This pride can become magnified by the long-term commitment many professionals have, at least until recently, made to their jobs. I have found many people who had worked in the public sector for their entire career, perhaps because such positions offered relatively stable and generous benefits (e.g., pensions and health care), predictable pay increases commensurate with training and experience, and job security (especially when these positions were unionized). These professionals and leaders constitute the backbone of a critical and persistently undervalued service to society, and this commitment helped them to weather many of the limitations and changes in the public sector.

- Any element that promotes an enduring commitment to the field is also important because years of training and experience may be necessary before professionals are comfortable working with a range of people living with ASD. For those not pursuing specialized postgraduate training, it may be difficult to accumulate this training within the private sector, unless the agency itself acts aggressively to train and retain experienced employees.

- This commitment is further magnified in programs that are closely tied to their communities: For example, a public school employee probably sends his or her own children to the local public school, pays a significant amount of taxes to support these schools, votes on school-district initiatives and for school board members, and lives in a community with friends and family who have done the same, perhaps for generations. Thus, public-sector programs may also be helpful in making people with disabilities integral to their communities.

Despite these many opportunities, I have also found that the distinct character of the public sector can also have a negative side. Although public agencies have a mandate to serve all those in need, the fact that the amount of funding received is not necessarily tied to the number of people served places pressure to reallocate resources creatively when there are spikes in need. In the case of early intervention and public education, additional pressures can arise because mandated services must also be provided with specific time frames. The long histories of many public agencies can also create an institutional inertia in which any change is met with skepticism. Without strong leadership and accountability, this history creates layers of policies and procedures (the original purposes of which are long since forgotten) that can create more barriers both to families trying to gain access to services and to advocates and leaders trying to change services. Change can also require coordination among the local, state, and federal agencies responsible for funding and oversight, a task made extraordinarily difficult when each layer views the other's role and contribution with suspicion. I believe that these factors have together slowed the response of public agencies to the explosion of need experienced since the 1990s.

Programs in the Private Sector   I believe that programs developed in the private sector can and should play a critical role in all aspects of services, training, research, and policy, when the right opportunities present themselves.

- The private sector does not have to rely on politics and taxes to raise money for new programs, and so, once a funding source has been identified, programs can grow as quickly as personnel can be hired. This is one reason for the explosion in private services since the 1990s, especially where the public sector could not respond swiftly to the need.

- I believe that private-sector programs probably have more discretion in the use and distribution of resources. This is tremendously helpful in the start-up of new programs, which can require a significant upfront investment in personnel, training, facilities, and other elements. Programs can also be more creative on the roles and responsibilities of key personnel, with no need to reference the often archaic lexicon of job descriptions in public-sector programs.

- Competition in the private sector can drive innovation and customer service, and when combined with a corporate culture that emphasizes integrity and careful planning that anticipates medium- to long-term needs, can create organizations that respond swiftly to emerging needs. Under these conditions, competition is an antidote to the institutional inertia that plagues the public sector.

Despite these strengths, I also think it is unrealistic to expect that the programs in the private sector will easily meet all of the challenges faced by people living with ASD. The lack of a few, stable funding streams means that private services have to devote more resources to securing support: They may find it difficult to confidently develop a more comprehensive, multiyear strategy, and may instead develop services for a specific niche. For families living with ASD who must cobble together different services from different agencies or transition frequently from one agency to another, continuity and coordination of care may become impossible. For private-sector programs themselves, increases in the number of different payers (e.g., insurance companies, school districts, other state or county agencies) with different fee structures and standards of care only complicates long-term planning. Reimbursement levels may be tied tightly to a per-head and per-service rate, and so programs may lack discretionary funding unless they plan carefully for this. For payers, assuring consistent, quality care becomes more challenging as the number of private-sector programs increases. Private-sector programs that chose to shave costs by reducing the pay or benefits of employees, or by increasing their caseload, will find it difficult to retain experienced professionals or justify long-term training strategies.

Other Considerations   Although I have attempted to broadly characterize some strengths and weakness inherent to public- and private-sector programs, I must offer some caveats. First, other general characteristics of the program will probably play a greater role in determining efficiency and effectiveness, such as reliance on data-based decision making informed by research and on processes that assure input from people living with ASD and other key stakeholders. Second, the quality of the program is ultimately limited by the availability and quality of its professionals and leaders. I am excited that the shift away from an economy based in manufacturing to one based in services could help to bring a new generation of professionals into the workforce. This new generation of professionals and paraprofessionals is ready to commit to a career of working in the front line with people with ASD, if the field can create positions that are fulfilling and rewarding and provide the necessary training. Third, I recognize that the future will probably bring an increasing number of programs that are neither public nor private, but hybrids that bring the best of both together. Finally, I believe that even greater progress can be achieved if all involved look beyond individual programs and look at the broader network of services, training, research, and policy to identify the most prominent gaps and promising opportunities. I discuss some of these ideas in greater detail in the final chapter of the book.

LEVELS OF PROGRAMS

In the United States, as in many developed countries, each element (e.g., services, training, research, policy) can often be found at three or four different levels: 1) a local level (e.g., site, town, school district), 2) a regional level (e.g., county, multicounty region, metropolitan, other area), 3) a state/provincial/department level, and 4) a federal/national level. The level here describes where programs are organized *and* delivered, although some programs might be provided at one level and organized at the next higher level. Even with some larger private-sector agencies and professional organizations, it is useful to distinguish between the functions and structure of different levels (e.g., headquarters versus specific sites of a company or chapters of an advocacy organization).

I believe that it is important to describe some characteristics of each level, and then provide examples of agencies. First, many readers might not grasp the tremendous range of agencies and organizations that potentially play a role in improving the lives of people with ASD. Second, where there are natural relationships across levels (e.g., when a site is part of or funded by a larger agency or organization), professionals might be able to more quickly establish common standards or strategies. Third, this may reveal levels at which different elements (i.e., services, training, research, and policy) naturally fit. For example, anyone seeking to improve services must understand the infrastructure and funding of these local, community-based agencies and organizations if these improvements are to be sustained.

Local Programs

Many different elements of services are delivered locally in the community where the person with ASD lives. Those not specially adapted to people with ASD may be delivered, funded, and organized locally; for example, primary care in a community-based medical practice, or typical child care in an after-school program, summer camp day care setting. Special educational services in a small- or medium-size school district would also be delivered, organized, and at least partially funded locally. Specialized, individualized care may be provided locally, although is often organized and funded at a regional level. Examples of such care include consultation provided in the home and/or school through early intervention, education, or consultation, as well as on-site job coaching or specialized respite. I argue that the majority of services needed daily or weekly by people with ASD should be provided locally.

In contrast to the large proportion of services provided locally, little or no specialized training, research, or policy (including decisions about the funding and infrastructure of services) occur primarily at the local level. This introduces a potential disconnect between services provided for people living with ASD and other activities intended to guide or support these services. One significant exception would be public education provided locally, which would include almost all educational programming except for placement in a private or certain specialized public school programs. Though many training programs and policy decisions are made at the state and federal level, school districts in the United States enjoy a remarkable degree of independence in the allocation of resources and the way certain programs are implemented. In some school districts, principals and special education administrators are also given significant latitude in the use of resources. I have seen significant program changes begin when parents and teachers recognize and then seek to address an unmet need with the support of school leaders. This kind of homegrown program development can sometimes generate more excitement and inspire greater ownership of change than recommendations from experts from the state level, recommendations that are often treated skeptically no matter how stellar their credentials or how compelling their presentations. Another significant exception might be a specific grant-funded program for training or research when the reach does not extend beyond the locality. Also note that some of the same strategies that regional agencies may use to influence training, research, and policy may also apply to local agencies. I discuss these next.

Case Studies   The case studies described here benefited most significantly from direct services.

- *Services:* All primary medical care, screening, paraprofessional support, and early intervention were provided locally. Most education and child care were also provided locally. Some diagnosis (Asif's pediatrician) and advocacy (i.e., Asif's community group) were also provided locally. Other local services were provided with consultative support from a regional program or specialist (e.g., Asif's seizure medication, Evan's diagnosis and medication treatment, Joshua's program to decrease anxiety associated with flying).

- *Training:* Asif's parents benefited from the training and support provided by a local community group (which also received some pilot funding through a local foundation).

- *Policy:* Evan's teacher was also motivated to complete a specialized certification when her school district changed its policies to recognize the certificate when awarding pay increases.

Regional Programs

Types of Regional Programs

- *County:* State agencies often allocate resources at the county level: This allows for greater local control over resources (e.g., in facilitating contracts with local agencies for the provision of services) and helps to accommodate variations from one region of the state to another. The size of counties can vary greatly, from small rural counties to metropolitan areas larger than some states (e.g., Los Angeles County).

- *Designated regional offices or sites:* In many states, state services and training are organized by regions that may encompass multiple counties—for example, an agency for developmental disabilities in a state with 60 counties may organize these into five regions for purposes of training. Large states (e.g., California, Texas, New York) will often have an intermediate, multicounty level for the organization of services and/or training because providing such support at the state level is simply unmanageable. State colleges often have multiple campuses at which different training programs might be offered. Similar arrangements are found with advocacy or professional organizations seeking to provide training or support below the state level.

- *Ad-hoc regional collaborations:* Sometimes, regional arrangements are made for specific initiatives: Several counties may collaborate to support a service or training program that is simply too specialized to be provided at the county level, or several school districts may collaborate to operate a separate school for students with disabilities.

- *Stand-alone agencies and programs:* Many different kinds of specialized service settings (e.g., hospitals, behavioral health facilities, vocational or residential programs) and university-based programs for research and training functionally serve a broad region. Unlike other arrangements described earlier, these agencies were not intentionally distributed so as to ensure consistent coverage across a state. This results in some areas (usually urban) receiving specialized services while other areas receive nothing, unless the person with ASD or the professional is willing and able to travel for services. There are also private foundations in many regions that provide funding for many different kinds of projects. Large private health insurance companies often operate via regional or state programs, some of which are part of a national organization or association (e.g., Blue Cross Blue Shield).

Elements Emphasized in Regional Programs

Many community-based professionals and organizations at the regional level are primarily focused on the delivery of services and supports (see the various case studies). In most cases, this service-delivery model simply reflects the nature or limitations of the service provided or population addressed: 1) it may be unrealistic to make more specialized support available in every community (e.g., residential programs, more specialized school programs), 2) it may not require day-to-day contact with a patient (e.g., advocacy, case management, specialized evaluation), or 3) it may be more flexible because the provider travels to the site (e.g., consultation in the home, school, or workplace; in-home respite). I return in Chapter 14 to discuss the factors that drive the regional development of services and training.

When the regional entity is part of a larger organization, it is more likely to disseminate than independently create programs of training, research, and policy, unless it is part of a specially funded project. In a similar fashion, funding might be disseminated by regional offices but cannot usually be significantly reallocated solely by them (e.g., to create entirely new programs). As in the case of local agencies, this creates a significant gap between those who deliver services and those who develop training, research, and policy intended to support these services. At the same time, regional programs are better positioned than many larger entities to straddle this gap, especially when seeking to change services. As compared to decision makers at the state level, those at the regional level are more likely to know those who are providing or utilizing services and perhaps who are increasing the commitment to change. I describe some other specific strategies next, and elaborate on these at the end of the book.

- Local and regional programs should take full advantage of any opportunities to provide input into training programs (e.g., when a state program is seeking a site to pilot a new initiative) and participate in research (e.g., when a research project is looking for participants or sites) and/or policy initiatives (e.g., when a state agency is seeking workgroup or committee members). Local and regional programs should also step forward to propose new programs, especially those that are funding-neutral or that target gaps already identified by the state agency. These recommendations also apply to a privately run organization, for individual sites seeking opportunities to develop new programs.

- A local or regional site can consider applying for pilot funding from a foundation, advocacy organization, or other entity. The application may be framed as a pilot project, demonstrating proof of concept, and framed as the first phase in a two-part strategy to implement more significant change. In this way, the stated goals for the project may be more realistic, especially when this pilot phase is described relative to a larger project unfolding over a longer period of time. For projects that will ultimately require active collaboration with multiple partners or a more substantial commitment from the state agency, the pilot phase can also serve to demonstrate the existence of such collaborations.

Case Studies   The cases presented here benefited most significantly from regional programs delivering more specialized services and managing locally delivered services. Some training was also disseminated locally.

- *Services:* Some assessment and treatment services were delivered locally but organized regionally (e.g., Asif's and Evan's early intervention [EI] services, Evan's behavioral health and rehabilitation services support). Other specialized services were delivered via regional centers such as case management (Evan), emergency care (e.g., Evan and Sofia), specialized medical care (e.g., Asif's neurological and gastroenterological evaluations, Joshua's and Chloe's psychiatrists, and consultation and a second opinion with a developmental pediatrician regarding Evan's diagnosis and treatment), higher education (Chloe), vocational programs (Liam), some special education programs (Sofia), and other programs (e.g., Joshua's summer camp, Chloe's college supports).

- *Training:* Much training was delivered regionally, including certificate and degree programs based at regional colleges and technical schools (e.g., for Evan's teacher, Joshua's speech language pathologist [SLP] and camp counselors); regional workshops offered privately (e.g., Picture Exchange Communication System [PECS] training for Asif's SLP); in-house ASD training (e.g., for Evan's case manager); and the introductory workshop in ASD for Joshua's teacher at a research clinic. Asif's parents received advocacy training via a program funded in part by a regional foundation.

- *Policy:* An ambitious regional workgroup was created to explore a new mixed-use development project including housing for people with disabilities such as Chloe.

STATE PROGRAMS

Types of State Programs

State Government   The executive and legislative branches serve many important functions, most notably proposing and approving new policies, laws, and funding related to services, training, and, in some cases, research. State agencies help to implement programs devised by the executive and legislative branches by allocating funding and resources agencies, collecting information contributing to policy decisions, developing the regulations for state laws, and interpreting and implementing regulations pertaining to federal laws. In some cases (e.g., Medicaid), states must commit to "match" a proportion of federal funding before any federal funds are released. State agencies often disseminate funding and programs across the state via county and/or regional offices (see earlier discussions), and are themselves often divided into different bureaus and offices. As with the executive branch, actions of state agencies are related to services, training, and, in some cases, research. In addition, there are some committees and workgroups that may cut across agencies (e.g., co-ordinating committees for people with disabilities). Some states create positions or bureaus specifically to focus on people with disabilities.

Other Programs

- *State chapters of advocacy and professional organizations:* These implement policies and programs developed by the national office (occasionally state-specific), usually focused on aspects related to training and policy. Many of those focused on professional affairs may also play significant roles in setting licensure requirements and other functions.

- *State colleges and universities:* These take leadership in higher-level education, research, and, to a lesser extent, policy development. In most medium to large states, they include several campuses.

- *Other programs:* Some states still operate state-level facilities (e.g., state schools for the deaf or blind, state psychiatric centers), although these are much smaller and likely to focus on training and support to community-based services centers, as opposed to providing direct services themselves. Although not designated to serve a specific state or region, other large or specialized private institutions (e.g., a children's hospital, a psychiatric hospital, a large vocational training program) or programs within an institution (a specialized inpatient treatment program in a psychiatric or a children's hospital) may essentially function as does a state center in a smaller state.

Elements Emphasized in State Programs   Virtually no services are directly provided at the state level, although agencies at the state level often play a critical role in defining the mandate, determining funding, and providing oversight. State-level agencies and programs also take a much more significant role in implementing if not developing training and policy programs. Even when training is devised or policy is set at the federal level, state-level agencies and programs play a critical role because the state is inevitably the intermediary in the delivery of these programs and because there is often considerable flexibility in how these policies and programs are implemented. This can include the distribution of federal funds and other resources allocated to states for services, training, and research. Although the federal government still provides much more research funding than the state government, there are examples of state governments who creatively target research funding by raising money themselves or reallocating federal funds: 1) beginning in 2003, autism research in New Jersey was funded through a $1.00 surcharge on all traffic tickets, and 2) in 2009, Pennsylvania designated almost $8 million from funds generated by the national tobacco settlement and distributed to each state.

Case Studies   The cases presented here benefited most significantly from state policy, funding, and oversight of services and training provided or disseminated by state or state-level programs.

- *Services:* Only highly specialized services might be available at the state or multistate level (e.g., Sofia's specialized inpatient treatment and Chloe's college program). Evan's parents were reimbursed directly with state funds for his respite services, which they found through listings provided by a state advocacy group. Expansions in Evan's services were made possible by insurance legislation for ASD.

- *Training:* Asif's pediatrician and Evan's practicing nurse practitioner (PNP) received training in identification of ASD through a state chapter of a professional organization and a state agency, respectively. Evan's case manager benefited from annual training conferences in ASD organized by the state departments of education and public welfare and the organization of teacher certification in ASD at the state college. Liam's teacher benefited from vocational training offered by the state department of education, the consultant-trainer for his sex education curriculum was a statewide expert, and the center of excellence in developmental disability at the state university provided training to public defenders.

- *Research*: Some research may also be funded by state agencies. For example, research funded by a state agency identified disparities in access to services and led to the program through which Evan's nurse received training in identification of ASD.

- *Policy*: Many significant funding and policy decisions are set at the state level. This includes the autism insurance legislation that benefited Evan (but not Sofia) and policies to support teacher training. States' policies and funding might also function to decrease service options (e.g., policy changes and/or decreased funding limited the options for Sofia's residential placement and Evan's respite and access to rehabilitation). States also monitored the ability of local and regional providers to adhere to state and federal regulations (e.g., with respect to Evan's EI services and his suspension from school).

National Programs

Federal Government   The executive and legislative branches serve many important functions, most notably proposing and approving new national policies, laws, and funding related to services, training, and research. Federal agencies and departments (e.g., health, education) help to implement programs devised by the executive and legislative branches by allocating funding and resources provided to the agency, collecting information contributing to policy decisions, developing the regulations for laws, monitoring the implementation of these regulations by states, and disseminating funding and programs across the state via county and/or regional offices. These agencies are themselves often divided into different entities (e.g., bureaus, offices, centers). In addition, there are some committees and workgroups that may cut across agencies (e.g., the Interagency Autism Coordinating Committee). Although most federal funding is disseminated via state agencies, families benefit from some direct payments (e.g., Supplementary Security Income), supplements (e.g., copays for medications), and tax breaks.

Other Programs

- *Headquarters of national professional and advocacy organizations*: These develop policies and programs usually focused on aspects related to advocacy, training, and policy. They sometimes disseminate information about these directly to interested parties, and other times disseminate these through state chapters. Many of those focused on professional affairs (e.g., American Academy of Pediatrics, American Psychological Association, American Speech-Language-Hearing Association) may also play significant roles in setting licensure requirements, accrediting training institutions, and so forth.

- *Headquarters of national foundations*: Foundations focus on providing significant funding for research and other projects. Other organizations may provide information and advocacy *and* fund research (e.g., Autism Speaks, Organization for Autism Research).

- *Headquarters of other agencies and organizations*: Large private health insurance companies often operate via regional or state programs, some of which are part of a national organization or association (e.g., Blue Cross Blue Shield). Other large for-profit and not-for-profit providers may have programs across many states (e.g., Easter Seals, Universal Health Services). Other national organizations play significant roles in specific autism initiatives: They may promote specific programs within the broad area of other services, as in the role of the Association of University Centers on Disability in the Act Early Summits (see Chapter 12), or they may take the lead in a specific national initiative, such as the National Autism Center's National Standards Project.

Elements Emphasized in National Programs   No services are directly provided at the national level. National programs may broadly determine the mandate and define standards through regulations where there is applicable federal law (e.g., Individuals with Disabilities Education Act [IDEA]) and provide a proportion of funding for services. National agencies and programs take the lead in developing policy and provide guidance and some funding for training programs implemented at the state level. National programs are unlikely to train providers directly, although they implement programs to train the trainers. Nonetheless, many state-level agencies and programs often have considerable discretion in the allocation and form of services and training whenever laws and regulations are not overly prescriptive. National agencies and organizations provide the bulk of research funding, as well as the infrastructure for the dissemination of research findings.

Case Studies   All of the cases benefited from public programs that benefited most significantly from national policy, funding, and research.

- *Services*: Although no services are delivered nationally, programs through federal agencies can still impact services quite directly; for example, Evan's pediatrician benefited from a federal program that offered reduced interest rates on student loans for rural professionals, while Joshua's parents were reimbursed with Medicaid funds for the costs of his summer camp. Federal and other national agencies may also provide pilot funding for a new service model before seeking to disseminate this model through a network, as was the case for the specialized inpatient program serving Sofia.

- *Training*: Federal funding contributed to training in identification of ASD for Asif's pediatrician and Evan's PNP. Programs providing information and advocacy were funded by federal programs (Asif and Evan) and national advocacy organizations (Asif's advocate/translator). Federal funding sparked the creation of introductory workshops that benefited Joshua's teacher and parents.

- *Research*: Almost all of the research was funded by federal programs and national foundations. This included the sleep protocol used for Evan, which drew from both federal and private foundation funding.

- *Policy*: Federal policy generally guided most services and set specific expectations regarding certain services (e.g., the rapidity with which Evan's EI was initiated and the need for a meeting following his suspension from school). The need to develop a pilot inpatient treatment program was developed at the national office of a large private health care provider.

EXAMPLES OF AGENCIES

I summarize here examples of agencies and programs. These do not capture the range of infrastructure possible, but do illustrate some of the possibilities and complexities.

A Public School Autism Spectrum Disorder Program

Specialized public school programs often begin as physically and operationally distinct entities; they consist of separate schools or classrooms, with little interaction and integration with regular education. Specialized public school programs are increasingly defined in terms of specialized personnel (including training) and approaches (e.g., specialized curricula and teaching methods). As a result, the boundaries of public school programs for ASD have become more permeable, now also including specialized instruction, training, or other support provided across a range of settings to better address the broad range of student needs: in regular education setting for those without significant intellectual disabilities; in community-based instruction for those with significant intellectual disabilities; in the home, to encourage generalization and promote breakthrough skills; and on the job to support the post-21 transition.

Elements

- *Services*: Programs for ASD primarily provide local services to students within that school district. Some districts may operate a special program that may accept students from another district, in which case they recoup costs by charging a special tuition to the school district of residence. Schools may also send students with particularly intense or complex needs to a specialized private school, or a residential program in- or out-of-state, but may delay or avoid doing so because of often-exorbitant costs. Sometimes states can help defray these costs by supplementing it from other funds.

- *Training*: Programs for ASD focus on training their own staff. They may supplement traditional teacher training in several ways: 1) with an in-house program of training and mentoring specific to ASDs, 2) by sending teachers and other staff to trainers provided by private or by other public agencies, and/or 3) by encouraging or supporting additional certifications. All of these are in addition to an often-intense schedule of mandated training for all educators. Programs for ASD may also provide practicum placements to future teachers.

- *Research*: Programs for ASD may partner with a university-based researcher around a specific project, may participate in other projects, or disseminate information to prospective participants, but rarely initiate projects themselves.

- *Policy*: The school district within which the program rests has some flexibility in implementing policies and standards developed at the state and federal level.

Infrastructure

- *Sector*: Schools operate primarily (90%) in the public sector, with the potential of some (10%) private services, contracting out for speech, occupational, and/or behavioral therapies, paying for private or residential school placement, and so forth.

- *Level*: In most school districts, a program for ASD would operate at the local level. A school district for a metropolitan area, or one that accepts students from outside of the school district, may operate at the regional level.

- *Funding*: Most (60%) funding may come from local taxes, some from state (30%), and relatively little (10%) from federal sources. Thus, significant program changes usually require the support of both local and state funding sources. Some costs are eligible for reimbursement from noneducation (e.g., medical) sources, when these are necessary for educational progress. This includes some therapies (e.g., speech, occupational), summer camps, and a portion of the costs for residential placement.

- *Mandate*: As an entitlement, education must be provided in a timely manner to all those eligible. This includes special education services to all those with ASD who need individualized objectives or educational accommodations to gain access to the regular education curriculum. Services cannot be delayed for even the most complex students, or families can petition for special services and/or compensation through due process.

- *Oversight*: Immediate oversight is provided by leaders (e.g., principals, special education directors) within the school district (sometimes referred to as the local education agency). The state department of education (state education agency) evaluates compliance with state and federal standards. Intense scrutiny by parents and their willingness to initiate formal proceedings via due process can be construed as a type of oversight.

- *Domain*: Although schools focus on education, they may collaborate with health and community providers and may be compelled to do so when reasonable progress cannot be assured.

A State Intellectual Disabilities Agency   As described earlier, states wield significant influence in setting policies and distributing resources. Once a bill is passed and overall funding levels are approved by the legislature, individual state departments are authorized to implement the relevant programs related to services, training, research, and policy. Different elements of these programs are further allocated across a complex bureaucratic hierarchy in which specific bureaus are nested within an office, which is itself nested within a department (see Figure 4.1, which describes the structure for the Commonwealth of Pennsylvania). Significant coordination of programs across bureaus, offices, or departments is very complicated and requires the support of the person overseeing the two entities. In Pennsylvania, for example, the Secretary of the Department of Public Welfare (DPW) would likely need to support any coordinated program across the Office of Developmental Programs and the Office of Medical Assistance Programs that involves any significant shift in the mandate, resources, or oversight. I have found that coordination across departments, offices, and bureaus will not happen naturally, but requires a specific initiative undertaken by committed individuals within each entity. Eligibility for services, or the types of service provided, is usually the critical component demarcating the boundaries of an agency: For example, all states have an entity responsible for services for people with disabilities (see example described later in the chapter), but people with ASD but not ID may be ineligible unless specific provisions for people with Asperger syndrome have been identified.

Only by appreciating the complexity of this government hierarchy can one begin to grasp the challenge of developing a comprehensive and coordinated approach to ASD, when the needs of people living with ASD are deconstructed and then distributed across multiple departments, offices, and bureaus. Consider the development of a coordinated strategy for addressing problem behaviors of people with ASD. In Pennsylvania, the Department of Education (DOE) and DPW each have offices and bureaus that have independently developed programs for training and services in schools and the community, respectively. Autism insurance legislation can significantly shift the availability of resources, but this is administered by the Department of Insurance. Within DPW, problem behaviors may be addressed within the Office of Developmental Programs (ODP), although in-home wraparound support is overseen by the Office of Mental Health and Substance Abuse Service (OMHSAS). Wraparound is a rehabilitative service, however, and so cannot address problems of habilitation: These are attributed to a fundamental skill deficit (e.g., the lack of toilet training), and are viewed as the sole responsibility of the educational system. Physical and behavioral health services that are Medicaid-funded are themselves administered by a different office. Licensing of hospital and residential providers of services for problem behaviors is a separate function.

The funding and management of paraprofessional staff working one to one in the classroom with a child with behavior problems illustrates these complexities. Such staff may be funded either through school districts or through behavioral health services (at least partially funded and/or managed by DPW). I have encountered countless classrooms in which paraprofessional staff funded through behavioral health services (sometimes from multiple agencies) work side by side with educators and school-based personnel, but do not report either to the teacher or the principal. When individuals and agencies lack the goodwill to collaborate under these circumstance, programming can quickly deteriorate.

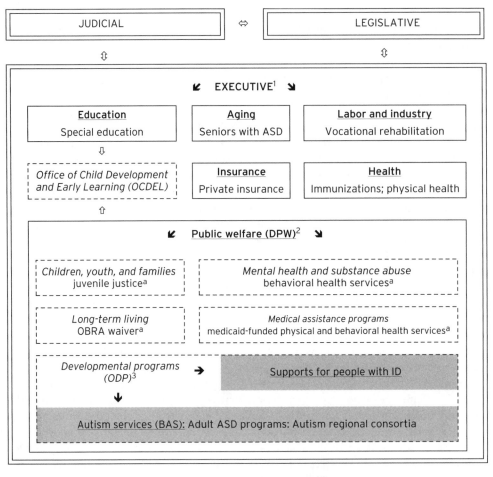

Figure 4.1. Structure of Pennsylvania state government. (*Key:* ASD, autism spectrum disorder; BAS, Bureau of Autism Services; DPW, Department of Public Welfare; ID, intellectual disability; ODP, Office of Developmental Programs.)

[a]ASD Programs coordinated with BAS.
[1]Other Departments in the Executive Branch: General Services; State; Revenue; Transportation; Corrections.
[2]Other Offices in DPW: Administration; Income Maintenance.
[3]Other Bureaus in ODP: Policy and Program Support; Financial Management and Budget.

There are ways to promote coordination across bureaus, offices, and departments. Many states have designated a type of specialist position for ASD within a department or office. Although this person can serve many important functions within the department or office (e.g., speaking for ASD in multiple committees, building bridges across multiple initiatives, funneling information to policy makers), he or she often functions in an advisory capacity and lacks direct authority over key policy or significant resources. In some cases, an office might be explicitly shared between two departments; for example, the transition from early intervention to education services is more seamless because DOE and DPW jointly run Office of Child Development and Early Learning, which coordinates related programs in both departments. Coordinating committees either focused on ASD specifically or on disabilities generally can also bring perspectives not only from multiple departments but also directly from advocates. These committees can have a greater impact when they include (or at least report directly to) the secretary of a department if not to the governor.

Pennsylvania took the unusual step of creating a Bureau of Autism Services (BAS) with the ODP in the DPW (see Figure 4.1). On the one hand, the creation of a separate bureau with its own personnel and budget has led to the initiation of many innovative programs (see Chapter 5) that have undoubtedly improved the lives of people living with ASD in the Commonwealth. On the other hand, the placement of BAS within ODP and DPW has perhaps limited its influence elsewhere: Housing BAS within ODP limits BAS to an advisory role with respect to DPW programs outside of ODP (e.g., wraparound, licensure), and housing BAS with DPW has led to a more prominent focus on people under age 3 or older than 21 so as to avoid overlap with education-based services and in response to the dearth of services for adults.

For bureaucrats, these distinctions make perfect sense and appear reasonable in the light of the government's many responsibilities. For those advocating for change, these distinctions between each of these entities appear bewildering, if not a deliberate obfuscation of accountability. For people living with ASD, these distinctions can lead to critical failures of care, unless either a knowledgeable caregiver or professional acts in a case-management capacity. At the end of this chapter, I try to illustrate how this worked in the case of Evan.

Elements   Note that the type of state ID agency referenced here is usually nested in a state department distinct from the department of education.

- *Services*: State ID agencies primarily fund services provided locally, either by other public agencies (often at the county or regional level) or increasingly by contracted private services. An exception might be information or advocacy services, which the ID agency might provide directly.

- *Training*: State ID agencies may offer training to service providers either through their own personnel or through consultants. State ID agencies can also influence the licensure set for different categories of recognized professionals.

- *Research*: State ID agencies may participate in research (e.g., by providing data regarding service utilization to other researchers) or partner with other researchers to conduct in-house applied research (e.g., into parent satisfaction). This process may be easier for states with a registry for ASD housed within the ID agency.

- *Policy*: Together with the executive and legislative branches, the state ID agency is often a principal driver of all aspects of policy, helping to advocate for new legislation, leading the development of regulations, and defining mechanisms of oversight. Examples of policy include determining eligibility for services, defining the types of services provided, seeking new programs eligible for matching funds from Medicaid.

Infrastructure

- *Sector*: State ID agencies are increasingly likely to contract out direct services to private agencies. Some training and program evaluation/research activities are also likely to be contracted out.

- *Funding*: The majority (perhaps 60%) of funding is likely to come from state taxes and the rest from federal sources (sometimes in the form of a Medicaid match). Thus, significant program changes usually require the support of both state and federal funding sources.

- *Mandate*: People with ASD are not entitled to receive ID services, although the agency is ultimately accountable to the government (and ultimately the voters) for fairly distributing public resources to those eligible. In some states, people with ASD but not ID may also be eligible for some supports through ID agencies.

- *Oversight*: The state ID agency provides oversight for the services it funds, including the licensing of eligible programs and facilities.

- *Domain*: State ID agencies focus on community-based supports (family support, residential, behavioral) and perhaps Medicaid-funded health services.

An Autism Spectrum Disorder Clinic in a Not-for-Profit Hospital   A clinic for ASD in a not-for-profit hospital illustrates one of the greatest challenges of providing private medical services: the reimbursement structure of managed care. Although the decision to offer a service may ultimately hinge largely on the ability to be appropriately reimbursed for it, the level of reimbursement is not always commensurate with the effort and resources to provide the service. Even for such essential services as identification, for which clear guidelines have been developed by multiple agencies, the mechanisms for reimbursement appear unclear. In the case of screening for ASD, for example, practitioners have continued to report that they are unsure how to appropriately bill for such activities. In the case of more comprehensive diagnostic evaluation, clinics have reported difficulties obtaining reimbursement for more comprehensive developmental evaluations, especially those including tools such as the Autism Diagnostic Observation Schedule (ADOS; Lord, Rutter, DiLavore, & Risi, 1999) or critical components such as psychological assessment. Regardless of the point at which the breakdown occurs, the result is unnecessary delays in critical services for ASD, such as identification. For a clinic in a not-for-profit hospital, this picture may be further complicated by the expectation that some services are provided at a loss to certain patients or under certain conditions.

A hospital-based clinic that does not resolve these problems is unlikely to survive, let alone thrive. Diagnostic evaluation is often central to a clinic's practice (perhaps as the primary way to recruit new patients) and so clinics may be compelled to become very creative: relying on a more cursory diagnostic evaluation, stretching the diagnostic process out over multiple visits to allow other kinds of billing, embedding diagnostic activities into a broader evaluation package that includes activities reimbursed at a rate that compensates for the "loss" incurred by diagnosis, or simply accepting that diagnostic evaluation will be conducted at a loss, but with the hope that other assessments and interventions in the clinic itself, or provided elsewhere in the hospital, as a whole will compensate for this loss. A hospital-based clinic for ASD itself is unlikely to meet all of the needs of people with ASD but can partner with other departments to deliver key services for co-occurring conditions: for example, neurology, genetics, speech pathology, psychology, gastroenterology, and so forth. A hospital-based developmental pediatrician can provide consultation for community-based providers throughout a region and can manage the majority of day-to-day concerns but seek more expert guidance for specific problems.

A creative and committed clinic for ASD successfully juggles these challenges to provide the right services needed by families. An clinic for ASD strategically positioned in a hospital and with active partnership with other departments can provide unparalleled care. For example, a hospital-based developmental pediatrician who understands and collaborates actively with community-based providers can provide careful monitoring, and shepherd people living with ASD through the most significant of crises. Otherwise, the mismatch between clinical activities and reimbursement rates or the failure to coordinate care across related specialists can lead to a tremendous waste of resources with relatively little benefit to people living with ASD. These conditions can emerge surprisingly quickly unless the hospital proactively adopts a strategy for coordinating care across departments for people with ASD. Once a hospital-based clinic strategically identifies a package of services that is relevant to the needs of people with ASD *and* is financially sustainable, other opportunities can arise: the creation of a critical mass of clinicians to support training or research activities; the development of new kinds of services; the ability to provide consultation to community groups or to other colleagues, and so forth. To the extent that these activities do not involve direct (and billable) clinical care, or are not subsidized via a grant, they are unlikely to be directly reimbursed by insurers.

The distinctions between for-profit and not-for-profit or public institutions are relevant here. Analyses by Horwitz (2005) suggest that reimbursement rates are beginning to subtly shift the general package of services offered by different types of hospitals. Whereas a government-run or not-for-profit hospital may provide a broad range of services regardless of their profitability, for-profit hospitals are more likely to offer more profitable services (e.g., open-heart surgery) and less likely to offer less profitable services (e.g., psychiatric emergency services). This same relationship was more pronounced over time within a service as reimbursement rates changed. For example, the likelihood that a for-profit hospital would offer home health care more than tripled over an 8-year period during which reimbursement rates increased, and then shrunk by more than 60% during a 3-year period after reimbursement rates decreased. Government-run and not-for-profit hospitals showed parallel but much less pronounced trends over this same period. Interestingly, these same trends were not evident for all types of services examined, which suggests that profitability probably interacts with other important factors to determine service availability. Nonetheless, these analyses reveal the potential for for-profit hospitals to respond quickly to emerging needs when services are potentially profitable, and how the range of services may vary depending upon hospital type.

Elements

- *Services*: A clinic can provide key diagnostic services, ongoing monitoring, and specialized treatment. It can also serve as a hub for more specialized evaluations by other departments, coordinating referrals and integrating findings.

- *Training and research*: A clinic must either be large and well established or affiliated with a university-based department or researchers before it is likely to engage significantly in training and research. Significant engagement can include providing placements, contributing actively to other structured training programs (see Leadership Education in Neurological and related Disabilities [LEND], described later in this chapter), partnering with other researchers to initiate projects, collaborating in a multisite study, and so forth.

- *Policy*: A clinic may participate in, or take leadership of, the development of a hospital-wide strategy for ASD. Individual clinicians may be enlisted as experts in the development of statewide policy.

Infrastructure

- *Sector*: A clinic resides predominantly in the private sector, although services might be reimbursed with public funds.

- *Level*: A specialized clinic for ASD often operates at the regional level (and sometimes the state level), and may serve patients from 100 to 200 miles away.

- *Funding*: The majority of funding comes from fees charged to Medicaid and insurance, with some private pay. The hospital itself may reallocate funds from other services to subsidize key clinic activities for ASD, or vice versa. Small grants from the institution itself, private foundations, or government sources may help fund specific training or research programs.

- *Mandate*: A hospital is obligated to provide emergency services to all people who enter the hospital, regardless of their ability to pay. In addition, a clinic in a not-for-profit hospital is typically expected to provide core services to families receiving Medicaid-funded services, even if reimbursement rates are such that these services are potentially provided at a loss.

- *Oversight*: Overall functioning of the clinic is subjected to oversight by the hospital, while individual clinical activities may be reviewed by insurance companies and other payers. The hospital is subjected to rigorous review by state licensing and national accreditation bodies.

- *Domain*: A clinic may provide a range of more specialized health services (identification of ASD, other specialized assessment), ongoing follow-up (including medication management), and may coordinate with other departments to provide other health-related assessments and treatments for co-occurring conditions (e.g., genetic, neurology, speech pathology, psychology, gastroenterology, occupational therapy).

A University-Based Center for Autism Spectrum Disorder   University-based centers for ASD can take many forms. Some "centers" may consist of little more than one or two faculty working on isolated projects whose activities are rebranded to create interest in ASD. Other centers may be physically and operationally distinct entities within the university, with a number of core faculty, dozens of trainees and supporting staff, millions of dollars of grants and institutional support, and active partnerships with clinics and schools. Some centers operate largely within a very restricted range of domains (e.g., predominantly medicine, psychology) and/or elements (e.g., focusing largely on one type of basic research). Other centers may be more multidisciplinary, include more research and policy initiatives, and training or research collaborations with affiliated hospitals or schools. The boundaries of the latter kind of centers are often fuzzy, reflecting that some faculty positions reside almost exclusively within the center, while other faculty may reside primarily with other departments but collaborate actively with the center on specific projects. This can be an effective way to leverage expertise elsewhere within the university.

Of all of the agencies described in this volume, university-based centers offer the greatest potential to develop and then demonstrate effective models of training and service delivery. These centers often fail to exploit this potential, however, because of the difficulty supporting the kinds of research needed and finding researchers to conduct it. Developing a program of research in the highly competitive academic environment requires the careful selection of an area of focus that yields publications in peer-reviewed journals and generates projects of potential interest to funding bodies. This pressure causes academics to err toward more narrowly focused research designs that favor simple hypotheses tested in highly controlled environments; hence the bias toward basic research. For the small proportion who elect to conduct applied research, this same pressure often causes them to favor designs that focus on a narrow sphere of intervention with a subset of the population, in a controlled clinical setting, and focusing on specific, short-term outcomes. Although these can contribute to the body of research used to determine if a practice is evidence-based, they may have little relevance to the challenges of providing services and related training in real-world settings.

The same pressure that fosters research rarely relevant to the challenge of scaling up services also forces researchers into career paths that can deprive them of the most relevant experience. Those seeking academic appointments must themselves begin to develop a program of research even prior to completing their doctoral training, and this pressure can push them away from the kinds of real-world experience that can inform this program of research. This pressure may cause them to narrow the range of potential collaborators, decreasing cross-agency and disciplinary collaboration, and reinforcing the silos that exist between different agencies and disciplines. At the same time, it is extremely difficult for those engaged primarily in training or service delivery in community-based settings to carve out the time needed to prepare a grant proposal or publish a paper, let alone develop a program of research. Together, this creates a cycle whereby the researchers recommending grants for funding or articles for publication have less and less knowledge of the day-to-day needs of people with ASD, and how this might be realistically improved through services, training, and policy.

Some centers have begun to break free of this cycle. They may not be a separate center for ASD, but an area of specialization in a broader University Center for Excellence on Developmental Disabilities (UCEDD). UCEDDs now constitute a network with vast experience in developing policy, connecting with the community, and promoting multidisciplinary collaboration. The centers may have specific funding to support community-based training and policy, such as the LEND programs. LENDs also constitute a network with a focus on training, policy, and community-based research. A center may develop relationships with specific academic departments to create a certificate or specialization in ASD, offer courses in ASD, or to simply weave content related to ASD into other courses. Similarly, a center focused on ASD may develop specific training arrangements to support practica with a rotation or emphasis on ASD, or other kinds of training or consultation. Faculty in the center on ASD may hold cross-appointments in a clinical setting to support translation of research into practice. Faculty may also be active in state and local advocacy organizations for ASD, or state-level committees on ASD. Few such initiatives will be actively supported—indeed, may be actively discouraged—in centers with a traditional academic focus, which ascribe little value to activities that do not contribute directly to grants or publications.

Elements

- *Services*: A small proportion of activities at a center may result in time-limited services provided to a specific clientele as part of a research project—for example, diagnostic evaluations as part of an assessment protocol or interventions as part of an outcome research study.

- *Training*: A center may provide a variety of training: Faculty may supervise the theses of graduate students, teach courses on ASD, offer workshops in the community, partner with a clinic on campus or an affiliated hospital or school to offer practica placements, and so forth.

- *Research*: In many centers, significant effort is dedicated to basic or applied research conducted by center faculty itself, in partnerships with hospitals, schools, or other agencies, in fulfillment of a contract with another agency.

- *Policy*: Faculty in a center may participate in policy initiatives, as a committee member or as the designated expert. When policy is part of the center's mission, faculty may take the lead in developing such initiatives.

Infrastructure

- *Sector*: Although centers can reside in universities that are private or public (e.g., a state college or university), activities draw on the full range of funding (see discussion later in the chapter).

- *Level*: A center on ASD often operates at the regional of state level, drawing students from hundreds of miles away and seeking to influence statewide policy.

- *Funding*: Funding may come from a variety of sources. Grant or foundation funding might support specific projects, while indirect costs built into a grant (up to 40% depending on the university and the grant competition) support the infrastructure of the university. Specific faculty positions (e.g., named professorships) or other general costs may be supported by interest generated from a designated endowment. The university might reallocate other general, institutional funds to support pilot projects, new faculty, or other operational costs. Some or all of a faculty member's salary might be generated by the tuition from the courses they teach. Public (and some private) universities may receive operating subsidies from the state.

- *Mandate*: A university center is only obligated to provide services to those paying for them (e.g., students, funding bodies).

- *Oversight*: Outside of the oversight provided by the university, and the obligations to granting agencies, a center is not subjected to external oversight.

- *Domain*: The range of domains addressed by a university center is limited only by the expertise of its faculty.

A Local Autism Spectrum Disorder Advocacy Organization   Advocacy organizations for ASD take many different forms. They may emerge as people living with ASD in an underserved region begin to meet over coffee to talk about how to get help, and then grow to focus on the activities of a small town or region. They may emerge as the local chapter of a national organization, extending the latter's reach to a new region. They may emerge as a spin-off or affiliate of another organization providing support to the community, such as a university-based center on ASD, of a parent information center for people with disabilities. Regardless of their origins, agencies and organizations focused primarily on advocacy have played, however, an increasingly important role in shaping services, training, research, and policy over the past decade, at the local, state, and national level, and across a range of issues. The Autism Society of America has continued to support a strong network of state chapters to raise awareness and mobilize resources at the local, state, and national level. Autism Speaks has emerged as a new and powerful force for change through its unprecedented contribution to research funding and the development of research networks, spearheading of state insurance reform to increase resources for services for ASD, and other initiatives. Other organizations have helped raise awareness and promote change in more specific areas, like early detection (First Signs), awareness of research (Organization for Autism Research), and participation in research studies (Interactive Autism Network). The increasingly articulate communities of caregivers and self-advocates put a face to ASD, ushering in a new era of accountability for program leaders. Together, these and other organizations have tipped the scales during the passage of the Combating Autism Act and other important legislation.

Several elements of the infrastructure and organization of advocacy organizations appear distinct. First, many advocacy organizations rely primarily on fund-raising from individuals and businesses to support their activities, and this is critical to building their growth. Caregiver-volunteers can devote extraordinary energy and creativity to establishing a new advocacy organization, but this is difficult to sustain for many years. The community-based activities intended to raise money and awareness can absorb much of this energy and creativity, leaving little for other kinds of activities beyond representation of the interests of advocates in the development of local, regional, and statewide policy. Unless the founders can pass the baton to a new generation of equally energetic caregiver-volunteers, or hire core staff to manage day-to-day operation if not provide other leadership, it is difficult for an advocacy organization to develop a multiyear strategy to grow beyond this core mission.

The fact that advocacy organizations are uniquely positioned to build consensus and coalitions is both a strength and a weakness. Advocacy organizations are unparalleled in their potential to generate awareness and harness the passion of caregivers and people with ASD. They can provide a forum for professionals and agencies to connect directly with those living with ASD. Under the right conditions, a coalition of advocacy organizations and other groups of academics and clinicians can generate significant momentum for change. Yet advocacy groups are, at their core, grass roots organizations. As such, they are compelled to fairly represent the many different points of view of their members, and to provide a forum for these views to be expressed. To lead an advocacy organization, a person living with ASD must not only be very driven, but have the personal and political skills to weave the opinions of others living with ASD and the coalition partners into a single message.

Elements

- *Services*: One primary mission of many advocacy organizations is to facilitate access to services by providing information to families about local resources. They may also organize activities during which families or people with ASD might socialize.

- *Training*: Advocacy organizations often sponsor individual presentations for parents and sometimes professionals. These may evolve into workshops or conferences.

- *Research*: Advocacy organizations may distribute information about research findings or research studies.

- *Policy*: A second primary mission of many advocacy organizations is to influence policy at all levels, by mobilizing people living with ASD to prioritize needs, advocate for new programs, and ensure representation to key committees and groups.

Infrastructure

- *Sector*: Advocacy organizations often exist as a not-for-profit, either standing alone or as a chapter of a larger organization.

- *Level*: Advocacy organizations must have a regional if not a local presence, to ensure grass roots participation and support campaigns for fund-raising and awareness. They may develop affiliations at the state level for the purpose of influencing policy, and at the national level for the local chapter of larger organizations.

- *Funding*: For most local advocacy organizations, fund-raising activities often support a core infrastructure (e.g., staff, office expenses), while specific grants from state, federal, and private sources may support specific initiatives.

- *Mandate*: Advocacy organizations are only obligated to represent their members and may struggle to find a common voice and specific focus for their work.

- *Oversight*: Except for its board of directors, or the monitoring of a local chapter by the national organization, local advocacy organizations are rarely subject to oversight.

- *Domain*: Advocacy organization may address concerns in all domains (e.g., health, education, community services).

CONCLUSIONS

Fitting Round Pegs in Square Holes: An Ad-Hoc Network Ill Suited to the Special Needs of Autism Spectrum Disorder?

Services, training, research, and policy in ASD are not developed in a vacuum but through an ad-hoc infrastructure of organizations that include public and private agencies at the local, state, and national level, focused on health, education, and community-based needs. I characterize this infrastructure as ad hoc because it was neither originally designed nor primarily mandated to address the specific needs of people with ASD. Instead, services, training, research, and policy must be built on an antiquated network of disciplines and agencies developed originally to serve the needs of related populations, most notably people with ID and those with psychiatric disorders. This legacy is evident in the current structure of public and private organizations and agencies divided between the traditional categories of education and mental/behavioral health, which often function in stubbornly independent "silos." Unfortunately, the needs of people with ASD resist such convenient categorization: Most children with ASD have significant educational *and* mental health needs, and these needs cut across home, school, *and* community settings.

The fact that the service needs of people with ASD span multiple service systems in this antiquated infrastructure is further complicated by the lack of coordination across agencies and a lack of understanding and collaboration between different domains that has persisted in practice despite an almost universal emphasis on a multi/transdisciplinary approach since the 1990s. Thus, relatively few programs are successful in effectively bridging these traditional categories and fully harnessing the power of multidisciplinary approaches. Children with ASD can receive excellent education services or excellent mental health services or excellent community support services, but rarely all three at once, and almost never through an integrated program. Because different programs often do not understand or effectively work with one another, they miss opportunities to create integrated networks that close gaps, or, worse still, may distrust other specific organizations such that they hesitate to collaborate.

The extent of these gaps should not be underestimated. I have found that most people assume that this network is inherently organized, evolving naturally to address most emerging needs and to bridge important gaps. The discovery of many unmet needs, shocking gaps, and inherent contradictions is usually met with disbelief, sparking a quest for a city, region, state, or country that must surely offer a more comprehensive and integrated network of services, training, research, and policy. I too embarked on this journey, and was disappointed (though perhaps not surprised) by the realization that such a place does not exist. By seeking leadership opportunities in different types of organizations, with the goal of promoting a more comprehensive and integrated approach, I discovered some of the reasons for remarkably—and frustratingly—consistent gaps and contradictions across regions and across elements of services, training, research, and policy, some of which I have already described. On the way, I have also been heartened by the many innovative programs, ardent advocates, and dedicated leaders seeking to improve this network, and inspiring this volume. In the final section of this book, I describe specific initiatives that can begin to bridge these gaps across disciplines and domains, in pivotal areas of service need that take advantage of new approaches to training and research.

The Perils of Expertise: When Autism Spectrum Disorder Is Neither Special nor Unique

It is perhaps ironic that the development of services, training, research, and policy, and their associated infrastructure, has also been hampered by the overwhelming emphasis on how ASD is "special" and different from other conditions. Although this focus on the unique characteristics of ASD has been important if not essential to increasing understanding and awareness, it has also blinded advocates, clinicians, researchers, and policy makers to equally important but less distinct features. Common co-occurring conditions—for example, severe aggression, self-injurious behaviors, or crippling anxiety—are important because they can, at certain points in the lives of some people with ASD, be more debilitating than the ASD itself. In addition, many of the services, training, research, and policy that benefit people with ID are just as important to those who also have ASD. For example, residential treatment programs originally developed for people with ID can extend their expertise to effectively serve some people with ASD and ID. Thus, many of the elements of services, training, research, and policy discussed previously are not—and need not be— specific to ASD. In the final section of the book, I return to discuss how the recognition of co-occurring conditions and the needs shared with other populations reveals important opportunities for growth.

The Labyrinth of the Autism Spectrum Disorder Service Infrastructure

For leaders, this fragmented infrastructure for ASD potentially creates inefficiencies because of gaps and areas of overlap across different agencies. For clinicians, this infrastructure creates hurdles when they are seeking to address needs than span multiple service delivery systems. For those living with ASD and seeking help, this fragmented infrastructure creates confusion and despair at multiple levels. For example, each organization may offer different services, rely on different inclusion and exclusion criteria, have different mechanisms for payment, and present different barriers to access. There is rarely a rhyme or reason for these differences—they reflect the vagaries of the infrastructure, not meaningful differences in the population served or the domain addressed. Even for the most confident and resource-ful person who has determined what he or she might need, this confusion compounds the search for providers. Providers themselves are often confused to some degree about any service that they do not provide, and so may not help families in their quest. For those who are less resourceful and confident, this confusion may render them almost powerless, compounding any helplessness they may already feel because of the perceived or actual disability conferred by ASD. It is truly a labyrinth: Those brave enough to venture inside to confront a service need they find overwhelming may become turned around so often and so quickly that they never emerge with a plan in hand.

I illustrate the challenging journey undertaken by people living with ASD by describ-ing what one set of caregivers—Evan's parents—might realistically face in searching for help during his early childhood years. I have expanded on the list of needs and services sought by his parents and describe the type (public, private) and level (local, regional, state, national) of agencies from whom they sought help when this might be relevant. I also rated whether the infrastructure was very (++) or somewhat (+) helpful or whether it somewhat (X) or clearly (XX) hindered their quest for help. I also mention which element (e.g., fund-ing, mandate) was most instrumental. Finally, I distinguish between those elements of the service infrastructure that helped Evan's parents directly, and those that helped more indi-rectly (e.g., supporting the professionals or agencies providing the services).

Elements that Directly Helped Evan

- *Early intervention*: Evan's primary care practitioner (PCP) was able to easily connect Evan's parents with general EI supports (a regional, publicly funded but privately con-tracted service). The service began quickly because of state and federal mandates stipu-lating that EI is free and easily accessible and because of state and federal oversight that monitors compliance.

- *Primary medical care*: Evan's parents initially had mixed experiences getting basic medi-cal care (especially for help with the ear infections possibly linked to tantrums and sleep problems). The lack of specialized mandates, oversight, and funding was a significant factor in the delivery of primary health care.

  - *Local PCP*: Evan's PCP was unable initially to make special accommodations because her practice was already overcrowded and she receives no additional reimbursement for case management of his unique needs. She took the initiative to hire a nurse prac-titioner who was able to provide more responsive and coordinated care.

  - *Regional hospital*: The long distance, long waits, and inability of the emergency ser-vices at a regional, privately run hospital compelled Evan's parents to look again elsewhere for his ear infections.

  - *Walk-in clinic*: Evan's parents were successful with a local, privately run walk-in clinic eager to accommodate to his needs and increase its clientele.

- *Case management*: Evan's parents benefited from some formal and informal case man-agement, primarily because of the initiative and goodwill of individual practitioners as opposed to programs that required cross-agency collaboration.

  - *ID case manager*: Consistent with her role as mandated by the ID agency, the case manager provided information and assistance to Evan's parents to gain access to funding and services in her agency and elsewhere. Her persistence and dedication was instrumental in advocating for the behavioral support ultimately needed to address persistent toileting issues.

- *Teacher*: The management of an individualized education program (IEP) (with local, state, and federal mandates, funding, and ultimately oversight) includes coordination of school-based services. The teacher's initiative in pushing for screening for ASD was pivotal to helping Evan gain access to more specialized support.

- *Nurse practitioner*: Coordination of medical care across agencies (e.g., for the confirmation of the diagnosis of ASD, treatment of co-occurring anxiety) was greatly facilitated by the nurse practitioner.

- *Child care*: There is little funding, and no mandate or specialized oversight for child care.

  - *Respite*: Although some public funds are available to defray the cost of respite, the lack of infrastructure and support will likely prevent the development of any real capacity for respite for Evan's parents.

  - *After-school care*: Multiple infrastructure barriers led to the failure to address problems that precluded after-school care and almost prevented Evan's father from returning to work.

- *Behavior support*: This was critical to Evan's education and after-school care (ultimately to his parents' ability to keep their jobs), but access to this support was especially tenuous because it depended on coordination among multiple providers.

  - *Behavior support (community based)*: Until Evan received an ASD diagnosis, and his family was able to navigate other service needs, access to behavior support was limited. Increased funding associated with an ASD diagnosis helped community-based behavior support develop across home and school. A rigid interpretation of state mandates almost prevented support to address Evan's associated toileting difficulties.

  - *Behavior support (school based)*: State and federal mandates were pivotal in ensuring that the behavior problems leading to Evan's suspension were quickly identified and addressed, at least in the school setting.

  - *Management of co-occurring conditions*: Difficulties gaining access to the developmental pediatrician delayed the identification and treatment of Evan's anxiety and sleep problems. Once identified, he enlisted the help of the nurse practitioner to intervene.

Elements that Indirectly Helped Evan Evan also benefited indirectly from help that the professionals around him received. Much of this took the form of training: 1) training in ASD offered to Evan's ID case manager as part of new employee orientation and annual conferences on ASD organized by the state departments of education and public welfare, 2) specialized certification in autism offered to Evan's teacher made more popular by tuition reimbursement and the promise of a pay increase, 3) the nurse practitioner's training in diagnosis of ASD. Information and advocacy was also important, when the case manager was able to direct Evan's family to resources assembled by the state chapter of a national advocacy organization listing respite providers.

Some of these initiatives were informed by research-based standards developed or adopted by national organizations: 1) autism teacher competencies shaped critical educational services delivered by Evan's teacher, 2) national standards guided the protocols for identification of ASD used by Evan's teacher and nurse, and 3) a national research network identified practices for sleep management. Research also revealed the underidentification of ASD in Evan's region, which led to additional training and support. Other forms of support were also important; for example, the federal program that offered reduced interest rates on student loans for physicians who set up practice in rural regions. Evan's case also illustrates how capacity grows more organically, through the many ways that practitioners might accumulate experience in ASD, including family members whose personal experience helps to drive innovation (e.g., the nurse practitioner).

Where to Start: Creating User-Friendly Directories and Road Maps

I believe that one way to counter this confusion and begin to map out strategies for eliminating gaps and barriers is to create road maps that inventory resources and define paths to pivotal services. I have participated in many groups who have sought to create directories that ultimately proved to become tremendously burdensome to develop and maintain, and ultimately failed to meet the needs of all potential users because the road maps lacked certain key elements. For those acting as case managers, a directory of practitioners searchable by profession, region, and types of services offered might be sufficient. For policy makers and program leaders seeking to identify areas of need, additional information about the waiting lists, caseloads, and costs of these services will be needed to develop a coherent strategy to increase capacity. In the final section of the book, I discuss how this information should ideally be combined with projections of total population need, and the training and other resources to develop expertise, to create an efficient and effective plan to scale up capacity.

These kinds of directories are rarely sufficient to help people living with ASD navigate the service labyrinth. First, such directories may rely on terminology that is familiar to service providers but confusing to laypersons, and so the directory must either be translated or accompanied by a glossary. Second, directories help professionals who already know what services they are seeking, but laypersons often need guidance to identify services they might need and the steps they must take to gain access to these services. By embedding the directory into a road map that describes which services are important and when, laypersons might be able to take greater initiative. A road map quickly becomes unwieldy as services become more specialized and individualized, and so I believe that road maps should perhaps initially focus on pivotal services likely needed by most people living with ASD. I elaborate on this recommendation in the final chapter of the book.

REFERENCES

Horwitz, J.R. (2005). Making profits and providing care: Comparing nonprofit, for-profit, and government hospitals. *Health Affairs, 24,* 790–801.

Lord, C., Rutter, M., DiLavore, P.C., & Risi, S. (1999). *Autism Diagnostic Observation Schedule (ADOS).* Los Angeles, CA: Western Psychological Services.

II

Exemplary Regional, Provincial, and Statewide Programs

5

Autism Spectrum Disorder Services, Training, and Policy Initiatives at The West Virginia Autism Training Center at Marshall University

Barbara Becker-Cottrill

The West Virginia Autism Training Center (WV ATC) is a statewide, state-funded agency housed at Marshall University. The primary mission of the WV ATC is to provide support to individuals with autism spectrum disorder (ASD) as they pursue a life of quality. This is accomplished through the provision of education and training for families, educators, and others significant in the life of the individual with ASD. Services are available at no cost for families of West Virginians of all ages with a primary diagnosis of autism, pervasive developmental disorder-not otherwise specified (PDD-NOS), or Asperger syndrome.

The WV ATC was established in 1983 through the diligent efforts of parents throughout West Virginia. The movement to close large institutions in the United States was prominent at this time and families were being encouraged to keep their children with disabilities at home. Dr. Ruth C. Sullivan organized a group of parents of children with autism to convince West Virginia legislators of the need for education and training for families and educators specific to the needs of individuals with ASD. The rationale was that in order for parents to keep their children in the natural home environment it was critical to provide them with education and training specific to their child's needs and strengths. The West Virginia legislature passed a bill establishing what we believe to be the first legislatively mandated statewide autism training center in the nation.

The way in which the mission of the WV ATC has been executed has changed over the course of time. West Virginia is one of the most rural states in the nation and providing individualized autism services statewide was and continues to be challenging. Originally, families were invited to come to Marshall University, where the main offices are housed, for up to 3 weeks. The education staff would conduct individualized assessments, develop training programs, and teach the child's parents to implement the programs through demonstration and coaching. Although a few families were able to participate, the majority of those needing services were unable to leave their jobs and homes for any length of time. Around

1988, the WV ATC changed the service-delivery model to a community-based model. The education specialist staff would travel throughout the state to conduct community-based assessments, develop training programs, and teach parents how to implement the programs. In most cases, with school-age children, the education specialist would also visit the child's school and offer training so that skills taught at home would generalize to the school setting. With a staff of five education specialists, caseloads of up to 50 families each, and travel times to homes and schools of up to 7 hours one way, services were diluted and follow-through was difficult.

In the early 1990s, when the increases in the prevalence of autism in California were making national headlines, the WV ATC also saw a significant increase in the number of families seeking services for their children. Direct services were becoming more and more difficult to deliver and waiting lists were getting longer. The administration and staff of the agency agreed that a different approach to delivering the agency's mission was needed.

In 1991 the WV ATC received training from the National Rehabilitation and Training Center for Positive Behavior Support. Education specialists were also trained to implement person-centered planning tools and began to infuse them in their work with families. Staff began to develop a comprehensive service delivery model based on positive behavior support. In 1996 WV ATC received a grant from the Centers for Disease Control and Prevention to pilot the Family Focus Positive Behavior Support (FFPBS) model of service delivery. The center's way of doing business was about to shift dramatically. The education specialist staff moved from being expert consultants (telling parents and teachers what to do) to being facilitators of a team (guiding and coaching team members as they developed a comprehensive positive behavior support plan for the individual on the autism spectrum). The new education specialist role entailed facilitation of collaboration among family and school and other team members. The new ideal was to empower the family and their team with the information, strategies, and techniques that they needed to fully support the individual with an ASD.

Education specialists were hired in regions throughout the state, providing for fewer travel hours to their assigned families. Additional funding from the West Virginia legislature in 2007 enabled the agency to hire 8 additional education specialists to total 16 full-time positions. The move from traditional consultative services to the FFPBS model increased both the quality and quantity of service delivery. More than 800 families and their teams in West Virginia have participated in the FFPBS model. More detailed information on the FFPBS model is provided in the following section.

In addition to the direct FFPBS service-delivery model, the WV ATC also provides a variety of nonindividual-specific services and resources. A lending library of books, DVDs, and audiotapes is available to all registered families at no cost. Lecture-style workshops on topics related to autism and education are conducted throughout the state, many supported by county schools. These include training for classroom aides seeking an autism mentor classification (described in the next section). Family coaching sessions are also offered on a variety of topics important to families (e.g., understanding the individualized education program [IEP] process, managing stress, guardianship, and supporting siblings). These are conducted by phone. The WV ATC also helps families connect with other local, state, and national resources. In addition, the WV ATC pioneered and operates a college program based on a model of positive behavior support for college-age students with Asperger syndrome who are seeking an undergraduate and/or graduate degree at Marshall University.

THE FAMILY FOCUS POSITIVE BEHAVIOR SUPPORT MODEL

The FFPBS model is the main direct service for families registered with the WV ATC. The structure of the model remains consistent for every participating family, but within the structure of the model, each positive behavior support (PBS) plan is highly unique for that child and each family plan meets the needs of the individual family. The process can last up to a year until the PBS plan is fully implemented and all team members are comfortable with it. Following are some key elements of the FFPBS model.

Key Elements

Family-Centered Planning Activities   In order to move away from an expert-driven and prescriptive consulting approach, the center's staff focused on the importance of developing not only technically sound behavioral intervention strategies but also behavioral interventions that fit well with the people and environments where implementation occurs (Albin, Lucyshyn, Horner, & Flannery, 1996; McLaughlin, Denney, Snyder, & Welsh, 2012). The importance of family context on improved child outcomes led us to incorporate family-centered planning activities from the start of our process. This planning incorporates activities that are modifications of activities developed within the context of person-centered planning (e.g., Bennazi, Horner, & Good, 2006; Falvey, Forest, Pearpoint, & Rosenberg, 1994; Kincaid, 1996; Mount 1994).

The process by which the facilitator (staff of the WV ATC) begins to understand family context includes the development of a series of frames that result in a family profile (Kincaid, 1996). The information communicated by families in a variety of topic areas is depicted through words and pictures on large pieces of paper or frames. Topic areas include family history, important people in the family's life, places in the community where the family goes, the family schedule for weekdays and weekends, family health, adaptive and challenging behaviors of the child, family fears, family choices, personal stressors, and strategies that work and do not work to reduce those stressors. The facilitator then assists the family in identifying themes that are common among the frames. The process concludes with the development of a family futures plan.

Planning Alternative Tomorrows with Hope   Planning Alternative Tomorrows with Hope (PATH) is a person-centered planning tool developed by Pearpoint, O'Brien, and Forest (1998). This tool is usually incorporated into the first family focus support team meeting and serves to provide direction for the entire team. The process begins with the individual or the family describing their dream for their child. The dream is depicted by words, phrases, and pictures that are displayed on a large piece of butcher paper in view of the support team members. The team then looks at the elements of the dream and determines goals that are positive and possible within a time period (usually 6 months up to 2 years). The process then works backward through time to determine how the team will reach those goals. For example, if the positive and possible goals are set to be accomplished in 1 year, the facilitator might then work on 6-month goals by asking the team, "What have we accomplished 6 months from today?" and "Who will help us accomplish this?" Once those goals are established, the facilitator continues with 3-month, 1-month, and first-step goals (those that will be accomplished in the next 3–5 days). Specific tasks toward reaching the goals are written on the PATH. The process includes the identification of people and agencies that will need to be enrolled to ensure the success of the plan. The PATH is reviewed at subsequent team meetings that are usually scheduled to occur on a monthly basis. Progress and/or barriers along with action plans to keep the process moving forward are discussed at these meetings.

Functional Behavioral Assessment   In situations where challenging behavior is a concern, the team conducts a functional behavioral assessment (FBA). An FBA is a process used to determine how challenging behavior is related to various environmental events. Using a variety of tools, including formal and informal interviews of care providers and educational staff, and direct observation data collection, the team determines how challenging behaviors are related to immediate antecedents and consequences, as well as broader setting events (e.g., medication, illness, predictability) and lifestyle issues (e.g., relationships with others, access to preferred activities/materials, opportunities for meaningful community-based experiences). Team members are actively involved in all components of the FBA process, collecting and providing interview information and direct observation data. The WV ATC facilitator assists in training and supporting team members during the FBA. The FBA is a hallmark characteristic of PBS and leads directly to the development of a comprehensive behavior support plan that addresses each of the factors related to challenging behavior.

Lecture-Based Training   A lecture series is provided for all team members. These lectures provide the educational background for the assessment, development, and implementation work in which the team will engage (Dunlap et al., 2000). The lecture series is based on the curriculum content recommended by the National Rehabilitation Research and Training Center on Positive Behavioral Supports (RRTC-PBS; NIDRR Cooperative Agreement H133B2004 and Grant No. H133B980005, 1989). The following topics are covered: overview of positive behavioral support; overview of autism, person-centered planning; support plan development; teaching alternative, replacement, and coping skills; crisis planning; and evaluation. Over the years, the lecture-based content has been modified to target topics that are most related to the training needs of team members.

Individualized Parent and Teacher Training   Training specific to interventions and strategies identified by the support team for the person with autism is provided to those team members who will carry them out across environments. The facilitator or a member of the team with experience in a specific area may provide this training. In addition, the team might enlist other qualified training personnel to ensure that appropriate training is provided in all areas of the support plan. This emphasis on the direct training of those involved in the individual's life is again consistent with PBS.

The Family Focus Support Team   The family focus support team provides the group action planning component of the model and is the driving force behind the success of the behavior support plan. Turnbull and Turnbull (1996) described group action planning as a tool for providing comprehensive supports to families. The team consists of people who are significant in the life of the focus child. They make a commitment to participate in team meetings, make contributions to the development of action plans, and help implement specific components of the plans.

The Behavior Support Plan   Consistent with a positive behavior support approach, the behavior support plan is a comprehensive plan that documents all of the action plans of the support team. Several authors (e.g., Bambera & Kern, 2005; Bambera &

Knoster, 1998; Dunlap, Sailor, Horner, & Sugai, 2009) have developed key areas that should be an integral part of any support plan. These include functional assessment plans and resulting data, targeted behaviors and strategies, alternative skill development, long-term lifestyle goals, and strategies to address quality-of-life issues.

Implementation of the Family Focus Positive Behavior Support Model

Families who are registered with the WV ATC are invited to apply to participate in the Family Focus Process. Participating families agree to commit to approximately 2 full days of planning and assessment during the first month, approximately 24 hours of lecture training, and at least 18 hours devoted to support-team meetings for approximately 6 months. They also agree to participate in home and community training specific to their child as determined by the behavior support plan. Team members determine meeting, lecture, and training schedules.

Phase I: Family-Centered Planning and Assessment WV ATC training staff coordinate and facilitate the PBS process. The process begins with an informal meeting between the facilitator, community partner, and family. The next step is to conduct family-centered planning and assessment. Usually, this activity takes place at the family's home but other arrangements are made depending on what is most comfortable and convenient for the family. The family is encouraged to invite anyone they wish to attend. Usually, only the immediate family is present. A family profile is completed through the development of the family "frames" and a family futures plan.

This phase sets the stage for the WV ATC staff to gain a more comprehensive understanding of the family's needs, priorities, and child-specific concerns. This information is used to develop an initial plan of action with the family. As well, the trainer talks to the family about who should be invited to future team planning meetings. At this time, the trainer and community partner also help the family learn more about autism and about other community, regional, and state resources, such as parent support groups and respite care providers.

Phase II: Team Training and Planning During this phase the trainer, along with the family, contacts individuals identified by the family who will become a part of the larger team (e.g., educational staff, behavioral health staff, day care providers, other family members, friends, neighbors). Approximately four 6-hour days (one per month) are scheduled for lecture training. An additional four to six 1- to 3-hour meetings are planned (at least one per month) for small-team meetings.

The first lecture is designed to provide an orientation about the process, information about autism, and an introduction to what will usually be the first action steps of the support team: the functional assessment. The support team then meets during that month to begin action planning. It is at this point that a PATH or other group action-planning tool would be used. For example, the PATH may list the need to complete a functional assessment to determine the function of "tantrumming." All members of the team have now received training through the lecture on how to conduct a functional assessment. The team now begins to plan the data collection method to be used, the frequency of collection, the settings in which data are to be collected, and who will be responsible for data collection and analysis.

Subsequent lecture training provides information specific to support plan development, including specific empirically derived strategies for teaching alternative behaviors.

Future support team meetings focus on the development of comprehensive plans to address the action plan. The team also discusses quality-of-life issues, and a variety of additional action plans may be developed each meeting. For example, a goal may be established to investigate summer camp opportunities and report back to the team at the next meeting. In summary, this part of the process ensures that all participants agree on a direction for training and program development and that each task developed by the team is implemented, modified, or reassigned if necessary.

In between lectures and formal support team meetings, members may meet in smaller groups to develop the specifics of an agreed-upon goal. Each day, members of the team are involved in some phase of the support activities. In addition, members may frequently call upon each other for assistance, feedback, and support.

Follow-Up   After 6 months to a year of actively building the support plan through team meetings, and implementing and modifying strategies, procedures, and action plans, the team selects a new team facilitator to replace the WV ATC facilitator. The WV ATC facilitator is available to the team as needed and continues to provide supports through phone discussions and less frequent visits for feedback purposes. If the team has been empowered through the process and has learned to function collaboratively and in a positive direction, the WV ATC staff is needed less often.

Revisions to the Original Model

In 2010 the center's staff began to look more closely at the fidelity of implementation of the FFPBS intervention. One inconsistent area was the amount of lecture-based training provided to each team. Particularly for school-age teams, the availability of school personnel to attend training became more and more limited. Some teams had to condense training modules based on the allotted time their supervisors would approve. The development of an effective PBS plan relies on team members that are educated in PBS, including functional behavioral assessment, proactive strategies, and behavioral principles. In order to achieve a consistent knowledge base among all team members, the lecture-based series was revised. We also developed it as a course to earn professional development credit. We hoped that educators would see additional value in the training if credit was available.

The new training curriculum is a 40-hour program, partly didactic and mostly work that is completed independently. Training DVDs and curriculum are provided through the Internet at a site for FFPBS team participants. The Autism Internet Modules (AIM) developed by the Ohio Center for Low Incidence and the Nebraska ASD Network are also incorporated into training based on the training needs of the individual team. Expected outcomes of the training are listed in Table 5.1.

Evaluation of the Family Focus Positive Behavior Support Process

Throughout the years, the WV ATC has conducted evaluations of the FFPBS intervention, most specifically with regard to the effects of the model on familial stress and quality of life of the individual with ASD. Data from the WV ATC study during years 1999–2004 showed that total stress scores on the Parenting Stress Index (Abidin, 1995) decreased significantly ($p < .05$) from preintervention to postintervention. Parents also identified personal stressors prior to intervention and after intervention. There were significant decreases in personally identified stress.

Quality-of-life changes for the individual with ASD were also reported. Team members (including parents) reported significant increases in 13 different areas (e.g., ability to

Table 5.1. Expected Outcomes for Family Focus Positive Behavior Support (FFPBS)

FFPBS TEAM MEMBERS will be able to	
Identify the key characteristics of positive behavior support (PBS)	Describe the goals of person-centered planning
Identify and define behaviors of concern	Collect data on behaviors of concern
Conduct data analysis	Identify functions of behavior
Identify desired and alternative behaviors	Develop hypotheses
Describe a functional assessment	Link interventions to functional assessment
Identify reinforcers	Develop lifestyle enhancements
Develop prevention (antecedent) strategies	Develop teaching strategies
Develop response (consequence) strategies	Recognize key elements of a PBS plan
Evaluate outcomes	Identify when strategies need to be modified
Work collaboratively with a PBS team	Access additional PBS resources for systems change

learn new skills; more time interacting appropriately with peers, family, and community members).

Questionnaires to assess team members' satisfaction and comfort with the process and the implementation of PBS plans were also a part of the evaluation process. All team members reported that they were able to work together for the benefit of the individual with autism and were able to agree on plans. They felt that the team facilitation process by the autism facilitator was effective and helped them meet time lines as well as consistently implement the strategies they developed. Families reported high levels of satisfaction with the family-centered planning phase of the process and the lecture series information. In particular, families felt that the positive behavior support plan helped them deal with inappropriate behaviors displayed by their child and helped them teach more appropriate behaviors. They also felt that it was helpful to have a team of people working together for their child and to support family needs as well.

Improving Evaluation Measures   In 2010 the WV ATC modified and added evaluation tools to assist in a more comprehensive analysis of the outcomes of FFPBS for the individual with an ASD and their families and team members. Again, with a focus on the effects of FFPBS on familial stress, quality of life, and behavioral changes for the individual with ASD, and team member satisfaction with the process, we instituted the measures listed in Table 5.1.

The Future of the Family Focus Positive Behavior Support Model   Staff at WV ATC find the FFPBS model to be a good fit for West Virginia's statewide mission and the organizational structure of the agency. Given that the PBS trainers reside in different regions of the state, they have been able to serve families even in the most rural parts of the state with positive outcomes. The goal is to build capacity to reach more and more families each year.

Modification and improvements to the FFPBS process based on the evaluation measures presented here will be an ongoing activity for the WV ATC. The center will also continue to improve the way in which it assesses family and child outcomes. Longitudinal outcomes for the individual with ASD will be addressed more specifically. It is known that from year to year support needs change as does the availability of those individualized supports. Ensuring that behavior support plans are continuously updated, implemented with fidelity, and modified based on the outcome data for the individual will be a primary focus for the agency.

AUTISM MENTOR TRAINING PROGRAM

In 1992 the West Virginia legislature established a school personnel class titled "Autism Mentor" (WV Code 18A-4-8). These individuals are experienced classroom aides (paraprofessionals) who work with students with ASD and meet the established standards and requirements. The requirements for this special credential include a minimum of 15 points (30 hours) of staff development training related to working with students with ASD and at least 2 years of successful work in the classroom with students with ASD. When these requirements are met, the paraprofessional submits evidence of his or her 30 hours of autism-specific training to the State Office of Special Education (OSE). The OSE verifies the evidence submitted and sends a letter to the local education agency (county school system) where the paraprofessional is employed.

The decision to hire a qualified autism mentor rests with the local education agency. The decision of whether a student requires an autism mentor is made during the student's IEP meeting. Typically, supporting data must be produced to justify why a student with ASD requires an autism mentor to be successful in the least restrictive environment.

When this new classification of classroom aide was added to the West Virginia personnel code, the OSE requested that the WV ATC develop training workshops that would help satisfy the autism-specific training requirements. The WV ATC developed and offered Autism Mentor Training Part I and Part II, totaling 24 hours. At the end of each 12-hour block of training, participants complete a written exam and must score 80% or higher to be able to submit the training hours to the OSE. An additional Advanced Autism Mentor 6-hour training program was added to the training sequence a few years later. Although it is not mandatory that classroom aides who are seeking this special classification take the WV ATC's training sequence, a majority of them do. Since 1992 the WV ATC has provided autism mentor training to hundreds of autism mentors throughout the state. Points can also be earned by attendance at other workshops related to working with students with ASD.

MODEL PROGRAM: THE COLLEGE SUPPORT
PROGRAM FOR STUDENTS WITH ASPERGER SYNDROME

The College Support Program for Students with Asperger syndrome (AS) was developed by the WV ATC to support students with AS through their college years at Marshall University. It was apparent that there were many high school students with Asperger syndrome that were experiencing academic success, but these students were not considering moving on to college. Navigating the social world of college life was reported by many parents and the individuals themselves to be an overwhelming thought. It was clear that social supports would be as important, if not more important, in the development of a model.

In 2002 a strategic plan was developed and presented to the president of Marshall University. The plan included the key elements of the program as well as plans to systematically expand the program across time. The WV ATC proposed that Marshall University begin with only one student the first year and then add additional students every year until 20 students were enrolled. No funding was requested. The WV ATC would dedicate one staff position to implement and oversee the program. A program fee charged to the student would cover the cost of a stipend for graduate assistants, who would work with the students enrolled in the program. The key elements of the program are listed next.

Use of a Positive Behavior Support (PBS) Approach PBS is a proactive, collaborative, and assessment-based process that is used to support students in reaching their goals. Each student, along with his or her family, participate in person-centered planning prior to the first semester, resulting in a PATH and/or a MAP (Making Action Plans).

Development of Individual Student Plans Plans are developed through a team approach and provide a framework for supports designed to assist students in reaching goals that may lead to competitive employment and independent living upon graduation.

Faculty and Staff Support Faculty, staff (including residence advisors), graduate assistants, and tutors receive training related to Asperger syndrome and specific information about the unique characteristics and learning style of the participating student they will be interacting with.

Academic Supports for Students Academic supports are highly individualized and include

- Course advising, based on the learning strengths, abilities, and interests of each student

- Students, program staff, and team members working together to determine reasonable accommodations beneficial to each student

- Individual and small-group tutoring or assistance with gaining access to tutoring

- Strategies designed to teach students organizational skills

- Consistent, periodic interaction with professors

Social Supports Social supports are developed to meet individual needs and interests. They are varied, with support staff providing assistance for student involvement in campus organizations, clubs, and extracurricular activities.

Independent Living Skills Supports Supports in this area are designed to teach effective adaptive living skills and are provided to assist students as they navigate through the day-to-day needs of a college lifestyle. They are available for supporting students as they become involved in both on- and off-campus communities.

THE WEST VIRGINIA AUTISM SPECTRUM DISORDER REGISTRY

In 2002 the West Virginia Health Commissioner received a proposal generated by the WV ATC to consider autism spectrum disorders as reportable conditions of childhood. ASD was established as a reportable condition of childhood in West Virginia as per Legislative Rule 64, Series 7, Category 11A, 3.5.b.2. In 2004 the West Virginia Autism Spectrum

Disorders Registry (WVASDR) began operations. The WVASDR is housed and managed by the WV ATC at Marshall University, as per protocol in the legislative rule. ASDs for the purpose of this registry are Autistic Disorder (299.00), Rett's Disorder (299.80), Childhood Disintegrative Disorder (299.10), Asperger's Syndrome (299.80), and Pervasive Developmental Disorder–Not Otherwise Specified (299.80).

Reporting entities include licensed psychologists, psychiatrists, and physicians. Within 30 days of making a diagnosis of one of the ASDs, the diagnostician is responsible for completing a report form and reporting the diagnosis to the WVASDR. Specific identifiers such as names or addresses are not required. In order to ensure there are unique identifiers, the county of residence and the last four digits of the child's Social Security Number are required. Other information required includes birth date, place of birth, race, age at which symptoms were first noted, the age at which the child was diagnosed, observed behavioral characteristics listed in the *Diagnostic and Statistical Manual of Mental Disorders, Fourth Edition, Text Revision* (*DSM-IV-TR;* American Psychiatric Association, 2000) upon which the diagnosis was made, and any comorbid conditions.

Reporting compliance has been problematic throughout the years. Based on an analysis of the number of individuals newly diagnosed in a given year who become registered for the services of the WV ATC compared to the number of children reported to the WVASDR in that same year, we estimate roughly 50% are not reported to the WVASDR. Efforts to increase reporting compliance are ongoing.

The WV ATC maintains a list of diagnosticians that have diagnosed individuals that are registered for services. These diagnosticians are contacted each year and are provided with updated information pertaining to the WVASDR and reporting forms. Presentations related to the mandatory reporting of West Virginians with ASD have been provided to psychology associations and the medical community. Additional mailing lists of diagnosticians have been obtained and information and reporting forms have been delivered to the individuals on these lists. We will continue to persist in our efforts to increase reporting compliance. Our data should give us important insight into trends related to age of diagnosis, type of ASD reported, associated features, and comorbid conditions.

REFERENCES

Abidin, R.R. (1995). *Parenting Stress Index: Professional manual* (3rd ed.). Odessa, FL: Psychological Assessment Resources.

Albin, R.M., Lucyshyn, J.M., Horner, R.H., & Flannery, K.B. (1996). Contextual fit for behavioral support plans: A model for "goodness of fit." In L.K. Koegel, R.L. Koegel, & G. Dunlap (Eds.), *Positive behavioral support: Including people with difficult behavior in the community* (pp. 81–98). Baltimore, MD: Paul H. Brookes Publishing Co.

American Psychiatric Association. (2000). *Diagnostic and statistical manual of mental disorders* (4th ed., text rev.). Washington, DC: Author.

Bambara, L.M., & Knoster, T.P. (1998). Designing positive behavior support plans. *Innovations* (No. 13). Washington, DC: American Association on Mental Retardation.

Bennazi, L., Horner, R.H., & Good, R.H. (2006). Effects of behavior support team composition on the technical adequacy and contextual fit of behavior support plans. *Journal of Special Education, 40,* 160–170.

Dunlap, G., Hieneman, M., Knoster, T., Fox, L., Anderson, J., & Albin, R.W. (2000). Essential elements of inservice training in positive behavior support. *Journal of Positive Behavior Interventions, 2*(1), 22–32.

Dunlap, G., Sailor, W., Horner, R.H., & Sugai, G. (2009). *Handbook of positive behavior support.* New York, NY: Springer.

Falvey, M.A., Forest, M., Pearpoint, J., & Rosenberg, R.L. (1994). *All my life's a circle.* Toronto, Ontario, Canada: Inclusion Press.

Kincaid, D. (1996). Person-centered planning. In L.K. Koegel, R.L. Koegel, & G. Dunlap (Eds.), *Positive behavioral support: Including people with difficult behavior in the community* (pp. 439–466). Baltimore, MD: Paul H. Brookes Publishing Co.

McLaughlin, T.W., Denney, M.K., Snyder, P.A., &Welsh, J.L. (2012). Behavior support intervention implemented by families of young children: Examination of contextual fit. *Journal of Positive Behavior Interventions, 14*(2), 87–97.

Mount, B. (1994). Benefits and limitations of Personal Futures Planning. In V.J. Bradley, J.W. Ashbaugh, & B.C. Blaney (Eds.), *Creating individual supports for people with developmental disabilities: A mandate for change at many levels* (pp. 97–108). Baltimore, MD: Paul H. Brookes Publishing Co.

Pearpoint, J., O'Brien, J., & Forest, M. (1998). *PATH: Planning possible positive futures.* Toronto, Ontario, Canada: Inclusion Press.

Turnbull, A.P., & Turnbull, H.R., III. (1996). Group action planning as a strategy for providing comprehensive family support. In L.K. Koegel, R.L. Koegel, & G. Dunlap (Eds.), *Positive behavioral support: Including people with difficult behavior in the community* (pp. 99–114). Baltimore, MD: Paul H. Brookes Publishing Co.

6

The Pennsylvania Bureau of Autism Services and the Department of Education

Providing Educational and Community Services Across the Life Span

Erica Wexler, Cathy Scutta, Michael Miklos, Nina Wall-Cote, and Peter Doehring

The Commonwealth of Pennsylvania presents unique opportunities and challenges to the development of services, training, research, and policy with respect to autism spectrum disorder (ASD). It is the sixth most populous state (12.7 million residents), covering more than 45,000 square miles, and including the fifth largest city in the United States (Philadelphia). After California, New York, and Texas, Pennsylvania is home to the largest number of institutions of higher learning in the United States. In this chapter, we discuss some of the autism-related activities of agencies within two state departments—the Pennsylvania Training and Technical Assistance Network (PaTTAN; within the Department of Education), and the Bureau of Autism Services (BAS; within the Department of Public Welfare [DPW]).

TRAINING UNDERTAKEN BY THE BUREAU OF SPECIAL EDUCATION: THE PENNSYLVANIA TRAINING AND TECHNICAL ASSISTANCE NETWORK

The Structure of Public Education in Pennsylvania

In general, the structure of Pennsylvania's public education system resembles that of other states: its 500 public school districts are operated and funded under the authority of the Commonwealth's general assembly and the locally elected school boards of directors; public schools include elementary, primary, intermediate, middle school, junior high, high, junior-senior high, area vocational-technical, independent, alternative education and charter schools, and each public school is headed by a school principal who is responsible for the day-to-day operation of the school and reports to the school district superintendent or assistant superintendent. Pennsylvania has also created a system of county or multicounty-level agencies (intermediate units) that provide consultation and training, and sometimes themselves operate special programs, schools, and classes for children and youth with special educational needs. Some intermediate units provide services to multiple counties, with the result that there are 29 intermediate units for the 57 counties of Pennsylvania. (For a more detailed description of the relationship of the department of education to other Pennsylvania agencies, please refer to Chapter 4.)

The State Department of Education sets broad policies consistent with federal and state law and coordinates programs across school districts. Notwithstanding state and federal laws and regulations governing public education, school districts retain considerable authority over the manner in which programs are implemented, in part because the bulk of funding for Pennsylvania public school programs comes from local property taxes.

PaTTAN is the training arm for the Bureau of Special Education within the Pennsylvania Department of Education. PaTTAN provides leadership for the direction of training and technical assistance efforts within Pennsylvania by remaining in a constant state of needs assessment by daily interaction with the professionals in the field. In the sections that follow, we discuss several initiatives undertaken by PaTTAN related to autism, beginning with the initial planning and analysis undertaken by the Autism Focus Group.

Autism Focus Group

The first autism-specific training initiatives undertaken by the Pennsylvania Department of Education, through the work of the Bureau of Special Education and PaTTAN, began in 1997 when the bureau assembled a group of cross-systems stakeholders for the first Autism Focus Group meeting. The Focus Group quickly agreed that the unique pattern of strengths and vulnerabilities in the areas of communication, social competence, and behavioral regulation that is characteristic of learners' ASD requires the development of specialized training supports that meet certain interrelated criteria. First, no specific strategy, approach, or curricular materials will be appropriate for all learners, given that ASD presents differently in each learner. Second, it is also critical to instruct across people, contexts, and with multiple examples, because these learners often have difficulty with generalization of skills, especially when participating and cooperating with staff or peers, or in independent learning situations. Third, educational staff must understand and apply the principles of behavior and learning across all educational situations and settings, and be able to make timely instructional adjustments based on strong observational skills. This includes using whatever motivates each learner and means constantly assessing and adjusting for variations in these motivators. Finally, staff needs to remain abreast of the professional literature because research in evidence-based interventions is in constant evolution.

Using these criteria, the Autism Focus Group identified strengths and needs in the areas of credentialing, training, service delivery models, funding/cost efficiency, diagnosis, and efficacy. Since 1997, PaTTAN has been charged with providing training and on-site technical assistance in various topics relating to assessment, curriculum and instruction, specialized interventions, and ongoing progress monitoring to the educational professionals supporting learners with autism in Pennsylvania's schools. PaTTAN autism consultants work with regional intermediate unit training and consultation staff to disseminate and support evidence-based practices to build the capacity of the local-level educational professionals.

Designing Professional Development Projects to Create Change

The ultimate goal for all of the work of PaTTAN is to operationalize training efforts that will build local capacity to implement and sustain evidence-based practices in real schools with real children and adolescents. The greatest challenge in professional development is to ensure, however, that whatever is being trained will actually be applied in the field (Fixsen, Naoom, Blase, Friedman, & Wallace, 2005). For this reason, we turn to the body of research related to systems change, organizational behavior management, organizational development, and sustainable implementation to guide our work. This body of research suggests that many factors must be considered when beginning to create change. This includes identifying, conveying, and convincing others of a need; establishing a sense of necessity and forming alliances with others who will help generate and sustain the change effort; creating a detailed, action-oriented plan of change while at the same time generating a plan to ensure the needed infrastructure for sustaining the change; educating, training, and coaching the implementers of the change; and developing methods of evaluation and ongoing progress monitoring of the change effort (Fixsen et al., 2005; French & Bell, 1999; Schwahn & Spady, 1998). In the initial stages of program innovation and implementation, stakeholders must be first involved in establishing the need for change and then in generating interest, consensus, and support for the proposed change. "Champions" for the innovation must be identified, with the recognition that the "right" champion at the state level must have the appropriate and necessary support. The infrastructure needed for change must be assessed and potential gaps must be identified in anticipation of potential barriers to moving forward (Fixsen et al., 2005). Finally, "purveyors" must be chosen, or those individuals who will represent the program or practice and actively work to implement with fidelity and good effect (Fixsen et al., 2005).

This body of work has also helped to identify factors related more directly to implementation. Implementation plans must specify all components of both the intervention and its implementation, including staff selection, staff training, staff coaching, and self-evaluation. Implementation plans must also specify measurable learner outcomes resulting from the intervention, as well as the fidelity of implementation. Plans must ensure and address how the fidelity of implementation will be assessed (Fixsen et al., 2005). Both measures are important at the clinician level and at the systems level in determining program adoption and sustainability (Fixsen et al., 2005).

The efforts described next are intended to embody these core training principles. It is also important to note that these include many overlapping elements. For example, techniques based in behavior analysis lie at the core of PaTTAN's Autism Initiative Applied Behavior Analysis Supports and the National Autism Conference. Training efforts also emphasize techniques based in direct instruction, and combine training and on-site coaching regarding key elements of the instructional environment, routines, and teaching strategies.

Autism Initiative Applied Behavior Analysis Supports

The PaTTAN Autism Initiative Applied Behavior Analysis Supports (PaTTAN AI ABA Supports) provides consultation and support to many classrooms serving a wide range of students with ASD and other special education needs from preschool through high school. Consultation is provided to participating classroom teams by behavior analysts hired and trained by the PaTTAN AI ABA Supports. On-site training is provided in a wide range of

techniques and targets, including those with a basis in B.F. Skinner's analysis of verbal behavior (Skinner, 1957), and is intended to remediate functional language deficits (e.g., mand
training, natural environment teaching, and intensive teaching of the verbal operants). Instructional efforts are also geared to training staff to teach critical social-communicative
skills including pragmatic skills such as requesting, labeling, conversational skills, and
responding as a listener. Programming is relevant to skill sets for a variety of social, academic, and communication repertoires, and for students who range from having minimal
verbal skills to students who are participating in general educational settings.

Formative assessments such as the Verbal Behavior Milestones Assessment and Placement Program (Sundberg, 2007) are used to initially establish a baseline and then to help in
the design of an individual teaching program that supports careful tracking skill acquisition
over time. Data-based decision making in the evaluation of student progress and the fidelity of program implementation is a central focus of staff training. Competency and fidelity
related to specific instructional skills are carefully assessed on-site, with results provided
to participating teachers and local education agency participants, and used to guide subsequent training efforts.

The goal of the PaTTAN AI ABA Supports is to train teachers and other school personnel in instructional and behavioral analytic skills and teaching protocols that are effective for students with various language and developmental delays. Project participants are
expected to develop not only specific instructional skill sets but also the ability to problem
solve when faced with instructional challenges. All components of the PaTTAN AI ABA
Supports are driven by an evidence base in the empirical literature of behavior analysis and
instruction. Individual student programs are verified through ongoing data-collection processes. The primary focus of the PaTTAN AI ABA Supports is derived from instructional
design components included in the site review process. Those instructional design components include classroom organization, data collection and analysis systems, consultation
delivery, instructional delivery, and behavior management. Staff training processes include
direct competency assessments.

The training framework includes systematic participant training delivered through
on-site consultation and specific competency checks. Direct measurement systems are then
used to assess the degree to which those skills are actually delivered in ongoing classroom
applications. Participating local educational agencies designate a staff person to be trained
by PaTTAN AI ABA Supports staff in order to establish local sustainability. With increasing
site competency, the level of PaTTAN AI ABA Supports consultative support is reduced.
The PaTTAN AI ABA Supports provides continued monitoring of implementation via the
site review process as sites obtain independent model status.

The PaTTAN AI ABA Supports system is primarily focused on intervention models
available in the public domain. However, various commercially available tools have been
utilized in public school autism programs in Pennsylvania. PaTTAN has provided training resources to assist school districts and intermediate units in the effective use of these
materials. Examples of a commercially available tool include the Competent Leaner Model
(Tucci & Hursh, 1991), Direct Instruction Programs (Science Research Associates, 1998),
and various social skills training models (Bellini, 2006; Goldstein & McGinnis, 1997).

National Autism Conference

The 4-day-long National Autism Conference provides an opportunity for professionals
and family members to attend invited presentations on comprehensive, evidence-based

information to assist educators, providers, and families in developing effective educational and therapeutic programming for all students with ASD. The conference has been held annually in early August for the past 15 years and draws on nationally recognized experts such as Brian Iwata, Vincent Carbone, Mark Sundberg, Jose Martinez-Diaz, Jerry Shook, and Ami Klin. Since the 2000s, conference attendance has ranged from 1,200 to 1,500 and has included educators, professionals, parents, families, and individuals with ASD from across the United States and from other nations.

The conference has evolved in several unique ways in response to the needs of its attendees. For example, the structure and content of the conference has been adapted to meet the needs of family members. A structured day camp experience (The Children's Institute) is provided free of charge to 100 children with autism and their siblings to allow parents to attend the conference and learn alongside professionals. Combined with the choice between specific topics and an introductory (Autism 101) track, this format makes information accessible to both new and more seasoned parents. The conference has also expanded the ways sessions are presented, used, and stored: 1) attendees can attend live or via webcasting, 2) the technology implemented to support webcasting has also allowed content to be archived as part of a state-of-the-art professional development website, and 3) Penn State students can attend the conference for course credit.

THE DEPARTMENT OF PUBLIC WELFARE: SERVICES FOR CHILDREN WITH AUTISM SPECTRUM DISORDER IN PENNSYLVANIA

In addition to services provided by the Department of Education, behavioral and physical health services are also frequently used by children with autism. These services fall under the jurisdiction of the DPW. Although this section focuses on programs and initiatives within the purview of the BAS in the Office of Developmental Programs within the DPW, many other important services are offered to children with autism through other offices in the DPW (see Chapter 4 for an overview of the structure of autism services in the DPW). In general, it is important to note that the system structure as described in this chapter reflects the recent history of Pennsylvania's service delivery system, but that this system is constantly evolving in significant ways. We recommend that readers refer to the DPW's web site (www.dpw.state.pa.us) for the most up-to-date information. It is also important to note that key elements of some services may depend on programs administered by other bureaus and departments. For example, important elements of the implementation of Pennsylvania's autism insurance legislation (Act 62) are administered by the Department of Insurance and not by the BAS (for a summary of some of the challenges and opportunities surrounding such legislation, please refer to Chapter 4). Before describing some of the initiatives and programs undertaken by the BAS, the following section highlights the activities of one of the other key services offered within DPW but outside of the purview of BAS: behavioral health and rehabilitation services.

Behavioral Health and Rehabilitation Services Offered Through the Office of Mental Health and Substance Abuse Services

Pennsylvania's children and teens with ASD who do not qualify for county mental health and intellectual disability services have been able to receive medically necessary behavioral health and physical health services through the Medicaid children's health care benefit package titled Early Periodic Screening, Diagnosis, and Treatment (EPSDT).[1] These services, referred to in Pennsylvania as Behavioral Health Rehabilitation Services (BHRS; and often referred to informally as *wraparound services*), are intended to provide trained professional support for children in home and community settings to reduce or replace challenging behavior. These services are overseen by the Bureau of Children's Health Services within the Office of Mental Health and Substance Abuse Services.

The implementation of BHRS illustrates how the rules and regulations needed to clarify and demarcate the boundary between service systems can unintentionally lead to artificial distinctions in programs. According to the Centers for Medicare and Medicaid Services (CMS) and Section 1905(a)(13) of the Social Security Act, "rehabilitation" services, such as BHRS, are meant to "reduce physical or mental disability or restore eligible beneficiaries to their best possible functional levels" (Binder, 2008, p. 2). In contrast, "habilitation" services are meant to "help individuals acquire, retain, and improve self-help and adaptive skills, but are not intended to remove or reduce individuals' disabilities" (Binder, 2008, p. 7). In other words, "rehabilitation" services focus on restoration of an assumed previous level of functioning, whereas "habilitation" services help individuals acquire new skills (Binder, 2008). Habilitation services are not covered under EPSDT, and, therefore, are only available to recipients of home and community-based services (HCBS) Medicaid waivers administered by the DPW's early intervention or intellectual disability systems (Human Services Research Institute, 2004; Thomson Medstat, 2006a). When the EPSDT entitlement ceases at age 21, individuals with ASD may continue to a receive services through HCBS waivers or through county mental health and intellectual disability programs, but many receive no services at all.

In Pennsylvania these distinctions are interpreted to mean that rehabilitation cannot focus on the acquisition of new skills. As a result, providers of behavioral health and rehabilitation services cannot teach but can only help to reduce problem behaviors. In practice, habilitation can sometimes be difficult or impossible to distinguish from rehabilitation. The reduction of challenging behaviors can certainly help to "restore . . . beneficiaries to their best possible functional levels"; however, the prevailing, evidence-based models for the reduction of challenging behavior now universally emphasize the reliance on proactive strategies. In most cases, these strategies include the teaching of essential communication skills to replace challenging behavior or the teaching of other self-management or social skills. Restoring the individual to the "best possible functional levels" may also be impossible in the absence of essential life skills, now that participation in the community to the fullest extent possible is universally recognized as essential to the quality of life of individuals with developmental disabilities. For example, the child who is barred from an after-school program because he or she is not toilet trained will never attain the "best possible functional level."

EXPANDED INITIATIVES UNDERTAKEN BY THE DEPARTMENT OF PUBLIC WELFARE: THE BUREAU OF AUTISM SERVICES AND ITS PROGRAMS

As policy makers consider the numbers and develop programmatic responses to address the need for appropriate supports, they struggle to overcome the following obstacles: 1) the

---

1. Children and youth, up to age 21, who qualify for Supplemental Security Income (SSI) based on their family's income and assets are automatically eligible for Medicaid, whereas those whose families exceed financial limits, but meet SSI disability criteria, can still receive Medicaid under Pennsylvania's "disabled child" or "PH-95" category. The PH-95 category considers only the child's income (Thomson Medstat, 2006a).

definition of ASD continues to be debated, 2) there are a limited number of applied research-based interventions to use (or fund) to appropriately support individuals with ASD, 3) there are limited resources to fund new or expanded services, 4) the increasing number of children with ASD are growing up and there are almost no long-term supports in place to care for or assist them as they transition into adulthood as entitlements fall away, and 5) individuals with ASD are served in multiple systems, which often leads to cost-shifting and a lack of coordination across service delivery systems.

This section describes the adult programs and collaborative partnerships that were established as a result of the recommendations of the Pennsylvania Autism Task Force. Overviews of the Pennsylvania Autism Census Study and Pennsylvania Autism Needs Assessment are also provided. This leads to considerations for future steps that will need to be taken by Pennsylvania and the nation at large regarding supports for individuals with autism and their families.

Existing Services for Individuals with an Intellectual Disability

To begin to understand the fragmentation of, and gaps in, services that led to the service delivery changes described in this chapter, it is important to first understand the preexisting service delivery systems offered through the DPW. Perhaps the most well-established and well-funded services are those offered to individuals with intellectual disabilities (ID). These programs were first established in 1966 via the Mental Health/Mental Retardation (MH/MR) Act, which required counties in Pennsylvania to establish mental health and ID programs using state-funded grants. The programs were intended to provide a comprehensive service delivery system. This included a full array of treatment and rehabilitation services in both institutional and community settings to eligible consumers of all ages (Pennsylvania Association of County Administrators of Mental Health and Developmental Services, 2002). Many individuals with ASD are also diagnosed with an ID and are able to receive supports through these county programs or through Medicaid waivers. Those with ASD but without a qualifying IQ (i.e., in the range of 70 or below) or a co-occurring diagnosis of mental illness do not, however, meet eligibility requirements for services through county mental health and ID programs (Thomson Medstat, 2006b). As a result, many individuals with autism have historically been left without appropriate supports. This has been especially significant after a person reaches the age of 21 and ages out of the educational system where services are an entitlement.

The Pennsylvania Autism Task Force and the Creation of the Bureau of Autism Services

In 2003 then-secretary Estelle Richman of the Pennsylvania DPW recognized that a plan for improving the organization, financing, and delivery of services to individuals with ASD in the Commonwealth was greatly needed. She convened the Autism Task Force, ensuring that family members constituted the majority of participants. More than 250 family members, advocates, medical and health care professionals, clinicians, researchers, educators, agency and legislative staffers, administrators, and provider professionals collaborated to produce the Task Force's final report, which was released in December 2005 (Pennsylvania Autism Task Force, 2004). The five primary recommendations made by the Autism Task Force (see Figure 6.1) incorporated major themes identified by the 12 Task Force subcommittees.

Although the Task Force identified micro-system challenges unique to the Pennsylvania service delivery system, the macro-system challenges and recommendations delineated in the report are not unique to Pennsylvania. Rather, they are challenges facing policy

1. Create an Office of Disability within the Department of Public Welfare that has a bureau or division of autism spectrum and related disorders.
2. Create a consumer-led organization that provides information about autism services in multiple systems and advocates for the needs of individuals living with autism.
3. Develop an autism-specific medicaid waiver to allow for greater flexibility and creativity in providing services for this population.
4. Situate regional autism centers across the state that provide high-quality services to individuals with autism, train professionals in the area to assess and evaluate the needs of people living with autism, provide education and supports to families, and create opportunities for research to continually improve treatment and supports.
5. Develop creative mechanisms for blending and braiding funding between education and medicaid to ensure coordinated, collaborative care across systems.

Figure 6.1. Recommendations of the Pennsylvania Autism Task Force. (From Pennsylvania Autism Task Force, Pennsylvania Department of Public Welfare. [2004]. *Autism Task Force: Final report.* Harrisburg, PA: Pennsylvania Department of Public Welfare; adapted by permission.)

makers that are being articulated nationally by the autism advocacy and self-advocacy communities. To date, the Commonwealth of Pennsylvania has fully addressed or made substantial progress toward the implementation of the Task Force recommendations, with the greatest progress made toward Recommendations 1, 3 and 4, which are described next.

Response to Recommendation 1: The Creation of a Bureau of Autism Services

The first recommendation of the Autism Task Force was to create an Office of Disability within the DPW, and a bureau or division for ASD within that office (Pennsylvania Autism Task Force, 2004). In May 2005 initial steps were taken to implement this recommendation and reorganize the management of Pennsylvania's waiver programs. By 2007 the Office of Mental Retardation (OMR) had been formally renamed the Office of Developmental Programs (ODP) to include a new BAS. The Bureau of Supports for People with Intellectual Disabilities was created within ODP to continue the work of OMR's oversight of the state centers and the two existing county-managed intellectual disability waivers: The Consolidated Waiver and the Person/Family Directed Support Waiver (PFDS).

The creation of a dedicated autism bureau was a crucial issue for many advocates in the autism community, because of the long-standing need to better integrate services and supports across different systems and to identify important gaps in the system of supports. For example, an individual younger than age 21 could be served through the mental health, mental retardation, early intervention, and education systems in Pennsylvania. However, the rules and regulations meant to clarify boundaries between these programs (sometimes dictated by the nature of funding) often created unintended barriers for the families who ultimately became responsible for crafting a coordinated system of care. Adults with ASD, absent additional qualifying diagnoses, were most often not served anywhere. An additional challenge voiced by the autism community was that when services were available, they were usually not autism-specific. As a result, the services were often mismatched or inappropriate and did not meet the needs of the individual with autism.

The Pennsylvania Autism Census Study

In 2005 the Pennsylvania DPW's newly formed BAS commissioned Dr. David Mandell and his team of researchers at the University of Pennsylvania School of Medicine's Center for

Mental Health Policy and Services Research to conduct a census of the number of individuals diagnosed with ASD living in Pennsylvania. The purpose of this study was to obtain an estimate of the number of individuals living with ASD in Pennsylvania as well as to learn about demographic characteristics of that population (Lawer & Mandell, 2009). The intention was to reveal the scope of need for autism-specific services and programs and to inform policy development and the design of effective services.[2]

Data for this study were gathered from the Pennsylvania DPW and Department of Education; county mental health, intellectual disability, and human services programs; children and youth offices; early intervention programs; Health Choices; county behavioral health agencies; and the U.S. Department of Education's Rehabilitation Services Administration. Individuals with ASD not receiving services through one or more of these program offices, and/or those who were misdiagnosed or were never formally diagnosed with autism, were unable to be counted. Due to these limitations, as well as other factors discussed in subsequent sections, the estimate is likely a dramatic undercount of the number of Pennsylvanians with ASD, particularly adults. Nevertheless, the census yielded important information about the population of individuals with ASD in the Commonwealth.

According to the study, in 2005 there were a total of 19,862 children and adults in the Commonwealth who were diagnosed with ASD and who were receiving services. Given trends, that number was estimated to have reached closer to 30,000 Pennsylvanians with autism in 2010. The report also illustrates that the number of adults with autism has begun to increase dramatically. In 2005 the census captured 1,421 adults with ASD who were 21 years of age or older, just 7.1% of the total ASD population in Pennsylvania. It is estimated that this number increased by 179% to 3,825 in 2010 and will increase by 621% to 10,140 by 2015. By 2020 the adult ASD population will reach almost 20,000, which is roughly equal to Pennsylvania's entire ASD population, children and adults, in 2005. The increase in Pennsylvania's numbers is supported by national trends and emphasizes the need for collaborative planning to respond to the complex needs of the thousands of children with autism who are transitioning into adulthood and the thousands more who will be transitioning in the future (for more discussion about the census and its implications for policy and planning, please refer to Chapters 3 and 14).

Response to Recommendation 3: The Creation of Adult Autism Programs

The third recommendation of the Autism Task Force was to create autism-specific programs for adults with ASD not served by any system. The first program developed by the BAS was the Adult Autism Waiver (AAW; Bureau of Autism Services, 2012a). In 2008 the waiver application was approved by the CMS and was launched statewide. The AAW is similar in structure to existing Pennsylvania waivers, such as ODP's Consolidated and PFDS waivers. In an effort to explore trends in innovative service models, the bureau also created a second model named the Adult Community Autism Program (ACAP; Bureau of Autism Services, 2012a). ACAP was designed to use a Prepaid Inpatient Health Plan (PIHP) model, which was very different in structure from traditional HCBS waivers. ACAP was approved in January 2009 by CMS.

The AAW and the ACAP were the first programs in the nation to be specifically designed to meet the unique needs of the adult autism population by incorporating a number

---

2. In 2012 an updated Pennsylvania Autism Census Study had been commissioned by the DPW and was underway at the time of publication.

	ADULT AUTISM WAIVER	ADULT COMMUNITY AUTISM PROGRAM
Availability	Available statewide, but individuals not receiving ongoing state/federally funded services prioritized	Avaiable in a limited number of counties
Breadth providers	Physical health services not included as a waiver service; participants retain existing medical insurance	ACAP becomes the participant's health plan, and integrates physical/behavioral health & community services
Providers	Choice of an enrolled provider for all services	One primary provider and its network of providers (e.g., primary care physicians) provide most services
Residential services	Does allow for residential 24/7 care if a need is determined through assessment	At intake, participant cannot require 16 or more hours of awake support

Figure 6.2. Examples of adult programs initiated and operated by Bureau of Autism Services (BAS).

of important features. For example, these programs are both administered not at the local level but at the state level directly by BAS. The programs provide specific clinical and technical assistance to enrolled providers, and providers are required to complete autism-specific training and demonstrate competence on the techniques before and after enrolling to provide services. These programs were also designed to enshrine several criteria and components increasingly recognized as important in other states. For example, they do *not* use IQ as an eligibility factor. Additionally, service planning and measures of success are based on individual goals, and the services provided are based on proven approaches to help individuals with autism realize their goals.

There are also important differences between these programs, as summarized in Figure 6.2. The AAW is a traditional HCBS waiver designed to provide long-term services and supports for community living. The AAW is available statewide and prioritizes adults not receiving any state-funded or state and federally funded home and community-based services. Services are based on assessments and are tailored to the specific needs of adults with ASD, but the waiver does not provide physician services. In contrast, the ACAP is not a waiver. It is a managed care program that is an integrated model of care reflecting trends that have wide appeal across the national human services landscape. The ACAP provides physician, behavioral, and community services through an integrated approach to create a coordinated system of supports. Initially available in a limited number of counties, ACAP was designed to be expanded across the Commonwealth over time.

It is important to note that this overview reflects the structure of the programs as they were initially designed, and that one of the fundamental values incorporated into their design was the ability for their structures to evolve over time. It was critical to create programs flexible enough to change as the programs began to serve more people and a better understanding was gained of what appropriate supports for adults with autism across the life span and across the spectrum entailed.

The programs were designed to be implemented to increase in capacity across a broader geographic region. The AAW, for example, was approved to serve 200 individuals, and in January 2010 it was approved by amendment to increase capacity to 300 participants. The ACAP was initially approved to serve 200 adults with ASD in three counties, and it expanded to serve a fourth county in the fall of 2009. At the time this chapter was written, both BAS programs had reached capacity. To make the most of limited resources, coordinated planning was underway to identify the means to serve additional participants on the growing interest lists for the adult autism programs, and more broadly support individuals waiting for services through ODP's intellectual disability waivers.

Expanding Pennsylvania's Professional Capacity

The BAS recognized the need for qualified, trained professionals to evaluate, treat, educate, and provide services to individuals with autism across the spectrum and the life span. In response to this need, the BAS has made training a priority across all initiatives. At the time of publication, more than 15,000 professionals, families, and individuals across the Commonwealth had been trained through BAS training initiatives.

The BAS provides ongoing live and web-based autism-specific training opportunities for a wide variety of audiences. Training topics are developed based on research-based best practices and emerging needs. AAW and ACAP providers must complete autism training prior to enrolling as providers and then complete additional training before providing specific services. Both required and supplemental training opportunities continue as the providers work with BAS program participants.

The BAS also offers a number of live training conferences and workshops. For example, each year BAS hosts the Pennsylvania Autism Training Conference (PATC), with multiple sessions providing emerging trends and practical strategies to help professionals acquire the necessary skills to support individuals with autism and their families. Sessions are presented by both national and local experts and include a wide breadth of topics, including employment, housing, evidence-based interventions, community inclusion, justice intersections, sexuality, emerging genetic research, anxiety and depression, self-advocacy, and supporting siblings. The conference has been designed to complement the annual National Autism Conference hosted by the Pennsylvania Department of Education, described earlier in this chapter. PATC builds on PaTTAN's support of early childhood and school-age children by providing additional considerations for the life span, with a concentrated focus on proven and emerging best practices for individuals from transition age through adulthood.

In addition to the annual conference, BAS has developed a cache of statewide trainers to conduct the BAS functional behavior assessment (FBA) training, using a combination of interactive activities, facilitated DVD instruction, and data analysis. In an effort to create consistent systemwide standards, the BAS FBA training has been designated as a requirement for professionals providing behavior specialist services within the AAW, ACAP, and the BHRS system described earlier.

Many BAS trainings are provided through virtual forums. The BAS online training system is a free comprehensive resource center designed to enable professionals and families to gain access to trainings, documents, and other resources in one convenient location (Bureau of Autism Services, 2012b). For example, many of the required trainings for providers are housed online, and select sessions from live trainings are recorded each year and are posted, along with the session materials, as a resource. A series of community DVDs is also available online and through state libraries.

Response to Recommendation 4:
The Development of Innovative Statewide Collaborations

The fourth recommendation of the Pennsylvania Autism Task Force was to create regional autism centers. To extend the reach of supports and services available to Pennsylvania's autism community beyond ODP's programs, in 2008 BAS funded the development of Autism Services, Education, Resources, and Training (ASERT) regional collaborations. ASERT is a statewide resource that was created to enhance the lives of Pennsylvanians with autism by promoting public-private partnerships and leveraging resources among the mental health, ID, early intervention, education, and medical systems across the Commonwealth (Pennsylvania Autism Task Force, 2004). The mission of the three regionally situated collaboratives is to enhance the lives of Pennsylvanians with autism of all ages and abilities by 1) improving regional access to quality services and interventions, 2) providing information and support to families, 3) training professionals in best practices, and 4) facilitating partnerships among providers of services throughout the Commonwealth.

Each regional ASERT collaborative is a partnership of medical centers, centers of autism research and services, community support groups, universities, and other providers of services involved in the treatment and care of adults and children with ASD. Through intraregional collaboration, ASERT is charged with implementing strategies that meet the needs of Pennsylvania's most underserved populations, including the Hispanic community and individuals living in rural regions of the state. ASERT projects are designed regionally with the goal of statewide expansion and focus on three major areas: clinical services, education and resources, and training. Specific examples include the creation of a staffed resource center with a statewide toll-free number and web site, adult diagnostic and assessment clinic with a focus on comorbidities, statewide emergency responders training, telemedicine, adult and adolescent multimedia social skills, and employment and college preparation programs for adults living with ASD.

The work of ASERT is driven by the findings of the Pennsylvania Autism Needs Assessment. As part of the effort to improve the care and quality of life for individuals with autism living in Pennsylvania, the BAS sponsored an in-depth assessment to answer the question: "How are the current public systems meeting the needs of individuals with autism and their families?" With more than 3,000 responses, the Pennsylvania Autism Needs Assessment is believed to be the largest and most comprehensive survey of individuals with autism and their caregivers to date in the nation. At the time this chapter was completed, the results of the assessment had been compiled and published in a series of reports available online, with additional reports under development (Bureau of Autism Services, 2011). Report topics available at the time of publication include Statewide Summary; Service Needs; Barriers and Limitations to Accessing Services; Unwanted Outcomes: Police Contact and Emergency Hospital Care; Getting an Autism Diagnosis and Follow-Up Care; Employment Challenges; Family Impact; and Report Recommendations (refer to Chapters 3 and 14 for more complete references and discussions of the results of the needs assessment). The information collected from the survey not only guides the work of ASERT, but it is also intended as a road map for policy makers, service providers, community organizations, and advocacy groups to guide the development and implementation of effective services and the efficient use of resources. Furthermore, the findings are informing the future direction of the BAS by providing a blueprint for strategic planning.

Concluding Thoughts

Although awareness of autism has increased in recent years, in large part due to widespread media attention, the public still rarely sees the face of an adolescent or adult living with ASD on magazine covers or news programs. The fact is that autism, in all forms, is a life-long developmental disability, and the majority of affected individuals live normal life spans and will continue to need significant supports as they age (Gajilan, 2007). Policy makers and public administrators across the country are already contending with a severe lack of appropriate services, trained professionals, and uniform standards around diagnosis and treatment for individuals with ASD. As the increasing number of children diagnosed transition into adulthood, there will be even fewer resources available to address these systemic challenges unless considerable changes are made to prepare for their needs.

Many steps are underway to move Pennsylvania toward a more integrated service delivery system for individuals with developmental disabilities. Designing programs that meet the complex needs of adults with autism has been instrumental in providing an understanding of appropriate and cost-effective supports. It is now equally important to identify the means to integrate services across systems and streamline resources. Toward this effort, Pennsylvania will continue to collaborate with other systems supporting individuals with autism in an effort to streamline information and resources. The autism community continues to advocate for increased capacity within the two innovative programs the BAS has designed to meet the needs of adults with autism, as well as for increased capacity within other state programs where individuals with autism are served. It is critical that we investigate innovative means to support individuals with ASD who do not meet the federal guidelines for existing programs. Ongoing support for the continued work of the regional ASERT collaborations is central to the development of statewide capacity to address the needs of individuals living with autism across the spectrum and across the life span.

Most important, however, is the growing recognition that the public sector cannot continue to shoulder the responsibility of meeting the needs of vulnerable populations. As revealed through the Pennsylvania Autism Census and Needs Assessment studies, the nature of future collaborations needs to be far reaching. If there is to be support for the increasing number of individuals with autism, in an environment where fiscal resources are becoming more limited, innovative and collaborative responses will be critical. Only through the combined support of public, private, and nonprofit sectors will the magnitude of this issue begin to be addressed (refer to Chapter 4 for an additional discussion of the role of public–private partnerships).

GENERAL CONCLUSIONS

It is believed that the initiatives described earlier represent excellent first steps toward improving services to individuals with ASD across the Commonwealth. Pennsylvania began by convening groups of stakeholders to identify priorities and strategies (the Autism Task Force and Autism Focus Group). Pennsylvania has sought to improve services across the life span and in multiple service systems by drawing on the latest research findings. Through the Autism Census and Needs Assessment, stakeholders have sought to gather empirical data to accurately identify the needs of individuals and families living with ASD so that long-term planning can address those identified needs. Training models have been developed to increase capacity across the Commonwealth, explicitly including intensive coaching (ABA supports, positive behavior supports, early identification). Conferences have been created to inform best practices and bring together state and national leaders through sessions that address needs across the spectrum and across the life span. State funds have been allocated toward innovative collaborations and service models, in many cases connecting public, private, and nonprofit sectors together for the first time. Pennsylvania has established stakeholders within education and public welfare agencies recognized for their expertise in key aspects of ASD services, training, research, and policy.

It is, however, recognized that much work remains to be done. The capacity of professionals across the Commonwealth has been increased through the implementation of specific training projects (e.g., ABA supports, positive behavior supports, early identification, functional behavioral assessment). However, additional training is necessary to provide tools to those supporting individuals with autism in all systems, at all levels. Some of the strategies Pennsylvania envisions, including the blending and braiding of education and Medicaid funding and the development of sustainable public-private partnerships, will require a commitment that spans multiple administrations and the inevitable economic cycles. Yet given the momentum seen in Pennsylvania since the early 2000s, including the recent passage of autism insurance legislation, it is difficult to imagine that improvement of ASD services, training, research, and policy in the Commonwealth will not continue.

REFERENCES

Bellini, S. (2006). *Building social relationships: A systematic approach to teaching social interaction skills to children and adolescents with autism spectrum disorders and other social difficulties.* Shawnee Mission, KS: Autism Asperger Publishing.

Bureau of Autism Services, Pennsylvania Department of Public Welfare. (2011). *Pennsylvania Autism Needs Assessment* (Needs Assessment Report Series). Retrieved from www.paautism.org/asert

Bureau of Autism Services, Pennsylvania Department of Public Welfare. (2012a). *Adult autism programs.* Retrieved from www.autisminpa.org

Bureau of Autism Services, Pennsylvania Department of Public Welfare. (2012b). *Virtual training and resource center.* Retrieved from http://bastraining.tiu11.org

Fixsen, D.L., Naoom, S.F., Blase, K.A., Friedman, R.M., & Wallace, F. (2005). *Implementation research: A synthesis of the literature* (FMHI Publication No. 231). University of South Florida, Louis de la Parte Florida Mental Health Institute, The National Implementation Research Network. Retrieved from http://nirn.fmhi.usf.edu/resources/publications/Monograph/index.cfm

French, W., & Bell, C. (1999). *Organization development: Behavioral science interventions for organization improvement.* Upper Saddle River, NJ: Prentice Hall.

Goldstein, A.P., & McGinnis, E. (1997). *Skillstreaming for the elementary school child: New strategies and perspectives for teaching prosocial skills.* Champaign, IL: Research Press.

Lawer, L., & Mandell, D.S. (2009). *Pennsylvania Autism Census Project: Final report.* Harrisburg: Bureau of Autism Services, Pennsylvania Department of Public Welfare.

Pennsylvania Autism Task Force, Pennsylvania Department of Public Welfare. (2004). *Autism Task Force: Final report.* Harrisburg: Pennsylvania Department of Public Welfare. Retrieved from http://www.dpw.state.pa.us/ucmprd/groups/public/documents/report/s_001624.pdf

Schwahn, C., & Spady, W. (1998). *Total leaders: Applying the best future-focused change strategies to education.* Arlington, VA: American Association of School Administrators.

Science Research Associates. (1998). *Reading mastery.* New York, NY: McGraw-Hill.

Skinner, B.F. (1957). *Verbal behavior.* Upper Saddle River, NJ: Prentice Hall.

Sundberg, M.L. (2007). *The Verbal Behavior Milestones Assessment and Placement Program.* Concord, CA: AVB Press.

Tucci, V., & Hursh, D. (1991). Competent Learner Model: Instructional programming for teachers and learners. *Education and Treatment of Children, 14,* 349–360.

7

Delaware Autism Program

Statewide Educational Services in the Public Schools

Peter Doehring and Vincent Winterling

The Delaware Autism Program (DAP) is a statewide network of public school programs designed to provide educational and related services that are individualized, highly specialized, full-time, and year-round. We begin by briefly describing the overall mission, and structure of DAP, with particular attention to the laws and regulations unique to Delaware. We then describe several elements viewed as contributing to DAP's success: An integrated program of training in three areas (the educational classification of ASD, teacher certification, and behavior support), and efforts to adapt a program of extended educational and support services within the community to the changing needs of the student population.

Though Delaware's population makes it smaller than some urban school districts, it can also be viewed as a natural laboratory for developing innovative public programs. As with other states, Delaware includes diverse populations. Its public schools must also operate within the same tangle of local, state, and federal agencies and regulations. But the smaller number of school districts makes relationships more likely to emerge between local universities, state agencies and legislators, and parent advocacy organizations. These relationships demonstrate the potential for collaboration in the creation and support of a network of services.

OVERALL MISSION, STRUCTURE, AND FUNDING

DAP is operated by, and for, the Delaware public school districts, in coordination with the state Department of Education. It is a consortium of formally affiliated programs that together serve the majority of students identified with the educational classification of autism across Delaware's 19 school districts. County Programs operate more specialized programs serving multiple school districts, District Programs serve students with autism only within that school district, and a Statewide Program provides training and oversight and operates DAP's extended educational services. In 2007–2008, DAP served almost 700 students across 6 different school districts and more than 40 community-based sites, with the support of more than 400 staff, making it one of the largest public school programs of its kind in the United States.

This chapter was begun while Peter Doehring was acting as Statewide Director of the Delaware Autism Program.

Structure

Three school districts (one in each of Delaware's three counties) currently operate county programs that provide services accessible to any student in that county regardless of the school district they reside in. Each county program operates a separate school for students with autism or other developmental disabilities. Each of these schools was established more than 30 years ago, when such centers were presumed to be the most appropriate educational alternative for students with autism, and each has evolved differently according to local opportunities. The New Castle County Program located at the Brennen School in northern Delaware (in Christina School District) serves exclusively children with autism, and as the largest also houses the Statewide Program. The John S. Charlton School operated by the Caesar Rodney School District in central Delaware (in Kent County) serves children with autism and other developmental disabilities and low-incidence populations, and collaborates closely with the adjacent Dover Air Base (the military air transport hub for the eastern United States). For example, the military frequently offers to redeploy military families of children with developmental disabilities to Dover because of the proximity and close collaboration with Charlton School. The Sussex Consortium operated by the Cape Henlopen School District in southeastern Delaware (in Sussex County) serves primarily children with autism, and was recognized as Program of the Year in 2002 by the Autism Society of America. Each of these separate schools has recently undergone major capital expansions to accommodate increased program growth. The principal for each of the separate schools has full supervisory responsibility for the staff and for the student's educational program.

Each County Program also offers the full range of classrooms and community-based settings within its school district, for students from across the county. These include separate classrooms, to partial and full inclusion, in elementary, middle, and high schools within that district. In some cases, the principal of the separate school has full supervisory responsibility for the staff and for the student's educational program regardless of which school the program is based in. In other cases, that responsibility is shared with the principal at the integration site. Each County Program has also established agreements with other community-based settings to support inclusion. For example, a private preschool operated within a school in Cape Henlopen School District provides integration opportunities for preschoolers at the Sussex Consortium, which operates classrooms in the same building. John S. Charlton School has arrangements with local colleges (Wesley College and Delaware State University) to operate classrooms for older students. The Brennen School has had contractual arrangements with the University of Delaware, which provides support, vocational placement, and access to recreational facilities to students with autism placed at a neighboring high school. Each County Center has also established relationships with local businesses, nonprofits, and providers of services to adults with autism, to support the transition into vocational programs and placements.

As is the case across the United States, the need for a referral to specialized programs is determined by the team responsible for the child's current educational or early intervention program. At this point, an evaluation for the educational classification of autism, required for admission to DAP, is undertaken by an interdisciplinary team within DAP (described later in the chapter). Although most students are referred before 5 years of age, this evaluation may take place at any point in a student's education; it is not uncommon for suspicions to first arise only in elementary, middle, or even high school, in the case of students with Asperger syndrome. If the evaluation results in the educational classification of autism, and the team determines that appropriate services cannot be provided in the home school district, the student is referred to DAP. For districts lacking a DAP affiliate, the student would be served at the County Program, in which case the local district pays the "local tuition" to the County Program (the cost of education not covered by state and federal funds, or typically about 30%–40% of the overall cost).

Since 2000, three other District Programs have emerged to provide services only for students residing in that district, via the full range of settings (except for a separate school). These district programs emerged because key personnel within the district advocated for developing more specialized autism services, and parents and educators expressed concern about the lack of community integration and long travel times to the county centers. Leaders at the county centers also recognized that the benefits of being bigger (e.g., more easily creating opportunities for students with similar needs, and building around a core of experienced staff) could quickly become a burden (e.g., assuring adequate space and staff) when faced with annual growth of 7%–10%. We learned, however, that good intentions are simply not good enough. Creating and sustaining district programs required careful attention to staff training, parent involvement/support, and program oversight. We also learned that this process is best undertaken by a team including program administrators, parents, and staff who crafted multiyear transition plans to build capacity gradually.

In addition to these programs, the largest school district operates the Statewide Programs under the leadership of the Statewide Director, through a contractual agreement with the state Department of Education. The Statewide Director provides specialized oversight to three statewide committees designated in state code. The Peer Review Committee (described later in this chapter) provides independent consultation for students with challenging behaviors, while the Monitoring Review Committee provides consultation and oversight on issues pertaining to best practice, and a Statewide Parent Advisory Committee advises the Statewide Director on several issues important to families. A Human Rights Committee also identified in state code originally helped to establish guidelines for behavior support when the program was first created and is convened currently on an as-needed basis. Although principals and local school districts have full legal and administrative responsibility for the day-to-day programming for their students with autism, the Statewide Director is recognized as setting standards for research-based practice specific to autism, via specialized training programs (an example of which is described in this chapter), and their role in the committees referenced earlier. The Statewide Director is directly responsible for a program of extended services that includes a 15-bed residential program in three homes in the community as well as in-home respite available statewide (also described in this chapter).

DAP's unique structure is the result of laws and regulations passed more than 30 years ago, and modified slightly since (see Figure 7.1). To our knowledge, some of these laws are unique to Delaware: the option to enter school-based programs prior to 3 years of age, the availability of community-based respite and residential services via the public schools, and the position of Statewide Director. Over the past 6 years, we sought to formalize the respective roles and responsibilities of the partners within the DAP via Memoranda of Agreement. Though complex and unwieldy, these agreements provided parents, staff, and leaders within and outside of the program an opportunity to seek consensus and obtain commitments regarding key elements of the working relationship between and among the county programs, affiliated programs, and the state Department of Education. In addition, the state Board of Education must review and formally approve a request from a district to house a DAP affiliated program, before the full range of services and supports can be made available.

State laws	State regulations
Staffing (certification, specialized staffing positions, unit funding ratios); Committees (SMRB, PRC, HRC, SPAC, PAC); Program (length of school year, in-school respite, age of students); Eligibility; Supportive services (EES, ESS); Other (special school construction)	Committees (SMRB, SPAC, PRC, HRC); Eligibility; Certification (for teachers of students with autism, residential advisors)

Memoranda of agreement state DOE ⇔ Christina School District/Office of the Statewide Director (Signed 5/2004)

DOE	Office of the Statewide Director
Coordinate development of practice guidelines; work with colleges and professional standard board to support teacher licensure/certification; review/take action on SMRB recommendations; provide state data when requested; maintain PRC contracts; help secure licenses for EES	Maintain statewide committees; maintain EES and ESS; coordinate professional development and specialized staff recruiting; liaison with DHSS; provide data to DOE

Figure 7.1. Summary of state laws, regulations, and agreements related to DAP. (*Key:* DAP, Delaware Autism Program; DHSS, [State] Department of Health and Social Services; DOE, [State] Department of Education; EES/ESS, Extended Educational/Support Services; HRC, Human Rights Committee; PRC, Peer Review Committee; SMRB, Statewide Monitoring Review Board; SPAC/PAC, [Statewide] Parent Advisory Committee.)

DAP's unique structure is also made possible by the funding formula in Delaware. Although education is funded by the Delaware public school system with the same combination of local, state, and federal support used for the public education in other states, the majority (60%–70%) of education funding comes from state and not local or federal sources (in most states, the bulk of funding is generated locally, often via property taxes). The significant financial load assumed by the state is particularly important to sustaining the high staff-to-student ratios in relatively poorer districts; even though such districts sometimes balk at the "tuition" (e.g., the local share of costs) paid to a County Program to serve their students, the costs were markedly less than would be the case in another state, and far less than costs associated with private placement or possible litigation.

Population Served

DAP serves students across the autism spectrum under the educational classification of autism. This was affirmed by changes to state regulations in 2004 that extended the definition of autism to include pervasive developmental disorder-not otherwise specified and Asperger syndrome (see discussion later in the chapter). Up until the beginning of the 1990s, most of students served in DAP also presented with intellectual disabilities and more classic autistic symptomatology. Full-time, school-based services can be provided to people with ASD as soon as they are identified (as young as 18 months of age), because of special provisions in Delaware state law. These services can be provided until the end of the school year during which the individual turns 21 years of age, or until he or she no longer needs such intensive and specialized educational support. As with many programs across the United States, DAP has experienced significant growth statewide in its student population over the past 10–15 years, with average annual growth of 7%–10% between 2000 and 2008.

We undertook analyses in 2008 to estimate the proportion of students identified and served out of the likely population of students, assuming a prevalence of 1/150 (Doehring, 2008) (see Table 7.1). Results indicated that about 50% of the likely children and adolescents with ASD in Delaware have been identified with an educational classification of autism, the vast majority of whom were served within DAP. Although the number of students without

Table 7.1. Proportion of the Likely Population of Students with Autism in Delaware Enrolled in the Delaware Autism Program (DAP)

Age range (years)	Proportion Identified	Enrolled in DAP	
		Overall	Identified
Preschool (birth to 5)	62%	55%	90%
Elementary School (6-11)	62%	57%	92%
Middle School (12-15)	56%	46%	83%
High School (16-21)	28%	23%	85%
Overall	52%	45%	88%

Reprinted from Doehring, P. (2008, May). *A model for regional training and service delivery for children with autism.* Presented at the meeting of the International Society for Autism Research, London.

an educational classification of autism appears high, several factors must be considered here. First, the majority of students enrolled in DAP beginning in 2003 were identified according to revised state regulations that align educational classification criteria with the *Diagnostic and Statistical Manual of Mental Disorders, Fourth Edition* (*DSM-IV*, American Psychiatric Association, 1994), that include all ASD, and that emphasize convergence in symptomatology across the Autism Diagnostic Observation Schedule (ADOS; Lord, Rutter, DiLavore, & Risi, 1999), Autism Diagnostic Interview–Revised (ADI-R; Rutter, Le Couteur, & Lord, 2003), and unstructured classroom observations. Students identified prior to 2003 were unlikely to have been identified using this protocol. Second, educational classification seeks to identify a primary condition based on educational need: Students may not have received a classification of autism if other possible educational classifications were preeminent in determining need, or of the autism itself was not judged to have resulted in significant educational needs. We suspect that the majority of those not identified are relatively higher functioning or have other significant co-occurring conditions. Many of these may require relatively less intensive and specialized services, and therefore are less likely to be referred to DAP.

Educational Model

DAP's educational model is based in the principles of applied behavior analysis (ABA), and has been described in a number of publications (Bondy, 1996; Bondy & Frost, 1994, 1995; Bondy, Tincani, & Frost, 2004). The core tenets of the so-called pyramid model were articulated most clearly by Dr. Andy Bondy during his 15-year tenure as state director (from 1982 to 1997), and subsequently captured in the Picture Exchange Communication System (Frost & Bondy, 2000) and the Pyramid Educational Model (Bondy & Sulzer-Azaroff, 2000). It has emphasized careful attention to reinforcement and communication skills, teaching strategies that support independence and generalization to natural environments, data-based decision making, and proactive behavior support driven by functional assessment. This ABA-based educational model has remained at the core of programming for more challenged students, and has been combined with a very functional, community-based approach to training from preschool through the early adult years. In recent years, some sites within DAP have sought to integrate elements of other program models (e.g., verbal behavior model, including the use of the Assessment of Basic Language and Learning Skills [ABLLS]), and have included ongoing systematic coaching to ensure maintenance. The pyramid model has also been supplemented by a much more diverse range of strategies to address the social, language, and other unique learning needs of the increasing population of students with Asperger syndrome (AS) and high-functioning autism (HFA). We believe such changes are necessitated by the range of students who are served in our programs statewide.

DAP has also emphasized an intensive team approach at the individual and the program level. Staffing levels defined by state law allows specialists to work closely and collaboratively with parents and classroom staff, such that, to a classroom observer, specialists are often indistinguishable from teachers and assistants. Unfortunately, rapid program growth, local staff reallocations, and shortages of trained staff have not always allowed high staffing ratios to be strictly maintained. We have also worked hard to provide parents with significant roles not just as individualized education program (IEP) team members but in program planning: Each DAP county and district program had parent advisory councils that played a role in all major initiatives and strategic planning.

The extent to which DAP continues to rely on specialized and segregated settings is somewhat unique, and runs counter to trends elsewhere in the United States. The demise of segregated settings across the country has certainly been welcome as it has spurred the development of more integrated settings, increased the awareness and acceptance of people with autism by other parents and educators, and ultimately improved the quality of life for many people with autism. Aside from the overall growth of the program and the increased accommodation of students across the autism spectrum, the greatest change in DAP within the past decade has been the increased integration of students into regular education settings. DAP's long history, including involvement with families throughout childhood and adolescence (for some, almost 20 years), provides us with a body of experience and lifelong perspective that regular educators are unlikely to accumulate, however. This has led parents, staff, and program leaders to recognize that, for a significant minority of students at some point in their education, the benefits of more specialized programs and settings will likely outweigh the benefits of a more inclusive approach. In this context, it is interesting to note that very few parents have pursued litigation to seek more inclusive settings over the 30-year history of the program.

INTEGRATED PROGRAMS OF TRAINING IN EDUCATIONAL CLASSIFICATION, BEHAVIOR SUPPORT, AND TEACHER CERTIFICATION

We describe next examples of training that illustrate some of the principles we have learned are important to creating and sustaining expertise in complex tasks across multiple programs. The general strategies and components of training are outlined in Figures 3.1 and 3.2 presented in Chapter 3, and in the following sections, we include detailed tables that illustrate how these strategies and components are specifically addressed in programs of training in educational classification and behavior support.

Educational Classification of Autism Spectrum Disorders

We began to substantially revise all aspects of the educational classification of autism in Delaware in 2001, in response to several factors. First, the National Research Council's research-based recommendations specified that educational services be broadened to encompass the entire autism spectrum (Committee on Educational Interventions for Children with Autism, 2001). Given the increased interest in programs for children with Asperger syndrome in Delaware, we sought to adapt our evaluation procedures to accurately identify higher functioning students.

Table 7.2. Components and Strategies in Delaware Autism Program's Training Program for the Educational Classification of autism spectrum disorder

	STRATEGIES					
Components	Based on legal and scientific best practice	Build knowledge and expertise	Create and promote a common vision	Assess resources and barriers	Considers entire network	Shaped by data
Activities		Extensive and ongoing training of core evaluation teams while talks to others promote common themes & vision	Themes in all trainings autism is a spectrum disorder with a core social deficit; is seen at all levels of functioning, and features change with development	Provide coaching and supporting materials, draft agreement commits districts to program of training	Training also includes referral agents and parents; common evaluation protocol helps with referrals between programs	Number of evaluation teams balances need to decrease wait time and assure enough evaluations to maintain expertise
Programs	Detailed regulations based on National Research Council report broadened criteria to include spectrum and define assessment protocol alligned closely with *Diagnostic and Statistical Manual of Mental Disorders, Fourth Edition* (American Psychiatric Association, 1994)					
Leadership	Expert workgroup drafts regulations					

Second, informal needs assessment had indicated a more general need to expand the number and expertise of evaluation teams. The steady growth in identification presents a particularly daunting challenge to public schools, which are legally obligated to conduct assessments and provide appropriate services within 90 days of a formal request for assessment. Thus, the development of an efficient and effective protocol for the accurate educational assessment of ASD became even more important, especially given questions in Delaware regarding the accuracy of some of the diagnoses accompanying these referrals. This prompted the interest in the potential utility of gold-standard diagnostic tools such as the ADOS and ADI-R. Nevertheless, the protocol described next has never been successfully challenged via due process since it was first implemented.

We describe next the program of training we undertook in educational classification. Table 7.2 aligns the specific components and strategies relative to the model of training presented in Figure 3.3 presented in Chapter 3.

Realigning State Regulations   We decided to also seek revision of state regulations when we recognized that both state and federal definitions of autism were outmoded. Both definitions failed to capture the broader spectrum and the level of detail embodied in the *Diagnostic and Statistical Manual of Mental Disorders* (*DSM-IV-TR,* American Psychiatric Association, 2000). We were also concerned that it failed to emphasize the social deficits at the core of the disorder.

We drafted revised state regulations for the educational classification of autism with a team that included parents, program administrators, and professionals experienced in issues of diagnosis and classification. After incorporating recommendations from two nationally recognized experts in diagnosis, the revisions were approved by the state board of education in 2004. These revisions were innovative because they aligned the educational definition closely with the *DSM-IV-TR* to explicitly include the entire spectrum, without contravening the federal definition. We also did not seek to distinguish between disorders within the spectrum, and instead simply required that the student present with two indicators within the social domain, and one indicator in the communication or unusual interests/behaviors domain. We felt that this provided more concrete criteria that emphasized the core social deficit. Consistent with federal definition, we retained the requirements of emergence prior to age 3, and results in educationally significant impairment in important areas of functioning.

Given this broadened definition, and continuing concerns regarding the accuracy of some of the evaluations received, we also sought to define a rigorous assessment standard. Impairments must be pervasive and persistent (i.e., part of a clear pattern of behavior that is consistently manifested across a variety of people, tasks, and settings, and that persists across a significant period of time) and do not simply reflect overall delays or intellectual disability. We also set standards regarding the tools used and the training and teams; that is, relying on specialized, validated assessment tools that provide specific evidence of the features of ASD by individuals who have specific training in the assessment of students with ASD in general and in the use of the assessment procedures referred to previously. Finally, we emphasized the reliance on converging observations; that is, that the classification should be based upon an observation of the student in a natural education environment, an observation under more structured conditions, and information regarding the student's behavior at home.

Developing an Assessment Protocol   We next constructed a more comprehensive assessment protocol closely aligned with these revised regulations (Doehring, 2006). In general, this protocol mirrored those in many research-based diagnostic teams, with one exception: We did not investigate possible causes or consider the concept of a lifetime diagnosis, because the determination of education need was based on current functioning levels.

We prioritized the use of standardized instruments for ASD that specifically mirrored *DSM-IV-TR* (American Psychiatric Association, 2000) criteria, with particular attention to the unique social deficits. Our protocol therefore included the ADI-R and the ADOS. For the ADI-R, we asked only the "Current" questions contributing to the algorithm because of our focus on present levels of functioning. Our choice to rely on the ADOS and ADI-R was subsequently reaffirmed by analyses that formally compared the extent to which individual items from popular instruments for ASD—the Childhood Autism Rating Scale (CARS), Gilliam Autism Rating Scale (GARS), ADOS, and ADI-R—could be mapped onto specific *DSM-IV-TR* criteria using blind raters by experienced clinicians (Ruhe-Lesko, Doehring, & Abel, 2007). These analyses suggested that the CARS and GARS are heavily weighted toward unusual interests and behaviors (about 50% of items mapped onto this domain), whereas the ADI-R is more balanced and ADOS is relatively focused on the social deficits. In general, the psychometrics (i.e., reliability, validity, and positive predictive value) of the ADOS and ADI-R are also clearly superior to that of the other measures.

We supplemented these measures of ASD with an observation in a community-based setting (school, day care, or home), and considered these results in the light of the most recent multidisciplinary evaluation. Consistent with revised regulations, the determination of educational classification ultimately rested not on the results of any single test, but on the clinical interpretation of the convergence of evidence for specific indicators. We sought evidence of persistent and pervasive deficits (e.g., across assessment opportunities, and apparent for a period of several months) that were clearly atypical relative to the student's developmental level.

We debated the place of screening instruments such as the Social Communication Questionnaire (SCQ; Rutter, Bailey, & Lord, 2003) in the assessment protocol. In general, the sensitivity and specificity of the SCQ did not appear strong enough at the time to warrant general screening of the population of students, especially as most parents, schools, and community-based practitioners did not hesitate to refer to DAP when there were any concerns about ASD. Requests for evaluation carry considerable weight, and so it was unclear that we could ever deny a more complete assessment based on a negative SCQ result. We did find, however, that the SCQ was useful in priming parents to consider behaviors subsequently queried via the ADI-R.

We sought to develop a parent-friendly assessment process. We recognized, for example, that a reliance on the ADOS supplemented by some general questions regarding ASD features may be sufficient to gather the kinds of converging clinical information needed for classification. We retained the ADI-R, however, because we recognized that many parents valued the opportunity to discuss their children's behavior in detail, behavior that had often been perplexing and troubling to them. The detailed discussions arising from the ADI-R questions also helped to establish a consensus regarding behavior that was important for families who were surprised by the conclusions. We also felt that the interview was important in establishing rapport with parents, which was especially important for parents whose concerns may have been minimized by other professionals and for whom this evaluation may represent the first step in a long and close relationship between the parents and the special education system.

Over time, we also found it helpful to adapt other practices in response to feedback from teams and informal reviews. Except for the ADI-R, the assessment quickly expanded to involve an interdisciplinary team that has always included at least a school psychologist and speech pathologist, and usually included a teacher and/or an educational diagnostician who often acted in a case management role. We have also generated other supporting documents, such as internal guidelines that captured core principles described earlier (and that drove the training activities described next), and practices for disentangling ASD in students with co-occurring and severe intellectual disability (Doehring, 2006). In response to disagreements regarding more complex cases, we introduced criteria for provisional classification, which included a commitment to reevaluate in 6–12 months time. This was particularly useful in the case of young children yet to benefit from services, for whom we could assess the response to intervention.

Other changes have also been considered. Although the assessment protocol described earlier is adequate for more complex cases, we recognize that the training is intensive for new clinicians (who may require a year or more before they feel comfortable with the instruments) and the full protocol is perhaps unnecessary when clear-cut cases are presented to experienced clinicians. We began to pilot a shortened protocol that dropped community observations when the ADOS and ADI-R yielded clear results that were consistent with reports from and expectations of parents and the referral sources.

Implementing a Program of Training   The development of assessment expertise in ASD took place in several stages. All teams initially participated in a 7- to 10-hour didactic overview, including: 1) the latest research on the characteristics, causes, and course of ASD; 2) the criteria for educational classification; and 3) the core principles outlined earlier. Team members responsible for the ADOS and ADI-R participated in 2-day clinical training workshops in each of these instruments. Every 1–2 years, teams also attended a 3- to 6-hour workshop providing a research-based update on identification and recommended procedures for ASD in Delaware, and to share concerns about the process. Every 2 to 3 years, these were supplemented by invited workshops on autism and Asperger syndrome conducted by internationally recognized experts, who were also sometimes tasked with reviewing portions of the protocol. When possible, coaching and case consultation by the State Director has supplemented the initial training, and served as an informal quality control. By 2008, multidisciplinary teams in all 6 affiliated programs had participated in this training, and were estimated to complete more than 200 initial ASD assessments annually.

We also found it useful to raise general awareness regarding these changes in practice, by weaving some of the broader principles of the revised classification protocol for ASD into more general workshops on ASD provided statewide. During these 1- to 6-hour "Introductions to Identification and Intervention of ASD," we present the broader spectrum, changes to regulations, and the need for rigorous assessment by a well-trained team. This information is particularly important for teams making referrals to DAP.

Creating Networks of Expertise   Given the level of commitment required by individual professionals and participating school districts, it also became evident that this program development might be viewed as the creation of networks. For individual practitioners, this included the recognition that more experienced staff could provide critical mentoring and support to less experienced staff, but only if the core principles were clear to all. We further developed the expertise of more experienced staff by involving them in conference posters exploring various issues in classification and assessment (Doehring, Donnelly, Wagner, & Myers, 2007; Doehring, Gigliotti, Calkins, & Cain, 2008; Doehring, Wagner, et al., 2008; Ruhe-Lesko et al., 2007).

For affiliated programs, the network included a commitment regarding the resources needed to conduct assessments, and a common set of processes. We developed an informal training and technical assistance agreement between the State Director and districts participating in agreement that, in exchange for the State Director's commitment to provide ongoing consultation and support, participating districts must: 1) commit to maintain a specialized interdisciplinary assessment team, 2) funnel referrals within the district to designated teams to maintain their expertise (e.g., by assessing students suspected of ASD at least monthly), 3) participate fully in initial and ongoing training, 4) maintain records that support statewide monitoring, and 5) accept the conclusions regarding educational classification from other districts within the network. With general agreement in these elements, we began to train public school professionals outside of DAP to use the same protocol to identify students with milder ASD who might not need DAP's highly specialized services.

Independent Peer Review of Behavior Support for Students with Complex and Challenging Behaviors

Students with ASD can present with behaviors that are dangerous, complex, and difficult to change. In some cases, these behavior problems significantly limit integration into typical community settings, severely limiting the quality of life, and, in extreme cases, resulting in lifelong institutionalization. For these children, their behaviors are more problematic for schools and families than are the core features of autism per se. It can therefore be very challenging to develop behavior plans that are effective yet minimally intrusive, and that safely support the student in the setting that is the most appropriate yet least restrictive. Nevertheless, there is a wide range of evidence-based practices for challenging behaviors, most of which rely on antecedent interventions (National Autism Center, 2009). For these and other reasons, a training program that focuses on teaching these positive and proactive strategies is one of the best places for a public school to start.

A recently published description of such a program at DAP (Doehring & Winterling, 2010) and its components generally mirror the program of training in educational classification described earlier. Table 7.3 aligns the specific components and strategies relative to the model of training presented in Figure 3.3 presented in Chapter 3. Similar to schoolwide programs of positive behavior support, multiple levels of training have been provided; half-day parent workshops have emphasized the reliance on simple antecedent interventions derived from a functional assessment approach; 2-day introductions to functional assessment and behavior support based upon positive and proactive strategies have been provided to DAP school psychologists statewide, and advanced seminars in data collection and functional analysis, plus the opportunity to develop intervention protocols, have been provided to more seasoned psychologists and behavior analysts. This training was sometimes supplemented by case consultation that provided a service to the student while also cementing new skills. The program also evolved as other data emerged: We recognized that behavior

Table 7.3. Components and strategies in Delaware Autism Program's training program for behavior support

Components	STRATEGIES					
	Based on legal and scientific best practice	Build knowledge and expertise	Create and promote a common vision	Assess resources and barriers	Considers entire network	Shaped by data
Activities		Full range of training: Introductory to train-the-trainer	Themes in all trainings: Need for functional approach emphasizing positive, antecedent interventions & ineffectiveness of punishment but need for safety training	Inter-agency agreements allocate responsibilities for training and support	Series of talks emphasizing common themes and vision to parents and full range of staff	Criteria set for frequency of independent peer review committee review; Use of safety techniques audited
Programs	Leverages state and federal laws encouraging functional behavioral assessment and positive behavior support; emphasizes evidence-based practice					
Leadership	Oversight by peer review committee with experts in autism and applied behavior analysis					

problems sometimes function as the "canary in the coal mine," signaling more fundamental shortcomings in teaching or staffing that were better addressed by a broader program in staff training and support.

Other components are, however, unique. One is the oversight provided by the independent peer review committee (PRC) that includes three experts in ASD, ABA, special education, and functional behavioral assessment. This committee conducts monthly reviews of all Behavior Support Plans that address potentially dangerous behaviors, necessitate consideration of intrusive procedures, and/or result in a recommendation for a more restrictive placement. Consistent with state laws, state regulations, and agreements, committee members are contracted by the state Department of Education.

We also implemented a train-the-trainer approach in the use of safety techniques to respond to students in behavioral crisis, including physical restraint if clearly indicated. We contracted with a national provider of safety training with specific expertise in safe and positive methods for treating severe loss of control. With their assistance, we increased the number of people able to train other staff in these techniques from one staff member, to more than 24 statewide, between 2000 and 2008. These trainers have been able to implement a tiered training and support for all 400 and more DAP staff statewide.

This program also illustrates the potential synergy between concrete guidelines, increased staff training, and close monitoring within and across programs. Safety training included practice in the use of the techniques themselves, and a review of the conditions under which their use was appropriate. These were supplemented by detailed written guidelines, such that direct care staff could act with confidence when these conditions were met, and school administrators were clearly justified in taking disciplinary action when these conditions were not met. Guidelines also described expectations for documenting the use of such techniques, and triggers for review by the classroom team and by school administrators. A final audit of the entire program of training and oversight by school administrators was conducted at each site under the Statewide Monitoring Review Board, which generated specific recommendations for school improvement. In total, this program of oversight helped to ensure that each instance of physical restraint was documented, communicated with parents and appropriate staff members, and reviewed for its appropriateness according to program guidelines (Doehring, 2008).

Postgraduate Autism Certification for Teachers

At the present time, most special education teacher undergraduate training programs provide a broad base of knowledge and experience, and with relatively little emphasis on understanding and working with students with ASD or other severe disabilities. The expectation that teachers become competent regarding the regular curriculum, and remain knowledgeable regarding the ever-changing rules and regulations surrounding IEPs, as well as the shifting expectation when new federal laws such as The No Child Left Behind Act of 2001 (PL 107-110) are enacted, is an even greater burden. In our experience, the lack of preparation and increasing expectations leaves newly certified teachers ill prepared to manage a classroom with students with ASD, let alone develop effective lessons. Even with the rigorous training and support described in the following sections, we find that teachers need 2–3 years of experience to become comfortable independently developing lessons for students within a specific age and functioning level.

In this context, Delaware's required postgraduate certificate in autism has helped to provide a foundation for training. For more than 25 years, Delaware has required that teachers working primarily with students with ASD complete a certificate consisting of five graduate-level courses in ASD within the first three years of hire. The certificate has always included three required courses (Introduction to Autism, Methods and Curriculum, and Functional Communication), and revisions in 2006 added a fourth required course in Applied Behavior Analysis. Electives must explicitly address ASD or severe disabilities in the course title. The majority of the County and District programs have rigorously enforced these regulations.

Most courses have been provided through the University of Delaware, although other regional colleges and universities (e.g., Johns Hopkins University, Wilmington University, Pennsylvania State University) have also begun to offer more courses as the need has increased. Over the years, the Statewide Director and other DAP staff have been extensively involved in both the design and the teaching of the courses. The University of Delaware recently created a specialized master's program and a more limited Course of Study in Severe Disabilities to encompass the certificate, and has expanded the number of courses sections accessible downstate via videoconferencing. Through a special legislative dispensation, public school teachers can take these courses for free at the University of Delaware in the summertime. This is in addition to significant (e.g., 25%–65%) reimbursement for these courses taken at any institution during the school year as part of a specific degree or certificate program, through training budgets allocated to local school districts.

Despite a 15% annual increase in the number of new teachers hired between 2000 and 2008, and the challenge of delivering courses statewide, about 50% of DAP teachers had completed the certificate as of June 2007 (Doehring, 2008). Compared to other states, we believe that this represents the highest proportion of teachers who have completed such a certificate. It has proven to be an invaluable base upon which mentoring and other specialized training has been founded. We have outlined some ways in which this training can continue to grow, through increased emphasis in specific teaching techniques in the course on Applied Behavior Analysis, the creation of a course or certificate in Asperger syndrome, and by establishing what kind of training/certification is required for teachers with more limited contact with students with ASD.

PREVENTING OR FORESTALLING PRIVATE PLACEMENT USING EXTENDED EDUCATIONAL AND SUPPORT SERVICES BASED IN THE COMMUNITY

Some students with autism require an extension of educational services beyond what is offered by public school programs designed for typical students. Some of these services are needed in order to continue to progress toward the educational goals set by the student's educational team and are therefore referred to here as extended educational services. For example, many school districts across the country offer an extended school year (ESY) in the form of a summer program in response to needs defined via each student's IEP, including the need to prevent regression and the opportunity to work on potential breakthrough skills. The total number of hours varies greatly from district to district, however, with some offering part-time programs, or including long breaks prior to or after the summer program.

In more extreme cases, when there are profound deficits in essential skills, or persistent and significant behavior problems such that educational progress is severely jeopardized, families may also seek more extensive in-home supports or a private residential placement. In some states, in-home supports (e.g., behavioral consultation or wraparound services) are provided by behavioral health agencies, but usually without funding education services.

Residential placements may be funded by the school district together with other public agencies responsible for health and welfare. The costs of such placements are staggering to the individual with ASD (who often loses regular contact with the family and the community), to the family (who experiences tremendous feelings of guilt and shame, and who often never have their child live at home again), and to the state (because these extremely costly services will likely be maintained through the rest of the individual's lifetime). As a result, seeking a private residential placement is often the most challenging and heartbreaking journey clinicians, educators, and families may ever take together.

Families may seek other forms of support in response to the additional burdens associated with the challenges of caring for an individual with a disability. Such services can include specially designed respite, after-school care, or specialized summer camp. These are not typically provided by school programs but by community-based private agencies, though some of the cost can be reimbursed via government subsidies (e.g., Medicaid). The availability of such services is highly variable, and the lack of such services (e.g., respite) can be a source of significant stress for the family.

In the next section, we describe DAP's efforts to adapt extended educational and extended support services to better meet the needs of Delaware's growing and changing populations. DAP has offered these services for almost 30 years, to one degree or another under the supervision of the Statewide Director (Doehring & Winterling, 2010), and fully staffed and fully funded via the public school programs.

In 2008, only 1% of students with an educational label of autism in the State of Delaware required private residential placement to address an educational need, and fewer than 18% attended the residences on an ongoing and part-time basis (Doehring, 2008). This is in marked contrast to rates of full-time private placement in other states that are reported to have reached 25% among adolescents with ASD (California Department of Developmental Services, 2003). We believe that the combination of a comprehensive day program, targeted parent training, in-home support, the option of part-time services, and close collaboration between day and residential programs has helped to prevent or forestall full-time placement in a significant proportion of cases, and in some instances allowed us to shift students back into their home full-time. Since that time, the growing needs of our population, and the complexity of running some of these programs within the public schools, has sparked a debate within Delaware regarding the most effective way to continue to deliver these services.

Extended Educational Services

Extended educational services have been offered primarily via up to three off-campus homelike environments (a total of up to 15 beds) in the state within which students can be provided with a range of education-based services that cannot be easily or effectively taught in a typical classroom setting. These services have been delivered to most students on a part-time basis—that is, students typically go straight from school to the residence several nights during the week, or over the weekend. In an increasing number of cases, the onset of these services has been preceded by an intensive, time-limited parent training program.

Extended Educational Services: An Example of a Regional or Statewide Need   Extended educational services is an excellent example of an infrequently needed and highly specialized service that could only be developed at the regional if not

the statewide level. On the one hand, the need occurs infrequently enough that smaller school districts do not see the benefit to developing a plan to address it, or appreciate the costs of failing to do so. On the other hand, we have learned that, even with the most intensive and individualized programming, a proportion of adolescent students will always benefit from—if not absolutely need—such a service if they are to have any chance of continuing to live more independently as adults. As a result, districts often scramble to find a full-time private (sometimes out-of-state) placement in a crisis, usually at an exorbitant annual cost. In our experience, it is rare for students to return home once they are privately placed, and so the resulting cost to the state and impact on the quality of life is permanent.

Better planning and coordination of such infrequently needed services could also help in their management, if undertaken at the regional or statewide level. For example, it may become possible to create groups of students who are reasonably homogeneous with respect to age, gender, and type of need, and potentially serve them more efficiently and appropriately. At various points, each of DAP's residential homes has served, for example, a different population (e.g., adolescent boys, adolescent girls, and a preadolescent mixed population). In some states, the management of such services is helped by the interagency committees or groups created, either at the county or state level, to support schools or families seeking such services. Although such committees can make private placements possible by coordinating funding from various sources, or occasionally drawing on other sources to support other kinds of interventions, they are often crisis- and not prevention-oriented.

Whether offered publically or privately, extended educational services for children and adolescents with ASD may also be too specialized to be developed effectively at the local level by building on other related services. Agencies offering residential placements to adults with disabilities can sometimes extend their services downward to address the needs of students, but then must undertake to develop a parallel school program, and do not always have extensive experience in more complex cases of autism. Such agencies may also be tempted to create heterogeneous groupings (e.g., serving students with varying diagnoses and levels of functioning), which, in our experience, can make it challenging to truly individualize programs. For example, community outings best suited to a student with relatively better social skills may be inappropriate for a student with more profound deficits. It can also be difficult to develop specialization and expertise among frontline staff when homes are scattered across a wide area.

Delaware Autism Program's Program of Extended Educational Services

History   A residential program was included in DAP from the outset, and, 30 years later, it is still, to our knowledge, the only such program operated by a public school system. DAP's residential program was initially housed in a single six-bedroom home and served students from 10–21 years of age. Staff ratios set in state law provide three professional-level positions and six assistants per house, assuring that two staff members are present at all times. Until 10 years ago, the residential program largely resembled other private placements; the placement was full time (e.g., 5–7 days/week) for the majority of students, and was frequently a substitute for foster placement (e.g., the student was making good or excellent progress in the day program, but the family could not cope for other reasons) or placement in a private residential facility.

Revisions and Modifications Undertaken Since 2000   With the addition of
a third residence in 2000, we sought to radically reorganize the residential program as

extended educational services. We began to focus on part-time services within an array of supports tied directly to the student's IEP, allowing us to titrate the level of service according to a student's progress. We also sought to forestall or prevent full-time placement by offering these part-time services to children as young as 8 years of age who were showing emerging signs of significantly challenging behaviors or pervasive deficits in life skills. Instead of immediately moving to an extension of the school day to include overnight stays, we also sought to work with the student's school to design intensive parent training and staff support in the family home, for up to 12 hours per week over a 4-month period. At the same time, we also sought to work with the IEP team to carefully determine if and how the student was failing to make reasonable progress, and to develop and implement a plan to maximize learning opportunities and/or behavior support in school. If overnight services were needed, we began with brief stays (2 nights per week, or 3 weekends per month), and then increased only when the data clearly indicate that problem behaviors were increasing and/or adaptive skills were stagnating despite implementation of all other supports.

We have since adapted the model in other significant ways. Up until 2003, some of the students were receiving services primarily because of the parent's inability to provide adequate support, and so we began to shift these students into foster care arrangements. However, part- or full-time foster placement placed us in a quasiparental role that we were not licensed, trained, or staffed to provide. We also began to explore the benefits of time-limited support (for intensive toilet training and life skills). We implemented a staggered schedule whereby students attending school in northern county locations proximal to the residences came directly from school from Monday to Thursday, while students attending programs in the southern counties were brought directly from school on Friday and returned directly to school on Monday morning. This helped to maximize the use of beds, while also providing parents with the break they needed to be able to provide the more intensive levels of support needed when their children were in their care.

The Benefits of a Close Relationship with the Public Schools   Other unique features of the program at DAP stem directly from the integral relationship with the day program in the public schools. DAP's extended educational services has been guided by the same curriculum and ABA-based methods for teaching and behavior support within the day program: Staff across both settings have participated in the same ongoing program of professional development, and teams have been led by teachers who all must complete the same postgraduate certificate in autism. The fact that staff from one setting may substitute in or transfer to the other results in a greater understanding of the work that goes in each. We have found that teachers are better able to identify students who may soon need some form of extended educational services, and can more effectively argue for changes in the school program that might prevent or delay such services (e.g., greater focus on key skills or behaviors, or increased parent training or in-home support). As described elsewhere (Doehring & Winterling, 2010), the shift to tightly frame such services around specific educational objectives makes decisions regarding the shift into and out of such services more data-based. With this level of integration, the program is almost seamless across sites.

Other advantages arose when we sought to maintain the program in the community where the students attend school and live. The most important benefit has been the potential for part-time programming; it is less costly, it ensures that students maintain significant contact with the family, and it offers a more realistic possibility that the students can be transitioned back to home. Students can be taught in the community settings (e.g., local stores, recreation sites) also used by their parents, and are more likely to transition into vocational and residential options in those same communities when they graduate from school. Locating the program close to the student's own community opened possibilities for the time-limited support described earlier.

Challenges and Lessons Learned   The challenges of operating a program of extended educational services are significant. By 2003, we had determined that it was impossible to operate such a program 24/7/365 within our existing public school model: Although it may be feasible to pool resources in larger programs to provide the necessary staffing and supervision for a year-round program, this was not feasible for a smaller program such as DAP's without dramatically increasing costs. Once we had shifted students whose primary need was foster care into more appropriate placements and began to focus on part-time programming, we were able to close for holidays (which sometimes were almost impossible to staff), to more easily undertake renovations, and provide staff training more efficiently. As a result, the program operated about 335 days per year.

Operating a program for students with such intense and complex needs is daunting. Students often require higher levels of staff experience and support than in the public school setting. For example, great attention must be paid to monitoring and preventing behavioral crises (e.g., aggression, destruction, elopement). Whereas extra staff can be brought in from other parts of the school to help manage a behavioral crisis in a traditional day program, this option is difficult to sustain in a community-based home without dramatically increasing costs, even though the student population is at significantly higher risk for such crises. Other specialized medical and behavioral supports are also more difficult and expensive to implement outside of the traditional workday. The operational needs of such a program often collided with the rules and regulations of a traditional public school system; working conditions were not always comparable to those negotiated by unions, the high levels of staff and administrative support must constantly be justified to sources used to funding a traditional school program, and a supervisor must be on call evenings and weekends 335 days per year. In fact, the program has only been maintained because individuals at all levels—paraprofessionals, teachers, specialists, school administrators, and school district officials—have been ready to make extraordinary accommodations to meet the needs of the students and their families.

On the rare occasion when a student exceeded our capacity to serve him or her, it has been very difficult to find other agencies to take over. Although this is a testament to the success of our program in serving all but the most complex students, the recommendation to shift a student into another placement placed us in a precarious position. Many traditional private placements excluded students with explosive episodes of aggression, or other behaviors that represented a clear and immediate danger (e.g., pica involving objects such as nails, batteries), and so the remaining options were often the farthest away and/or most expensive. During this period, we were compelled to take extraordinary measures to ensure the safety and well-being of the student concerned, and, in many cases, the other residents and staff. Compared to other public school programs, we experienced much greater pressure from local and state education administrators, who were sometimes surprised by our concerns regarding who we could accept because of our success in meeting the needs of almost all students over the years.

The kinds of supports needed by families of these students also require exceptionally skilled and understanding staff. Families were often under great stress because of the presenting behaviors and skill deficits themselves, the uncertainty about their future needs and programs, and guilt and fear that often arose when residential services were considered.

Families were more likely to struggle with burnout because their child's behavior(s) had often deteriorated over a period of months or years, and to be reluctant to invest energy in new strategies or programs (e.g., more intensive parent training) because of past failures. Families had sometimes clashed with the public school program over their child's needs, and so needed frequent and open communication with staff to rebuild trust. We found that the behavior of students often deteriorated at home before deteriorating at school, and so less experienced teachers of these students tended to display less empathy for the family's concerns, further widening the rift.

Supervising such a service within a public school program has also been very challenging. The training traditionally required for public school administrators capable of acting in a supervisory role (e.g., principals, special education directors) rarely prepares them for the highly specialized oversight role in a residential program, although we have usually had the fortune of drawing on administrators who began as teachers at DAP. In the private sector, behavior analysts with good organizational and customer relation skills can transition into a supervisory role, *and* continue to develop and monitor the behavior plans that are often so important to the student's success. Behavior analysts are not, however, a category of professional currently funded with the Delaware Public School system, nor could they easily complete the coursework needed to become certified as a public school administrator. Aside from the difficulty staffing the position, it is a highly demanding job: One must be prepared to respond to emergencies 7 days per week, evenings and weekends, 335 days per year.

Future Directions   Given the challenges listed earlier, we understand why public school programs would be reluctant to step forward to develop extended educational services in the manner described earlier. In many respects, this is a shame: The number of students requiring such services is likely to increase at the same rate as the overall populations of students with autism, and the costs of private placement are unlikely to decrease. Although the kind of program operated by DAP is a natural extension of the day program with respect to the educational services provided, issues related to licensing of these quasiresidential facilities, supervision, and the need for behavior analysts make such services difficult to operate for public schools. At the present time, the manner in which the DAP's program of educational services will continue to be operated is being debated.

Nevertheless, there may be other options that are less challenging. For example, we think that schools should begin to anticipate the need for residential services, and begin to plan accordingly. This could include establishing contractual relationships with private providers for more than one student at a time. For example, we have successfully negotiated part-time services in the student's home community, such that students can continue to attend a public day program, and have a common set of educational methods across school and residential settings. We were also delighted to discover that highly specialized behavioral programs are eager to collaborate with public school programs to anticipate and better respond to this need. For example, we have worked closely with specialists at the Kennedy Krieger Institute to help provide training and oversight to facilitate transition for students returning to school and home after short-term hospital stays. As a result, we were able to work much more effectively with them when we required their services, and we believe that the experience gave them a new insight into the challenges faced by public schools.

We also think that schools may consider easier ways of extending their school program beyond the traditional day or year. We have made concerted efforts to shorten the breaks before and after the summer school program, and found that students were able to recoup lost ground more quickly, while their families do not have to face the additional stress associated with securing child care for lengthy school breaks. We have also successfully negotiated with a local summer camp to more closely align its schedule with school breaks, to the benefit of the camp and our families. Schools may also consider the benefit of a community-based site simply as another educational site that is occasionally used for time-limited after-hours programs. For example, the DAP site at the Sussex Consortium built a house on its campus that is a training site for the day program but also can function for short-term overnight programs (e.g., toilet training).

Extended Support Services

As described in Chapter 2, caregivers of people with ASD seek many other kinds of support from other agencies. One of the most common forms of support is respite, or periodic breaks from caregiving that can vary from an hour or two for dinner with a spouse, to a family vacation of a week or more without the person with ASD. Although other activities and services may provide a respite function (including the example of extended educational services described previously), we are focused in this section on specific respite services as defined earlier, and referred heretofore as extended support services.

The DAP Statewide Director has also overseen a program of extended support services that offers respite to DAP students through a network of providers drawn from DAP's affiliated school programs, with respite occurring either in the provider's home or in the student's home. These services were made possible because of a reference to respite as a form of educational service in state law. Any family with a child or adolescent enrolled in DAP has had access to up to 19 days of respite per year. Respite providers are drawn from among DAP staff (see discussion later in the chapter), and in the majority of cases are familiar to the child and the family. A respite coordinator in each district program received requests from families and distributed them to potential providers, beginning with the family's top choices. In 2006, after looking closely at how respite was used, we significantly revised and updated our internal guidelines to make respite accessible in four of six DAP sites (and 90% of eligible students) in the state.

As we have discussed elsewhere, it is difficult to assess the optimal amount of respite, because we know of no program in the country that has made respite easily accessible to a wide range of families over a long enough period to gauge the depth of the need. Following our attempt in 2006 to increase access to respite statewide, we found that about 20% of families used respite, and for an average of 19 hours/month. Although the need for respite varies greatly from one family to another, we did not find it easy to establish and implement criteria without collecting significantly more information. We therefore decided to establish a set amount for all families that could be increased only for families in which there were two children with ASD, or other specific circumstances. The cost of respite was rarely a barrier to its use—the family is responsible for a nominal copay which, in more extreme or urgent cases, has been eliminated or eased through the contributions of other parents.

Trust in the system generally and in the provider specifically appeared to be one of several factors affecting the use of respite. With some exceptions, use of respite grew slowly when first introduced into a program, but, once established, became central to the well-being of the subset of families who used it regularly. We believe that the use of DAP staff was critical in this and in other regards. By using DAP staff, we could ensure that they had completed not only the health and background checks required of all public school employees, but also completed additional training in safety and behavioral assessment required of all staff. Caregivers were much more comfortable when they knew the provider, and some grew comfortable enough over time to leave their child with a provider for up to a week at a time while they took a vacation. It was interesting to note that caregivers in southern Delaware appeared to use respite less, because they were more likely to have extended family in the community to whom they could turn.

We have also learned that respite takes careful planning to do well, and we have useful lessons for others considering establishing a regional network of respite. For example, we required that all respite be planned at least 24 hours in advance and did not, as a rule, accommodate "emergency" respite, for a variety of reasons. Prior to this requirement, we found that providers lacked critical, up-to-date contact information about the student (e.g., medical or behavioral conditions that required accommodations, emergency contact information, permission to seek medical treatment in an emergency). Although significant issues arose rarely during respite, the lack of such information was extremely problematic during these rare instances. When the emergency respite was requested because behavioral issues made it difficult for the student to stay at home, we did not want to put the child or the provider at risk by expecting the provider to address the challenging behavior. When emergency respite was requested because a parent was suddenly taken seriously ill, we wanted to avoid creating a temporary or quasifoster placement in which the provider ended up making decisions on the student's behalf. In these situations, we sought to at least identify another family member who could assume that role. When the "emergency" really reflected last-minute planning, we found that the other important information listed earlier was not up to date. In general, we also found it helpful to formalize these rules in guidelines shared with all parents and providers. These guidelines saved providers from being placed in an awkward situation in which they genuinely would have liked to help a parent in need, but felt uncomfortable because of the extenuating circumstances.

For families, the greatest problem was the lack of providers. Our primary solution has been to make respite easy and attractive to providers. For example, we have made payment for respite generous enough such that, for some providers, it became an important supplement to their salary. Clarifying rules and expectations also helped potential providers overcome their initial hesitation. But respite remained difficult or impossible to assure for families of students with more challenging behaviors or skills deficits, even though these families were the ones in the greatest need.

Few public school programs will have the means to develop the kind of program described earlier, but might consider other ways of achieving similar ends. Summer programming remains a great source of stress for families, especially those with adolescent children who might display problem behaviors as typical summer camps can no longer accommodate older, more challenged students. Aside from extending the school year as long as possible, schools can seek to coordinate with other summer camps to cover these gaps. We had learned of a summer camp in a neighboring state that had already sought training from staff at the Kennedy Krieger Institute. This camp then sought to adjust its schedules to better align with our school calendar, closing the gaps for DAP families, while significantly increasing its enrollment. Some DAP sites sought to establish agreements whereby community-based organizations (e.g., Boys and Girls Clubs, Variety) can establish on-site after-school care. A number of sites have offered specific evening or weekend respite—for example, opening the school on a Saturday in December for 3–4 hours to allow families to prepare for the holidays. Though the amount of respite provided is minimal, it has been greatly appreciated by our families.

CONCLUSIONS

Public schools are mandated, among other things, to provide an appropriate education to all eligible students regardless of their age or background. We think that the results of DAP's collective experiences and its willingness to pursue "out of the box" solutions to diverse student needs have played a large part in creating some of the unique programs described in this chapter. Unlike private schools and other settings, we cannot focus on a specific age range or small slice of the autism spectrum. This has led us to appreciate how the needs of our students change from the preschool years into the onset of adulthood, and how the extraordinary needs of some of these students requires equally extraordinary programming, such as extended educational services. As we have worked closely with families over the years, we have seen how the growing demands on the family's time and resources can wear down even the most committed of families, and make the educational benefit of extended support services even clearer. As a public school program, we also cannot bar anyone from our services because we are full or they cannot pay. This has compelled us to respond to the rapid growth of the program, in terms of the number and the range of people served, and so we learned that training programs were essential to scale up capacity to meet the exploding population of students without completely sacrificing quality.

But our status as a public school program has also limited our flexibility in responding to the changing needs of our student population. The need to keep pace with our exploding population has focused and shaped, if not dominated, our priorities. Whereas early intervention programs have emphasized in-home services and parent training, we have been unable to successfully challenge the prevailing expectation that education is always something provided by teachers and always occurs in schools. As we move forward into the future, our challenges remain and are intensified by persistent concerns regarding costs for education of students with needs for specialized services and by our quest for excellence in the services provided to each student and his or her family. We must provide an expanding range of education-based services to children with an array of complex needs. To address this dilemma we will need to continue to work to develop an effective system of personnel preparation, provide ongoing professional development to hone performance, and continuously look to modify how our services are provided, all to ensure our learners are effectively supported in the range of environments in which they will live and prosper.

REFERENCES

American Psychiatric Association. (1994). *Diagnostic and statistical manual of mental disorders* (4th ed.). Washington, DC: Author.

American Psychiatric Association. (2000). *Diagnostic and statistical manual of mental disorders* (4th ed., text rev.). Washington, DC: Author.

Bondy, A. (1996). What parents can expect from public school programs. In C. Maurice, G. Green, & S. Luce (Eds.), *Behavioral intervention for young children with autism: A manual for parents and professionals* (pp. 323–330). Austin, TX: PRO-ED.

Bondy, A., & Frost, L.A. (1994). The Delaware Autistic Program. In S.L. Harris & J.S. Handleman (Eds.), *Preschool education programs for children with autism* (pp. 37–54). Austin, TX: PRO-ED.

Bondy, A.S., & Frost, L.A. (1995). Educational approaches in preschool: Behavior techniques in a public school setting. In E. Schopler & G. Mesibov (Eds.), *Learning and cognition in autism* (pp. 311–333). New York, NY: Plenum Press.

Bondy, A.S., & Sulzer-Azaroff, B. (2000). *The Pyramid approach to education.* Cherry Hill, NJ: PECS.

Bondy, A., Tincani, M., & Frost, L. (2004). Multiply controlled verbal operants: An analysis and extension to the Picture Exchange Communication System. *Behavior Analyst, 27,* 247–261.

California Department of Developmental Services. (2003). *Autism spectrum disorders: Changes in the California caseload.* Sacramento: California Health and Human Services Agency.

Committee on Educational Interventions for Children with Autism. (2001). *Educating children with autism.* Washington, DC: National Academies Press.

Doehring, P. (2006). *Improving the educational classification of autism: Recommendations for school psychologists.* Anaheim, CA: National Association of School Psychologists.

Doehring, P. (2008). *A model for regional training and service delivery for children with autism.* London, England: International Society for Autism Research.

Doehring, P., Donnelly, L., Wagner, B., & Myers, K. (2007). *How are diagnosis and cognitive status reported in autism intervention studies published in* JABA? Boston, MA: Association for Behavior Analysis.

Doehring, P., Gigliotti, D., Calkins, H., & Cain, D. (2008). *The utility of the ABLLS in comprehensive assessment and educational planning: A comparison of instruments.* Atlanta, GA: Association for Behavior Analysis.

Doehring, P., Wagner, B., Ruhe-Lesko, L., Peters, K., Abel, J., & Myers, K. (2008). *Where are the data? Publication profiles of articles on autism in* JABA, JADD, *and* JPBI. Atlanta, GA: Association for Behavior Analysis.

Doehring, P., & Winterling, V. (2010). The implementation of evidence-based practices in the public schools. In B. Reichow, P. Doehring, D.V. Cicchetti, & F. Volkmar (Eds.), *Evidence-based practices and treatments in autism.* New York, NY: Springer.

Frost, L.A., & Bondy, A.S. (2000). *The Picture Exchange Communication System training manual.* Cherry Hill, NJ: PECS.

Lord, C., Rutter, M., DiLavore, P.C., & Risi, S. (1999). *Autism Diagnostic Observation Schedule (ADOS).* Los Angeles, CA: Western Psychological Services.

National Autism Center. (2009). *The National Standards Project: Addressing the need for evidence based practice guidelines for autism spectrum disorders.* Randolph, MA: Author.

No Child Left Behind Act of 2001. PL 107-110, 115 Stat. 1425, 20 U.S.C. §§ 6301 *et seq.*

Ruhe-Lesko, L., Doehring, P., & Abel, J. (2007). *The psychometric properties of commonly-used instruments for assessing autism, and their correspondence with the* DSM-IV. Boston, MA: Association for Behavior Analysis.

Rutter, M., Bailey, A., & Lord, C. (2003). *The Social Communication Questionnaire.* Los Angeles, CA: Western Psychological Services.

Rutter, M., Le Couteur, A., & Lord, C. (2003). *ADI-R: The Autism Diagnostic Interview-Revised.* Los Angeles, CA: Western Psychological Services.

8

Indiana Resource Center for Autism

Promoting Local Capacity Statewide Through Research, Education, and Policy

Cathy Pratt

IN THE BEGINNING . . .

In the 1970s, little was known or understood about autism. Still grappling with the belief that autism was caused by cold and uncaring mothers that were depicted as "Refrigerator Mothers" and struggling with the trend toward institutionalization, the Indiana Institute on Disability and Community (IIDC; n.d.) was built. At that time it was called the Developmental Training Center. The concept was to build a facility that could house students with some of the greatest needs in the state and provide 24-hour programming and care. Students included those who had been in trouble with the criminal justice system and children who had mental illnesses, including schizophrenia. One of the groups to whom the program catered was students with autism. At that time, little was known about autism or effective treatments. There was no real rush to find out because the incidence was between 1 in 10,000 and 1 in 5,000. It was truly a rare disability. Under the leadership of Nancy Dalrymple, innovative programs were created and opportunities were provided for some of the state's most challenging individuals. At this time, very little was written about autism. Conferences were not available. Information was scarce. Much of that early literature came out of the work of Dalrymple and her team, including Sheila Wagner and Michelle Garcia Winner.

As the years continued and community options were made available, it was decided that the IIDC facility would move from being a residential facility to an outreach and training program. In 1985, House Enrolled Act Number 1003 established the Indiana Resource Center for Autism (IRCA) with goals specifically aimed at helping individuals with autism and their families. These activities included training, information development and dissemination, research, and individual consultations. In this same bill, a state plan was also mandated that would organize various state entities to perform various activities, and Indiana's Legislative Commission on Autism was established. In 1986 a mandate requiring IRCA to conduct a Needs Assessment survey every 3 years was added. In 1992 the Indiana Legislative Commission on Autism unanimously passed a resolution that the IRCA remain at the IIDC, and be recognized as an irreplaceable institution in Indiana. In the 1980s, the IIDC became the state's University Center for Excellence in Disability and Community and part of the Association of University Centers on Disabilities (AUCD). AUCD grew out of what is now know as the Developmental Disabilities Act (PL 88-164) of the Kennedy administration, which promoted statewide centers that would focus on taking research to practice. And, although located at Indiana University, the classroom for the institute became the state of Indiana.

PRESENT DAY

For several years, the IRCA maintained a foothold in residential school programming and community outreach as individuals transitioned back into the community. The IIDC continued to evolve in the challenging climate of disability issues. Realize that during the tenure of this organization, the trend in the United States has been from no mandated educational services to inclusion, from institutions to supported and community living, and from sheltered workshops to competitive employment. Today, the IIDC consists of seven centers that are guided by one mission. The mission of the IIDC, according to its website is "to work with communities to welcome, value, and support the meaningful participation of people of all ages and abilities through research, education, and service. The institute collaborates with community agencies, schools, advocacy organizations, government, institutions of higher education, and other community partners to effect improvements in quality of life. This is the core of our mission. It defines outcomes for diverse individuals, including people with disabilities, in all life spaces: schools, employment, home, and community settings."

The IIDC of today is a life span program that adheres to clear values and principles. Undergirding the IIDC's mission statement are the values held by the faculty and staff who are employed there. The following values permeate all of the institute's activities:

- Those with disabilities must have opportunities to become full, contributing members of their communities—at school, work, home, neighborhood, spiritual, and recreational settings.

- It is essential that people with disabilities be active, well-informed decision makers about quality of life, services, and supports.

- All community members must be educated, enabling them to support the full and active community participation of those with disabilities.

In addition to the aforementioned value statements, institute faculty and staff also hold to organizational principles that define the manner in which we conduct our activities and that promote a life span focus, a holistic approach, a focus on systems change, and other important principles. These principles can be located at www.iidc.indiana.edu.

This history, mission, values, guiding principles, and evolution are important to understand because these factors have created opportunities and direction for the state and for IRCA. It is also important to understand the longevity of the IRCA. In truth, IRCA came into existence long before the dramatic increase and heightened focus on autism. Because of this longevity, Indiana has been better positioned in many ways to address the growing needs of this population. No longer a residential program, the IRCA of today focuses on building statewide infrastructures and capacity that promote successful life outcomes for individuals across the autism spectrum. These activities become even more critical as the incidence of autism spectrum disorders (ASD) in the state has reached 1 in 77 according to our child count data collected through the Indiana Department of Education.

ROLES AND RESPONSIBILITIES OF THE INDIANA RESOURCE CENTER FOR AUTISM

The IRCA staff conduct outreach training and consultations, engage in research, and develop and disseminate information focused on building the capacity of local communities, organizations, agencies, and families to support children and adults across the autism spectrum in typical work, school, home, and community settings. IRCA staff strive to address the specific needs of the individual by providing information and training on a variety of strategies and methods. Specifically, the IRCA staff engages in the following activities:

- Conduct outreach training (e.g., conferences, regional and statewide workshops, university courses, practicum opportunities, parent support groups) regarding positive behavior supports and evidence-based practices for teaching and supporting individuals with ASD across community, home, work, and school settings.

- Engage in individual consultations with the goal of facilitating an understanding of the issues, promoting collaboration among team members, and suggesting services and resources.

- Train and provide ongoing support to school teams to enhance programs and build local capacity to better educate individuals across the autism spectrum.

- Conduct research that provides information to enhance quality programming for people on the autism spectrum and that informs policy decisions.

- Maintain relevant databases and utilize them for documentation, research, and evaluation purposes.

- Serve as a state clearinghouse for information about ASD by responding to individual requests for information, maintaining a library collection of relevant books and videos for public distribution, and monitoring current information on external resources, trends, policies, services, current treatments, workshops, and so forth.

- Produce and disseminate information for professionals and families on ASD through newsletters, brochures, print, videotapes, and via the web.

- Evaluate materials and training to determine impact and need for change.
                    (Indiana Institute on Disability and Community, 2011)

Please visit the IRCA web site (www.iidc.indiana.edu/irca) for a full description of its activities.

These activities target family members, individuals on the spectrum, professionals, and community members. A professional staff of 10–12 is funded by state appropriations, and at various times by state and federal contracts and grants. Staff have expertise and credentials in early intervention, applied behavior analysis, positive behavior support, social skills instruction, adaptive physical education, school psychology, social work, education, professional development, and speech therapy. Graduate students, high school students, and volunteers also assist with the various activities.

Understanding the history of IRCA is important, because it has contributed to the opportunities that are available today. The overwhelming task of the IRCA is to adopt strategies and methods that result in change and expanded opportunities for individuals of all ages and across the entire spectrum.

Some believe that change is an event. However, at IRCA we have come to realize that it is a process that is more like an evolution. This evolution never ends because the needs of this population continue to grow, and our knowledge continues to expand and shift. Others believe that change happens top down, whereas others believe it happens bottom up. The evolution of change in our state speaks to the importance of addressing change at many levels and in many arenas at the same time. Change has happened in Indiana for many reasons. A few that are highlighted here include IRCA's relationship with Indiana's Legislative Commission on Autism, a focus on statewide infrastructure and local capacity building, and relationship building and collaboration with other programs. Each of these components of change is explained in detail next.

INDIANA'S LEGISLATIVE COMMISSION ON AUTISM

Under the legislative mandate, IRCA reports to Indiana's Legislative Commission on Autism annually about the status of activities and trends in the state. Perhaps the most valuable mandated activity has been the Needs Assessment Survey. Although it was not mandated who would be surveyed, a decision was made to gather information from families. Every 3 years, a survey is sent to all Indiana families in our database asking them about access to Medicaid waivers, insurance coverage, private therapies and associated costs, employment outcomes, interactions with the criminal justice system, quality of educational program, and other topics that may be relevant to families. Family members are also able to submit comments or letters as part of this process. Every 3 years the needs assessment survey is adjusted to reflect current issues, but many questions remain the same. This allows for comparison data through the years. This information is presented to the Legislative Commission on Autism and potential areas for legislation are identified. As a result of the momentum of advocates and legislators and the information obtained via the surveys, Indiana has an insurance mandate, an Autism Medicaid Waiver, and mandated training of first responders and school safety officers. Additionally, Indiana was able to add autism to the list of disabilities covered by the Children's Special Health Care program. In the early 1990s, autism was also defined across state statutes as a neurological disorder. The goal was to open access to various services. At times, the work of the IRCA is defined by legislation that is passed, such as training of school safety officers and first responders.

The Legislative Commission on Autism has also addressed training of medical providers, employment outcomes, and quality educational programming. The members of the commission act as the House and Senate champions of people with autism and their stakeholders. Representative Vanessa Summer, who often chairs the commission, comments that their job is to continue to chip away at the rock that reflects the needs of this population (personal communication). Although some have argued that this commission should be combined with the generic Developmental Disabilities Commission, having a separate commission insures families and individuals that autism issues will not get lost.

There is one other feature that has been critical to the success of legislation in Indiana. The autism community has generally worked as a cohesive unit. The Arc of Indiana, the Autism Society of Indiana, and every other statewide entity that affects individuals on the autism spectrum have gone to the commission with a common voice. The Arc of Indiana has provided tremendous leadership and advocacy. Before promoting legislation, there is a process of checking to make sure that our legislation does not work against legislation in other disability areas.

LOCAL CAPACITY BUILDING/STATEWIDE INFRASTRUCTURE

When IRCA moved from a residential school program to community outreach, many of the requests were in the form of individual consultations. Staff were typically called upon when a crisis occurred. Two things became obvious during those consultations. First, oftentimes educators and other school personnel did not have the skill or knowledge to implement recommendations. At that time, there was very little training in autism. Second, the focus was solely on changing the individual and not on changing the behavior of others or the environment surrounding the individual. By the time IRCA staff were called in, behaviors had often reached such a crisis level that real change was difficult to impossible. Staff and families were in a reactive rather than proactive mode.

With the numbers of individuals increasing and the spectrum becoming more diverse and challenging, it became important to take a statewide perspective on change. It is also important to note that as the incidence of autism increased, so, too, did the agencies and professionals who were interested and established businesses and programs. Some of the treatment approaches they promoted were evidence-based, some were not. As such, the IRCA strove to be an honest broker of information and training. Today, IRCA does not promote any one model or approach, but instead believes in individualized solutions that work for the context in which the individual lives, works, or learns.

As the IRCA staff considered how to effect change statewide, it was clear that a multitiered approach would be needed. Workshops and conferences were organized in which professionals from around the world were brought to teach on topics that included applied behavior analysis, Picture Exchange Communication System, medications, assessment, Treatment and Education of Autistic and related Communication Handicapped Children, verbal behavior training, social skills, and almost every treatment approach that appeared on the horizon. Regional workshops were organized featuring IRCA staff to discuss topics that included communication, social skills, behavior, educational strategies, early intervention, education, and transition. The goal was to create a common language and understanding around autism and the various treatment approaches. Another goal was to provide access to information about the treatment methods, so that professionals and family members could make informed choices.

Other strategies included creation of a library collection, and the development and dissemination of a newsletter. The IIDC maintains a library collection that covers a range of topics related to ASD, including early intervention, social skills, behavior supports, and others. The collection on ASD has been widely circulated. In Indiana, any resident can check out a book or video/DVD, and it will be mailed to them at no cost. This library is continuously stocked with current publications. In response to our legislative mandate, a newsletter, the *IRCA Reporter*, was created. By 2010 the circulation of this newsletter had quadrupled. For those in Indiana, the newsletter was free. In 2010 the newsletter went electronic and so is free internationally. Articles are written by IRCA and are practical and accessible to readers of all levels.

Perhaps one of the most important aspects of these multitiered approaches was the decision to train autism teams in special education planning districts across Indiana. Realizing that students on the spectrum were being educated in a range of settings from self-contained to general education classrooms, parents expressed an interest that every school in Indiana have someone with expertise in autism. In 1993 three school districts were invited to the IRCA to go through 6 days of training. After this initial training, the possibility of future interest was in doubt. However, the interest has been overwhelming and for many years the IRCA has had to turn away teams. As of 2010, IRCA staff have trained over 380 teams (more than 3,000 family members and professionals) from local special education planning districts across Indiana to address the diverse learning needs of students across the autism spectrum. Overall goals of the training have been to

- Build local capacity to establish and implement proactive and positive programming for students with ASD.

- Foster the development of observational skills for working with students/individuals with ASD and to provide current information about the diverse range of individuals who exhibit characteristics associated with ASD.

- Assist local teams to work in a collaborative manner and as part of the IRCA team.

Still today, team members attend three 2-day training sessions conducted in Bloomington. Teams represent general and special educators, related services personnel, general and special education administrators, and family members. The main components of the training include but are not limited to

- Educational programming and instructional strategies

- Characteristics of autism/Asperger syndrome

- Teaming

- Curriculum development and classroom modifications

- Diagnosis and assessment

- Functional assessment of challenging behavior

- Positive behavior support

- Communication strategies

- Transition planning

- Sensory issues

- Early intervention

- Social skills development

As part of the training, teams are asked to submit plans that articulate next steps and also clarify how IRCA can provide ongoing support. As the number of teams trained increased, it became apparent that another infrastructure needed to be created to continue to support local teams.

In 1996, local directors of special education were asked to hire, appoint, or in some way identify a staff member who would serve as an autism leader/mentor/coach in their district. Every special education planning district responded. Still today, autism leaders meet monthly in seven regions across Indiana. Twice a year all autism leaders are brought together to learn from a national leader in the field of autism. And a listserv is maintained allowing autism leaders to share resources and information, and to problem solve difficult situations together. IRCA remains committed to this network of autism leaders. In truth, they have become organizational colleagues across Indiana. The expert model is not the IRCA's preferred approach, and the organization believes that each person brings an important talent and skill to any issue. In situations that are highly problematic, IRCA may still be called in. Once its representatives leave, there is an enduring infrastructure that ensures that recommendations are followed. This group has also created innovations that have been shared statewide and nationally. For information about these innovative programs, visit the articles on the IRCA web site called "Hats Off" at http://www.iidc.indiana.edu/index.php?pageId=298.

In 2008 an effort was made to train teams in adult services. Unfortunately, this initiative did not continue. Although the need to prepare adult service providers is great, no clear course for support and training is apparent. The systems that support adults are more complex and layered than those that support students. The ultimate goal is to create a seamless system of autism leaders from school to adult services that makes services seem less fragmented to families and individuals on the spectrum.

RELATIONSHIP BUILDING/ COLLABORATION WITH OTHER ENTITIES

Relationship building and collaboration have occurred in various ways both statewide and nationally. First let's begin with a conversation of the statewide collaboration. Part of the legislative mandate under which IRCA was formed was to create a state plan. This was to be guided by a state agency. Through the years and changes in state administration, the plan got lost. In 2006, the Legislative Commission on Autism requested that the Autism Society of Indiana work toward the re-creation of a plan. The result has been a state plan that brings together numerous autism organizations, university programs, provider agencies, and state agencies across Indiana, such as Indiana Department of Education, Riley Hospital, Autism Society of Indiana, and so on. The group meets monthly and provides the opportunity for agencies to move forward on common goals. A challenge for this group is the lack of funding to fulfill the activities of the plan. However, it is a plan that can serve as a boilerplate for each agency as it develops business plans.

In the late 1980s, there were few statewide or university-based programs that addressed the needs of those on the autism spectrum. As a result, IRCA staff began hosting a meeting at the national conference of the Autism Society to allow university and statewide programs to share information and coursework information. This group formed under the name of the Network of Autism Training and Technical Assistance Providers (NATTAP). The group would meet annually at the Autism Society conference to update each other on activities. A directory was created that described each program in more detail. This allowed members of NATTAP to refer professionals and family members to programs in their state. Beginning in 1993, this program was codirected by Dr. Barbara Becker-Cottrill from the Autism Training Center at Marshall University and Dr. Cathy Pratt from IRCA. In the late 1990s, NATTAP was recognized as a formal program under the Autism Society. What is significant is that this group has allowed members to gain access to strategies and resources across the country. And, although the autism team leaders in Indiana serve as a tremendous statewide network, the NATTAP partners have provided a national network of like-minded professionals who share a common goal. What is significant is that these collaborations have provided the opportunity for national initiatives and efforts to be brought to Indiana. And in every sense, IRCA has a national infrastructure that both supports and informs its efforts.

In addition, IRCA staff serve on committees, task forces, and work groups locally, statewide and nationally. This allows us to continue to learn from new initiatives and to be in touch with the realities that families and individuals with ASD face. One of these national initiatives was the National Professional Development Center on Autism Spectrum Disorders. It was a multistate federal grant that focused on implementing evidence-based practices in schools. Serving on the advisory board of this grant provided IRCA with the opportunity to be one of the first of 12 states to receive technical assistance of this grant. The goals were to implement evidence-based practices in schools and to measure outcomes by determining whether students achieved individualized education program goals. As such, IRCA staff have moved toward a coaching model that promotes universal design in the use of evidence-based practices. Students with and without disabilities have benefited from this program. An important lesson that IRCA staff have learned from this grant is that often we confuse activities with outcomes. IRCA staff train more than 20,000 professionals and family members a year. Our web site gets around 5 million hits a year. We spend hundreds and thousands of hours via e-mail, phone calls, and direct consultations connecting with families and individuals on the spectrum. However, this project has helped us to better articulate the need for focusing on the tangible outcomes of our activities. Increasing numbers are not the important outcomes; changes in lives are. We will use the lessons learned from this grant to inform future practices.

Through the years, IRCA has had many partners that have contributed to achieving important goals in Indiana. These partners include Easter Seals Crossroads, Logan Center, The Arc of Indiana, Autism Society of Indiana, Indiana Council of Administrators in Special Education, Riley Child Development Center, and many others. Perhaps our most important collaborators have been the other centers at the IIDC. Although there are seven centers with different areas of focus, each of us contributes to the process of change that other centers can build upon.

CHALLENGES AHEAD

As the country faces economic crises, IRCA continues to try to address the needs of individuals across the life span and in all settings. Web sites, social networking, and other technology provide options for us to reach a greater audience. At the same time, we must remain mindful of those who technology has left behind. Although many are using modules, podcasts, and webinars, IRCA staff realizes that strategies are often not truly implemented with fidelity without coaching and ongoing support. Technology expands, but IRCA staff also realizes the importance of the relationships that are nurtured through conversation and direct interaction. As an organization, we realize the need to continue to reinvent and challenge ourselves. New programs will continue to be added as they fit within our mission and become relevant: For example, IRCA became engaged in training for first responders and has worked with police, fire, and other emergency departments; has created a self-directed club, called Students on the Spectrum at Indiana University, that is staffed by IRCA, and provides a support organization for university and college students; was part of the creation of a research and social skills clinic in conjunction with the Indiana University School of Education that allows students to receive training in assessment strategies and in conducting social skills; and topics have become more diverse to address sexuality and interpersonal skills of individuals on the spectrum. The reality that we face is that more individuals are being diagnosed and that some of this population is aging. Some present with multiple or complex issues, such as mental illness. No easy answers will be possible. And, although this increase is dramatic, we are only beginning to see the impact this increase of ASD will have on our adult service agencies. As with all organizations, IRCA will need to work in collaboration with agencies, build local infrastructures, promote policies that create opportunities for families and individuals, and be responsive to the changing political and economic climate. The goal is to stay true to our overarching beliefs. Although our activities may change and shift, we will continue to strive to insure that all individuals statewide regardless of the economic level, race, location, or any other factors have access to high-quality services. Indeed, this has been our driving force for more than 25 years.

REFERENCES

Indiana Institute on Disability and Community. (n.d.). *Mission, values statement, and guiding principles.* Bloomington, IN: Author. Retrieved from http://www.iidc.indiana.edu/index.php?pageId=37

Indiana Institute on Disability and Community. (2011). *Indiana resource center for autism.* Bloomington, IN: Author. Retrieved from http://www.iidc.indiana.edu/styles/iidc/defiles/2011IRCAIU.pdf

9

Regional Autism Intervention Program and Related Research Activities at McMaster Children's Hospital in Ontario

Jane Summers, Jo-Ann Reitzel, and Peter Szatmari

The Autism Spectrum Disorder Program at McMaster Children's Hospital (MCH) provides assessment, treatment, and consultation services to children and youth with an autism spectrum disorder (ASD), along with their families and caregivers. MCH, which is located in Hamilton, Ontario, is one of the top pediatric academic health science centers in Canada and the second busiest children's hospital in the province of Ontario. The hospital was founded in 1988 and serves a broader community of more than two million people. More than 140,000 children and their families receive services annually from the hospital.

The origin of specialized services for children with ASD can be traced back to 1984, when an intensive preschool program and regional diagnostic service was started for a small number of children with pervasive developmental disorder (PDD) in what was then known as Chedoke-McMaster Hospitals. It is worth noting that up until the establishment of this preschool program, there were no children diagnosed with autism. All children basically received a diagnosis of "developmental disability" and were treated on a functional basis, not a diagnostic one. In other words, their level of functioning in a variety of developmental domains was identified and a treatment program devised that focused on areas of significant delay. Once services that were targeted to a diagnosis became available, then the number of children with autism increased dramatically; today, more than 400 children and youth are in one of the autism treatment programs. Initially, children in the so-called PDD Program received individualized treatment geared specifically toward improving their social-communicative functioning. This usually took place in community day care programs or preschools once the children graduated from the hospital-based program. Parent training and education for community service providers were additional components of the program.

In 1990 services were expanded to include school-age children and adolescents with ASD up to the age of 18 years. This made the McMaster program the only one in Canada that provided services to children and youth with ASD from the point of diagnosis until adulthood. A multidisciplinary team was established to provide input from child psychiatry, developmental pediatrics, psychology, speech-language pathology, and early childhood education. In addition to direct intervention for preschool-age children, the team provided assessment and treatment services to growing numbers of older children with ASD in close collaboration with their families and community service providers.

The ASD programs currently in place at McMaster include 1) the ASD Pathway Service (the evolution of the PDD Program described earlier), 2) the Hamilton-Niagara Regional Autism Intervention Program, and 3) the ASD School Support Program. These are all funded by the Ontario Ministry of Children and Youth Services, which has responsibility for a variety of programs and services for children up to the age of 18 years, including early child development and children with special needs such as autism and developmental disabilities. We discuss each of these programs in turn, but begin by describing the provincewide Intensive Behavior Intervention (IBI) initiative. We then set the Hamilton-Niagara Regional Autism Intervention Program in the context of the provincewide IBI initiative and discuss other ASD-related programs at MCH.

THE ONTARIO INTENSIVE BEHAVIOR INTERVENTION PROGRAM

Responding to pressure from parents and professionals for access to evidence-based early intervention, the Ontario government announced plans in 1999 to implement a provincewide publicly funded initiative to provide IBI to children with autism who were between the ages of 2 and 5 years. Although initially conceived as a pilot project, it was to become the largest and most comprehensive IBI program in the world (Perry et al., 2008). The government plan called for high-quality assessment and intervention services to be delivered by a network of regional programs throughout the province. Preschool-age children with a diagnosis of autism or a disorder that would be considered "toward the more severe end of the autism spectrum" (Ontario Ministry of Community, Family and Children's Services & Integrated Services for Children Division, 2000, p. 8) were eligible for the program, and could receive IBI until they entered school at the age of 6 years. Services were to begin as soon as possible after children received a diagnosis. A "direct funded option" was also available to families who preferred to hire their own private therapy team using government funds that were administered through regional programs. Parents always had the choice to fund their own program of intervention, although this could run into hundreds of thousands of dollars.

Program guidelines specified that intervention was to be provided by staff who were trained in the principles of applied behavior analysis (ABA) and closely supervised by psychologists with extensive clinical experience in IBI for young children with autism. More recently, many IBI programs have begun to hire Board Certified Behavior Analysts (BCBAs) or individuals who are eligible for certification, and are encouraging their staff to pursue the necessary education and certification. At the same time, Ontario is developing a certification process and certifying body for behavior analysts.

Services were required to be intensive in nature (at least 20 hours of direct intervention per week), based on up-to-date scientific evidence, comprehensive in scope (addressing multiple domains of children's development), and linked with existing community supports. Moreover, there was an expectation that children in the IBI program would demonstrate "measurable gains and improvements by age six" (Ontario Ministry of Community, Family and Children's Services & Integrated Services for Children Division, 2000, p. 6). Program evaluation was identified as a key component of the Ontario initiative, and regional programs were mandated to provide statistical and clinical data to the provincial government to enable them to assess, among other things, children's short- and long-term outcomes in IBI in relation to factors such as their pretreatment characteristics and the timing, intensity, and duration of IBI. Although the intent of the program has been to work toward a common standard of care, there are nonetheless important differences between the programs offered by different regions.

Many challenges had to be overcome in the initial phases of implementation of the Ontario program, not the least of which was to recruit and train large numbers of frontline therapists and supervisory staff to ensure that high-quality IBI services were delivered consistently across the province. A private agency was initially contracted to develop a teaching curriculum and train large numbers of staff at the nine regional centers across the province. Training consisted of didactic instruction (classroom lectures and a knowledge-based written exam) and hands-on practice working with children. Successful completion of training was dependent upon therapists achieving a passing score on the written exam and on a live evaluation of their implementation of individualized IBI/discrete trial teaching programs. After the first 2 years of the provincial program, the responsibility of training and evaluating new therapists was shifted to the regional programs.

There have been many positive developments since the start of the Ontario program. Government funding to provide services to children and youth with ASD and their families increased from $44 million to $158 million over a 5-year period. The ASD School Support Program was started in 2004 to provide consultation to school boards about the educational needs of their students with ASD. In 2007, more than 1,400 children with ASD received IBI and many more children have done so in the past. The service system has been expanded to assist children and families while waiting for IBI and during and after their discharge from the program. By highlighting the needs of individuals with ASD in general, the IBI program has led to the creation of other training and employment opportunities that have boosted capacity for diagnostic and intervention services. This includes the grant assistance program that provides financial support to staff from autism intervention programs at publicly funded agencies who want to pursue educational opportunities to improve their credentials and qualifications. Due to the requirement for programs to provide assessment and intervention data to the government, opportunities for researchers to conduct large-scale evaluations of treatment effectiveness have also been created.

Soon after its inception, the Ontario IBI program started to engender intense public interest and government scrutiny. As a result, social, legal, and political forces have played a major role in shaping the program, not always to its benefit. The government removed age as a criterion for discharge from the program in 2005 as a result of a court decision (which was subsequently overturned by the Superior Court of Ontario) arising from a class action lawsuit over IBI because of the requirement that it end by age 6. Without clear discharge criteria or a specified limit on the duration of IBI, children can now stay in the program much longer. This has decreased the capacity of the system to absorb new referrals, and resulted in a dramatic increase in the waiting lists for services. Increased government funding has helped to reduce these waitlists, but the program's initial goal—to provide early intensive intervention to preschool-age children during critical periods of their development—has become more elusive, and its empirical base of support more tenuous.

Other important changes have yet to be fully implemented. In 2006 the government established an expert clinical panel for the autism intervention program. The panel was given the task of developing a set of clinical practice guidelines to assist IBI service providers to make consistent and transparent decisions about children's continuation in or discharge from the program. The panel recommended in 2007 that more precise inclusion criteria for the IBI program be developed to supplant the criteria that only those "at the severe end of the spectrum" be served because a review of the treatment literature showed that in fact these children made the least progress. For those admitted to IBI, the panel recommended the use of clinical benchmarks that could be used to monitor children's progress in IBI and to provide a means to evaluate whether they had achieved expected benefits in the program and should continue or be discharged. Accordingly, the Benchmark Development Expert Committee was formed in 2007 to operationalize these clinical benchmarks and reported its recommendations in 2008. These recommendations have not yet been implemented by IBI service providers because they are still awaiting endorsement by the government.

AUTISM SPECTRUM DISORDERS PROGRAMS AT MCMASTER CHILDREN'S HOSPITAL

Hamilton-Niagara Regional Autism Intervention Program

In 2000 MCH at Hamilton Health Sciences was selected by the Ontario provincial government as the lead agency to provide IBI to eligible children whose families lived within the geographic boundaries of the Hamilton-Niagara Region of Southern Ontario. Within the region, four agencies were contracted to deliver IBI services to children in their respective local communities under the leadership of MCH. Since the early 2000s, the program has been expanded to include pre-IBI (child and family support services), post-IBI (transition support services), and school support services that collectively make up the autism intervention program. A flowchart summarizing these programs is provided in Figure 9.1.

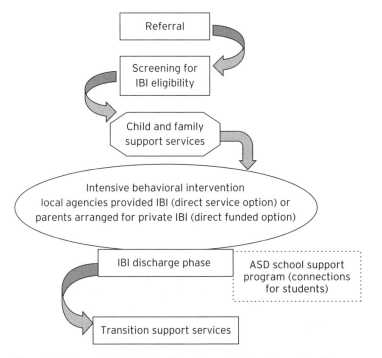

Figure 9.1. Care path for the Hamilton-Niagara Autism Intervention Program. (*Key:* IBI, Intensive Behavior Intervention; ASD, autism spectrum disorder.)

Referrals and Eligibility Children are typically referred to the IBI program after undergoing a diagnostic assessment in their local community; however, decisions about which children are eligible for the program are made at the regional level for consistency. In order to be screened for eligibility, the child must live within the geographic boundaries of the local agency and have received a diagnosis of an ASD from a qualified professional. Once a child is referred for screening, the waitlist coordinator meets with the family to provide an orientation to ASD services and arranges to observe the child, either at home or in another setting such as a day care or at school. At a subsequent clinical appointment, a psychometrist from the regional program conducts an assessment of the child's adaptive functioning using the Vineland-II Adaptive Behavior Scales, Second Edition, Survey Interview Form (Sparrow, Cicchetti, & Balla, 2005), confirms the clinical diagnosis, and evaluates the severity of the child's symptoms. At the same time, the waitlist coordinator gathers information about the child's language, imitation, and play skills during a semistructured play session. This information is reviewed by the regional eligibility committee to determine whether the child meets the criteria for admission to the IBI program.

Once children are deemed eligible for the IBI program, they are placed on a waiting list until a therapy spot becomes available in their local community. Within its first year of operation, the regional IBI program received more than 200 referrals. Approximately 70% of all children with an ASD who are referred for IBI are determined to be eligible for the program and the waitlist has grown steadily over the years. In some localities within the region, children have waited up to 2 years to receive IBI, and about 80% of families are on a waitlist for at least a portion of their care.

While on the waitlist, families are offered child and family support services. These include a variety of services (individual or group intervention, consultation and parent education) provided by a speech-language pathologist, behavior therapist, and/or an early childhood educator to help enhance their children's skill development, address problem behaviors, increase their knowledge about their children's disorder, and assist them to gain access to different types of supports. Although every effort is made to maximize these services for the families who are on the waitlist, these services often fall far short of the intensity the families seek. Some children do not receive services until they are 6–7 years of age, at which point they may become less responsive to treatment.

Intensive Behavior Intervention Once children come to the top of the waiting list, parents can choose to receive IBI through their local program ("direct service option") or to obtain government funding to purchase the services of a private therapy team ("direct funded option"). Four different agencies are contracted by the Hamilton-Niagara Regional IBI Program to provide the direct-service option. Each of these four agencies hires its own administrative and IBI staff to implement teaching programs for the children in its community. IBI teams function in a similar manner across the region and are staffed clinically with one senior therapist for approximately seven instructor therapists and an equal number of children. The senior therapist is responsible for conducting curriculum and behavioral assessments, developing and modifying children's teaching and behavior programs, supervising the implementation of programs by the instructor therapists, meeting with parents regularly to review children's goals and progress and to provide them with training in the principles of applied behavior analysis. At the parents' request, the senior therapist may share IBI reports with school staff and observe children in class to obtain information about school-related expectations and behavior. In the event that school staff would like to observe children in IBI sessions, the senior therapist helps to facilitate this arrangement. An individualized service plan (ISP) is developed for each child and family and is updated every 3–6 months.

Instructor therapists carry out IBI and parent coaching programs under the direction of the senior therapist. They are in direct daily contact with families and caregivers and share information about the children's health and other factors that may impact therapy such as scheduling changes. When not working directly with children, they prepare programming material and data summaries for the senior therapist. An instructor therapist can work with one child at a time or provide small group instruction. IBI sessions can be implemented in a variety of locations (center, home, and/or a community setting such as a day care) but are not permitted to take place within schools. In order to accommodate the 20 or more hours of therapy per week that children are required to receive while in IBI, most children who attend school do so on a part-time basis. In the last year, more than 80 children received IBI through the regional program. This translates into approximately 80,000 hours of direct therapy provided. This figure does not reflect indirect hours, which include supervision, program development, report writing and feedback, goal setting with parents, preparation of data summaries, parent training, and travel if sessions are held outside of the center.

Within the regional IBI program, intervention is conceptualized as occurring along two dimensions or spectra (see Figure 9.2). One dimension of the model encompasses a continuum of teaching approaches, ranging from discrete trial instruction (DTI) at one extreme to activity-based interventions at the other extreme. DTI is often used in the initial stages of IBI to strengthen children's key learning skills such as attention, motivation, and compliance as well as specific classes of behavior that include verbal and motor imitation and visual discrimination skills. Verbal behavior (VB) methods can build on DTI to focus more on language and related skills, using teaching methods that are often more natural than DTI but that nonetheless incorporate essential components of ABA such as reinforcement, prompting, and task analysis. Activity-based teaching approaches become more important for the development of broader skills such as language, play, and socialization, especially in more natural contexts during later phases of the program.

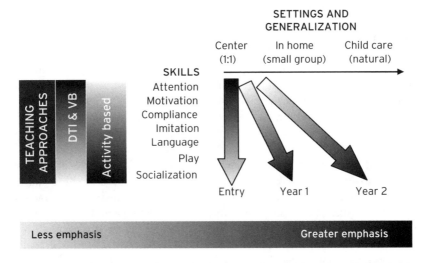

Figure 9.2. Hamilton-Niagara Intensive Behavior Intervention: 2-Spectra Treatment Model. (*Key:* DTI, discrete trial instruction and VB, verbal behavior.)

The other dimension of the model pertains to settings and children's generalization of skills across different people, environments, activities, and material. At one end of this continuum, center-based intervention involves specific staff and carefully controlled environmental arrangements that may initially include a reliance on one-to-one instruction. Intervention in community settings incorporates a diverse range of individuals and circumstances. Many different combinations of teaching approaches and settings are possible, allowing for maximum flexibility and individuality when designing children's treatment programs. For most children, however, early learning goals such as motivation, compliance, and attention will likely be the initial focus of a center-based program relying more heavily on DTI and VB, eventually building toward the use of activity-based methods in community-based programs to teach more complex social and play skills. In all cases, decisions about the nature, scope, and setting of children's IBI programs are based on data from IBI sessions and curriculum and psychometric assessments that are conducted at regular intervals.

Composition and Role of the Regional Team   A regional team that includes an executive director, clinical director, and manager provides leadership to the entire IBI program at MCH (see Figure 9.3). The team develops and implements administrative and clinical policies, performs a number of centralized functions (e.g., making eligibility and discharge decisions), and initiates an independent review process when parents do not agree with clinical decisions. The executive director and manager are part of the management structure within MCH and are also connected with their administrative counterparts in the other regional programs throughout the province. The clinical director is a Ph.D.-level registered psychologist who holds a faculty appointment within the Department of Psychiatry and Behavioural Neurosciences at McMaster University. The clinical director is responsible for ensuring that all clinical services—including those provided directly by MCH staff and those provided by agencies contracted by the program—are delivered in a manner that is consistent with program guidelines and that conform to ethical and professional standards for psychological services. Other members of the MCH regional clinical team consist of the clinical supervisors (also registered psychologists who hold university-level faculty appointments), clinical coordinators (master's level, BCBA), psychometrists, and the training coordinator.

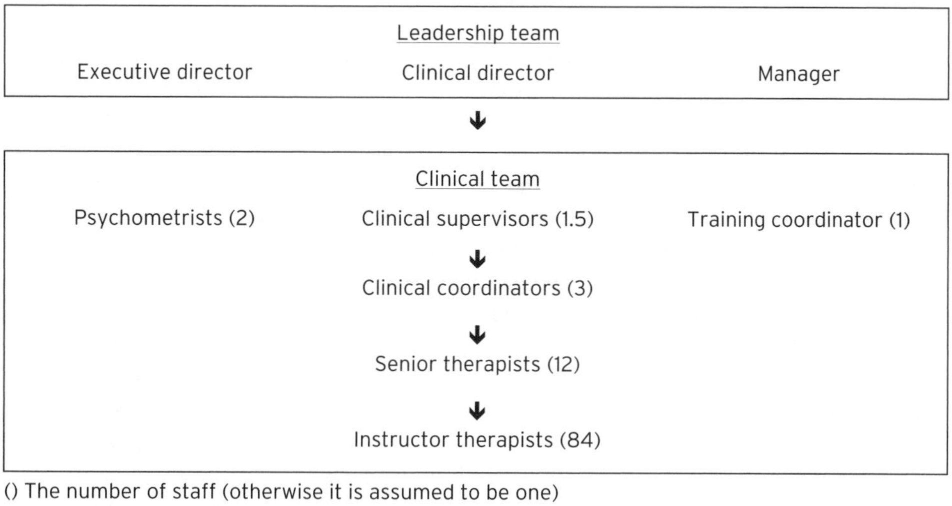

() The number of staff (otherwise it is assumed to be one)

Figure 9.3.   Regional team for Intensive Behavior Intervention, direct service option.

Psychometrists conduct standardized assessments of children's cognitive, adaptive, and/ or language functioning at predetermined time points (entry to and exit from the IBI program and every 6 months during IBI), under the clinical director's supervision. This assessment information is combined with data from children's IBI programs into a comprehensive, integrated report that is presented to families by members of the children's clinical team every 6 months. These clinical data are used to evaluate children's response to IBI, assist with treatment planning, and make decisions about when discharge from the program should occur.

Clinical coordinators work under the direction of the clinical supervisors and are responsible for overseeing the provision of IBI by teams within all four local agencies. The regional trainer works with all newly hired instructor therapists who must each successfully complete the IBI training program. The training program consists of daily quizzes and a written exam along with a live evaluation of therapists' skills implementing teaching programs. A yearly evaluation is also completed to ensure that staff continue to meet expectations. The trainer joins with clinical coordinators and senior therapists to train parents in the use of behavior analytic approaches so they can be more active participants in their children's IBI and also provides staff training to assist with ongoing professional development and support new clinical initiatives.

The clinical standards team was developed by the clinical director to ensure that consistent, high-quality, and equitable services are provided across the region in accordance with government guidelines for IBI programs. The regional team gives input to the clinical director concerning the development and potential impact of new policies and models of service delivery. The clinical director in turn is able to bring a provincial perspective to the discussions by virtue of being a member of a network that consists of the clinical directors from all nine regional programs.

Transition Support Services   Transition support services are notified when a decision is made to discharge children from the IBI program. The transition coordinator (who has a background in behavioral consultation) meets with families to provide an overview of the service, explaining that it is consultative in nature, geared toward family goals at home and in the community, and is available for up to 1 year following discharge from IBI. If parents are interested in pursuing services, the transition coordinator arranges to observe children during IBI sessions and obtain information about their treatment goals and teaching programs. Once children have been discharged from the IBI program, the transition coordinator works with families to prioritize their needs and develop a schedule for consultation visits. Transition support services may be very specific and short-lived in nature, such as assisting a family to apply for recreational programs or summer camps. Other goals may require ongoing involvement, such as assisting parents to continue to teach self-help and functional communication skills to their children or to help them deal with problem behaviors. Visits by the transition coordinator may occur frequently at times (as often as every 1–2 weeks) or occur on an as-needed basis at the request of the parent. Parents are informed about educational workshops that are offered on a variety of topics, and opportunities for both children and their parents to participate in transitional groups (such as a functional skills group) are made available. Transition support services are an important "step down" from IBI and assist parents to make the adjustment from very intensive to consultative services. Beyond this point, children are eligible for services from the ASD Pathway team and continue to be followed by their developmental pediatrician or child psychiatrist up until their 18th birthday.

Autism Spectrum Disorder Pathway Service

To our knowledge, the present ASD Pathway Service is the only diagnostic-specific program in the province that follows children from the point of diagnosis until their 18th birthday, when they enter the adult service system. Children who are initially referred to McMaster Children's Hospital go through a central intake process to identify their clinical and service needs and are assigned to a physician who coordinates their plan of care. The diagnostic process typically involves a physician (developmental pediatrician or child psychiatrist) who may utilize information from other disciplines and request additional assessments. Once a child has received a diagnosis of an ASD, he or she becomes a Pathway client and remains with the service until being discharged from the hospital.

Pathway services are organized into preschool and school-age groups. Parents are provided information about the IBI program and may choose to have their child screened for eligibility (more detailed information is provided in the section on IBI). Preschool-age children who are not eligible for IBI or whose parents do not wish to be considered for the program may receive services from a speech-language pathologist to address communication issues, or from an early childhood educator to address behavioral issues at home, in day care, or in preschool. Some children with ASD are with the "preschool" team until they turn 6 and formally enter school (school attendance is not mandatory in Ontario until the year during which children turn 6). Other hospital-based services may be used as needed, including neurology, genetics, physiotherapy, and occupational therapy.

Once they enter the school system, children and youth are linked to the ASD team within their respective school boards and receive therapeutic and assessment services at school (Ontario and other provinces have retained parallel catholic and non-catholic publicly funded school "boards," or districts). The Pathway team consults directly to families of school-age children about behavioral issues at home and in the community and helps link them with additional services and supports. Medical, mental health, and social work services are available to families of children from both age groups. Speech and language services are provided by the school system and not the Pathway team, which results in some discontinuity in services. The Pathway team serves more than 200 clients annually.

School Support Program

The ASD School Support Program was created provincially in 2004 by the same ministry that funds the regional Autism Intervention Programs. At the request of local school boards, consultants from the program can provide educators with information about effective, evidence-based teaching strategies for students with ASD, including ABA approaches. Until the announcement of the new Connections for Students Program in 2009, consultants were not permitted to provide services to identified students with ASD. The Connections Program is jointly mandated by the Ministry of Education and the Ministry of Children and Youth Services, and provides for School Support consultants who help to coordinate the transition in programming from IBI to school. These consultants act as a bridge between the ABA specialists in the school boards and staff in the IBI program to assist children who are being discharged from IBI to school. The School Support Program at McMaster Children's Hospital serves more than 7,000 professionals annually.

AUTISM SPECTRUM DISORDER RESEARCH ACTIVITIES AT MCMASTER CHILDREN'S HOSPITAL AND MCMASTER UNIVERSITY

One of the key components of the McMaster program is the integration of clinical service, research, and training for health care professionals. This is possible due to the close linkages among the hospital, university, and the Offord Centre for Child Studies. Some of the internationally renowned research to come out of the program has focused on the basic causes, characteristics, and outcomes associated with ASD. This includes investigations of the diagnosis of Asperger syndrome (Szatmari, Archer, Fisman, Streiner, & Wilson, 1995), and longitudinal studies of high functioning children with autism and other types of pervasive developmental disorder (Starr, Szatmari, Bryson, & Zwaigenbaum, 2003; Szatmari, Bryson, Boyle, Streiner, & Duku, 2003). Other research has examined developmental trajectories of children with ASD (Szatmari et al., 2009) and sought to identify susceptibility genes for autism (Liu, Paterson, Szatmari et al., 2008; Szatmari et al., 2007).

Other lines of research have developed specifically to address the needs of children in the IBI program, particularly children with ASD who are older when they start treatment and are more severely impaired. These children have often been excluded from research on the effectiveness of IBI, and so little is known about variables that may predict their response to treatment. In one study (Reitzel et al., 2012), children's mastery of skills on the Early Learning Measure (a tool developed by Smith, Eikeseth, Buch, & Lovaas [1995] to assess verbal and motor imitation, expressive labels, and receptive instructions) predicted their overall adaptive functioning and communication skills after 12 months of IBI. This finding is important because a full cognitive assessment can be difficult to complete for some of these children, especially prior to IBI. By contrast, the Early Learning Measure was relatively quick and easy to administer, and all children could be evaluated successfully. A better understanding of the relationship between children's early learning characteristics and developmental outcomes could improve efforts to identify children who are responding slowly to intervention. This could also help identify other strategies to help these children learn more effectively, or criteria for shifting the focus toward improving their functional independence and basic communication skills.

Along these lines, a randomized controlled trial (Reitzel et al., 2012) is currently underway to evaluate the effectiveness of a functional skills group intervention for children who do not benefit from IBI or are not likely to benefit from IBI. Children in the treatment group participate in a functional skills training group once a week over a 16-week period. They receive individualized and group instruction that is geared toward improving their functional communication and self-help skills and reducing problem behaviors. Parents meet with a parent coach each week to review principles of applied behavior analysis and how they can be used to teach functional skills to their children. They also have an opportunity to observe the group and to implement teaching strategies with their child while a therapist provides assistance and feedback. A secondary area of interest is whether parents who participate in the functional skills group have less stress and a greater sense of personal competency than parents of children in the control group.

Two recent studies to come out of MCH that involve children with Angelman syndrome, a neurogenetic disorder that often overlaps with autism, may be informative in relation to children in the IBI program. The first study provides evidence that discrete trial instruction (DTI) can be used successfully to teach functional skills to children with Angelman syndrome who have severe cognitive, speech, and motor impairments (Summers & Szatmari, 2009). The second study demonstrated the utility of a training manual for enhancing parents' ability to implement ABA procedures to teach a new skill to their child with Angelman syndrome (Summers & Hall, 2008). Taken together, these two studies provide information that can help in the development of services for children with ASD and severe impairments.

Since the early 2000s, there has been unprecedented interest in ASD in the province of Ontario. The Autism Spectrum Disorder Program at McMaster Children's Hospital, with its strong traditions of service, innovation, and discovery, will continue to play an important role in enhancing the lives of children and youth with ASD.

REFERENCES

Benchmark Developmental Expert Panel. (2008, September). *The development of benchmarks for the delivery of intensive behavioural intervention for children with autism spectrum disorders in Ontario.* Autism Ontario web site. Retrieved from www.autismontario.com

Expert Clinical Panel. (2007, September). The development of clinical practice guidelines for the delivery of intensive behavioural intervention for children with autism spectrum disorders in Ontario. Unpublished report to the Ministry of Children and Youth Services.

Liu, X.Q., Paterson, A.D., Szatmari, P., & the Autism Genome Project Consortium. (2008). Genome-wide linkage analyses of quantitative and categorical autism subphenotypes. *Biological Psychiatry, 64,* 561–570.

Ontario Ministry of Community, Family and Children's Services & Integrated Services for Children Division. (2000). *Program guidelines for regional intensive early intervention programs for children with autism.* Toronto, Ontario, Canada: Author.

Perry, A., Cumming, A., Dunn Geier, J., Freeman, N.L., Hughes, S., LaRose, L., . . . Williams, J. (2008). Effectiveness of Intensive Behavioral Intervention in a large, community-based program. *Research in Autism Spectrum Disorders, 2,* 621–642.

Reitzel, J., Summers, J., Szatmari, P., Zwaigenbaum, L., Georgiades, S., Duku, E., & Lorv, B. (2012). A pilot randomized control trial of the Functional Behavioural Skills Training Group for young nonverbal children with severe autism. Manuscript in preparation.

Reitzel, J., Summers, J., Vaccarella, L., Frei, J., Duku, E., Lee, D., . . . Lorv, B. (2012). Early learning measure as a predictor of adaptive outcomes for children with autism and intellectual disability after 12 months of Intensive Behavioral Intervention. Manuscript in preparation.

Smith, T., Eikeseth, S., Buch, G., & Lovaas, I. (1995). Early Learning Measure. Unpublished test available from first author.

Sparrow, S.S., Cicchetti, D.V., & Balla, D.A. (2005). *Vineland-II Adaptive Behavior Scales: Survey forms manual* (2nd ed.). Circle Pines, MN: AGS Publishing.

Starr, E., Szatmari, P., Bryson, S., & Zwaigenbaum, L. (2003). Stability and change among high-functioning children with pervasive developmental disorders: A 2-year outcome study. *Journal of Autism and Developmental Disorders, 33*(1), 15–22.

Summers, J., & Hall, E. (2008). Impact of an instructional manual on the implementation of ABA teaching procedures by parents of children with Angelman syndrome. *Journal on Developmental Disabilities, 14*(2), 26–34.

Summers, J., & Szatmari, P. (2009). Using discrete trial instruction to teach children with Angelman syndrome. *Focus on Autism and Other Developmental Disabilities, 24*(4), 216–226.

Szatmari, P., Archer, L., Fisman, S., Streiner, D.L., & Wilson, F. (1995). Asperger's syndrome and autism—Differences in behavior, cognition, and adaptive functioning. *Journal of the American Academy of Child and Adolescent Psychiatry, 34*(12), 1662–1671.

Szatmari, P., Bryson, S.E., Boyle, M.H., Streiner, D.L., & Duku, E. (2003). Predictors of outcome among high functioning children with autism and Asperger syndrome. *Journal of Child Psychology and Psychiatry, 44*(4), 520–528.

Szatmari, P., Bryson, S., Duku, E., Vaccarella, L., Zwaigenbaum, L., Bennett, T., & Boyle, M.H. (2009). Similar developmental trajectories in autism and Asperger syndrome: From early childhood to adolescence. *Journal of Child Psychology and Psychiatry, 50*(12), 1459–1467.

Szatmari, P., Paterson, A.D., Zwaigenbaum, L., Roberts, W., Brian, J., Liu, X.Q., et al. (2007). Mapping autism risk loci using genetic linkage and chromosomal rearrangements. *Nature Genetics, 39*(3), 319–328.

10

The University of Utah and the Utah Department of Health

Collaborating to Implement Community-Based Systems of Care for Children with Autism Spectrum Disorder

Paul S. Carbone, Sarah Winter, Harper Randall, and Judith M. Holt

A strong partnership between academia and public health has led to improvements in community systems of care for children with autism spectrum disorder (ASD) and their families in Utah. In this chapter we begin by describing the mission, structure, and function of the University of Utah Division of General Pediatrics and the Children with Special Health Care Needs (CSHCN) Bureau of the Utah Department of Health. Several aspects of these two programs have led to collaboration on initiatives designed to build systems of care for children with ASD. We highlight two of these. The first provides training and support to medical homes to implement surveillance and screening programs specific to ASD. The second is a statewide network of multidisciplinary evaluation clinics for children who are identified as being at risk. Because the average age of diagnosis of ASD in the United States is significantly older than the age at which intervention is available and effective (Autism and Developmental Disabilities Monitoring Network, 2009; Dawson et al., 2010), the overall goal of these two initiatives is to achieve early identification through universal screening and access to multidisciplinary diagnostic teams. These programs will ensure that the newest generation of children with ASD will have every opportunity to reach their potential.

OVERALL MISSION, STRUCTURE, AND FUNDING

University of Utah, Division of General Pediatrics

Many of the initiatives and activities for the early identification, diagnosis, and ongoing care of children with autism in Utah involve the faculty of the Division of General Pediatrics (DGP) at the University of Utah. The leadership of the division has a strong focus and skill set in CSHCN. Therefore, the faculty has become, both through recruitment as well as interest, leaders in the field of developmental disabilities. Strong relationships with partnering agencies as well as other departments of the university have enhanced the ability of the faculty to carry out the special activities related to children with ASD, which are described in this chapter.

The University of Utah Department of Pediatrics has a three-part mission: service, education, and research. The DGP emphasizes all three parts in its activities surrounding ASD and related disabilities. The division chief for the last 17 years has long been a champion of CSHCN. The expression of this interest has been the pursuit of grants related to CSHCN, the development of programs to serve these children, and recruitment of faculty with either board certification or special focus in their care. Given the geographic location of Salt Lake City and its surrounding population, the university's Department of Pediatrics and its facility partner, Primary Children's Medical Center, provide the only comprehensive medical care system for children in Utah and parts of four nearby states. Of the 17 faculty members in the Division of General Pediatrics, 6 have expertise in developmental pediatrics. Working in a variety of settings, described in detail next, these individuals play leadership roles in the initial evaluation, diagnosis, and ongoing care of children suspected of having an ASD. They are also involved with colleagues at the university and at other institutions in research regarding ASD and in advocating for improved and expanded services.

The Division of General Pediatrics is the administrative home of the Utah Pediatric Partnership to Improve Healthcare Quality (UPIQ) (University of Utah Department of Pediatrics, 2010). UPIQ is a collaborative effort to promote evidence-based best practices and assists physicians in implementing quality improvement at the practice level. Support comes from both private and public funds. The director of UPIQ is the chief of the DGP. As of 2012, 40% of the pediatricians in Utah and a growing number of family medicine physicians and dentists have been involved in UPIQ projects. In 2010 UPIQ organized a learning collaborative for dentists to assist them providing a dental home to children with ASD. Later in this chapter we describe a UPIQ project to improve early identification and referral of children with an ASD within the medical home.

Also housed in the DGP is the Medical Home Portal (www.medicalhomeportal.org), a web site that aims to help families, physicians, and others find reliable information and access to valuable professional and community resources to improve the care, health, and long-range outcomes of CSHCN, including families and providers of children with ASD (The Medical Home Portal, 2010). The portal is unique in its focus on both primary care physicians and families and in integrating comprehensive information about local resources. It has extensive information on ASD, their diagnosis and treatment. The portal includes more than 420 content pages, more than 800 links to other valuable sites, more than 600 scientific citations, and receives more than 7,000 visits per month. Funding for this effort is both public and private with medical direction provided by the DGP chief.

Utah Department of Health, Children with Special Health Care Needs Bureau

The CSHCN Bureau resides within the Utah Department of Health. With the Maternal and Child Health Bureau, the CSHCN Bureau is the Title V agency for Utah. These two bureaus receive funding through the Maternal and Child Health Block Grant, a public health program that reaches across economic lines to improve the health of all mothers and children. The goals of the block grant funding are to build capacity and systems, conduct public education and outreach, train providers, and provide support services for CSHCN.

The mission of the CSHCN Bureau is to facilitate access to comprehensive, community-based, culturally effective and appropriate health care and related services for Utah children and youth with special health care needs. The bureau serves children and youth, from birth to age 18, who have developmental delays and physical and emotional disorders. The services provided for children with ASD and other developmental disabilities are divided into direct clinical services and nonclinical services and programs.

Children with Special Health Care Needs Bureau Structure

The bureau is located on the University of Utah campus, literally a short walk from Primary Children's Medical Center, a large tertiary care children's hospital that serves Utah and surrounding intermountain states. The location provides an ideal opportunity for collaboration with the University of Utah Department of Pediatrics and the Division of Child and Adolescent Psychiatry. In addition, the bureau houses ample clinic space, allowing University of Utah physicians convenient access to clinics for children with ASD and other developmental disabilities. For the developmental clinics in Salt Lake City, nurses/care coordinators, physical and occupational therapists, audiologists, speech therapists, and child psychologists are housed within this same building and provide ready access to these services.

Direct Clinical Services

Children with chronic illnesses or disabling conditions need access to community-based systems of care, which include a medical home, specialty services, and other formal and informal supports. Because of the complexity, families need support in navigating this system in order to gain access to the services they need. The CSHCN Bureau offers support in the form of specialty and multidisciplinary diagnostic clinics for those with developmental delays. The clinics bring together teams of specialists, minimizing the challenges families face in gaining access to them separately and fostering collaboration in the diagnostic process.

The Child Development Clinic: Located within the bureau in Salt Lake City, the Child Development Clinic provides comprehensive diagnostic evaluations for children from birth to age 8. The multidisciplinary team is highly skilled in providing comprehensive evaluations for young children with a suspected ASD. Several psychologists, for example, are trained in the administration of autism diagnostic tests such as the Autism Diagnostic Observation Schedule (ADOS; Lord et al., 1989). Pediatricians are skilled in evaluating for medical conditions associated with ASD and can refer on to specialists in neurology or genetics as needed. Other members of the multidisciplinary team (audiology, speech and occupational therapy, and social work) perform evaluations and provide treatment plans. The goal of the clinic is to provide timely comprehensive evaluations and to coordinate these services with the medical home and local agencies. The waiting time for a new evaluation at the time of this writing is between 1 and 2 months, significantly less than in many parts of the country.

The CSHCN Satellite Clinics: A lack of local specialized pediatric services for children with complex health care needs living in rural areas presents an access barrier to needed health care services. To address this need, the CSHCN Bureau provides multidisciplinary clinics for families that live in and around eight rural communities in Utah. Most locations hold clinics three to four times per year and provide comprehensive evaluations and assistance with ongoing care for children, birth to 18 years old, with developmental disabilities. These satellite clinics offer a statewide system of community-based care for approximately 2,400 CSHCN and their families. All but one location requires transportation of contracted physicians and staff to be transported via state planes. The satellite clinics are described in detail later in this chapter.

Nonclinical Autism Spectrum Disorders–Related Services and Programs

In addition to providing direct clinical services the CSHCN Bureau provides leadership and oversight to a number of diverse programs that support the health of children with ASD and other developmental disabilities.

ASD System Development: The CSHCN Bureau provides state leadership to bring together the many agencies and advocates who influence the statewide system of services for children with ASD and their families. The bureau hosts the Utah Autism Initiative (UAI) Committee, a multi-agency, governor-appointed workgroup that advises the state legislature on issues pertaining to autism. The medical director of the CSHCN Bureau is an active participant with the Autism Council of Utah, an independent council working to foster collaboration, communication, and learning among families and agencies. The state-funded Utah Registry for Autism and Developmental Disabilities (URADD) collects and manages prevalence data on Utah children with ASD and other developmental disabilities. Under the direction of URADD, Utah is 1 of 14 sites that constitute the national Autism and Developmental Disability Monitoring (ADDM) Network. Administered by the Centers for Disease Control and Prevention, the ADDM Network is providing population-based estimates of the prevalence rates of autism and related disorders in different sites over time (Centers for Disease Control and Prevention, 2010).

Autism Infrastructure Grant, Health Resources and Services Administration/ Maternal and Child Health Bureau
In September 2008 the CSHCN Bureau received funding as the lead agency for an ASD systems development project entitled "Utah's State Plan for Improving Outcomes for Individuals with ASD and Developmental Disabilities." This plan is the product of a collaborative effort from parents of children with ASD and key individuals representing state agencies that serve children with ASD and other developmental disabilities. The activities under this plan address five identified needs: infrastructure development, early identification and diagnosis, children and youth services, adult services, and research. The first phase of this grant has allowed Utah to implement a number of initiatives including establishing family navigators throughout the state, providing support for Utah's Family-to-Family Health Information Center, and providing medical and dental home training to 24 practices across the state.

Utah Regional Leadership Education in Neurodevelopmental Disabilities
The Utah Regional Leadership Education in Neurodevelopmental Disabilities (URL-END) Program is a collaboration of the CSHCN Bureau, the Center for Persons with Disabilities at Utah State University, and the DGP at the University of Utah. Funded by an MCHB Leadership grant, URLEND provides opportunities for students and professionals from a variety of health-related disciplines to increase their leadership knowledge and advocacy skills for the provision of services for children with developmental disabilities. Trainees participating in URLEND rotate through the multidisciplinary clinics held at the bureau and benefit from the teaching of faculty that staff the clinics.

Funding
Current and recent funding to support clinical services for CSHCN clinics is shown in Figure 10.1. The recent downturn in the economy has resulted in cuts in state funding over the last several years and federal funding has been slowly declining over the last four years, making the continuation of these essential clinics an ongoing challenge. The CSHCN Bureau director has been active in educating members of the state legislature of the benefits of clinical services delivered by the CSHCN Bureau. Several federal grants support the other services and programs for children with ASD and other developmental disabilities described earlier.

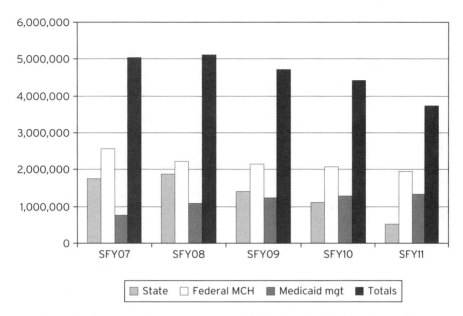

Figure 10.1. Funding sources for Children with Special Health Care Needs Bureau direct clinical services. (*Key:* MCH, Maternal Child Health block grant; SFY, State Fiscal Year.)

INITIATIVES

Early Autism Detection and Referral in the Medical Home

The American Academy of Pediatrics (AAP) has advocated for a "medical home" for all CSHCN. Rather than simply a place to receive primary medical care, the medical home represents a process of primary care that emphasizes comprehensive medical treatment that is fully integrated with other community systems, insuring coordinated care that is tailored to meet the needs of the child and family ("The Medical Home," 2002). Nationally, parents of children with ASD are less likely than parents of children with other disabilities to report a medical home model of primary care. More specifically, they perceive that the care their children receive does not meet all their needs, is not coordinated with the rest of the treatment team, and that a partnership in decision making is lacking (Brachlow, Ness, McPheeters, & Gurney, 2007). Among Utah parents of children with ASD, we identified similar dissatisfaction with primary care services, especially in the area of recognition of early signs. Parents perceived that physicians dismissed their initial concerns about behavior and development, resulting in delays in diagnosis. In the same study, Utah pediatricians acknowledged the importance of listening to parent concerns and moving away from a "wait and see" approach to developmental concerns, yet most do not adhere to recent AAP recommendations for universal autism screening of toddlers at 18 and 24 months (Carbone, Behl, Azor, & Murphy, 2010). These national and local data provided a rationale for undertaking a project to improve the quality of early identification within the medical home as a central theme within Utah's State Plan for Improving Outcomes of Children with ASD.

In 2009, the UPIQ designed and began implementation of a learning collaborative (LC) titled "Early Autism Detection and Referral in the Medical Home." The LC utilized established methods of quality improvement, such as Plan-Do-Study-Act cycles (Institute for Healthcare Improvement, 2010), that had proven successful during previous LCs on obesity prevention, asthma management, and preventive services (Young, Glade, Stoddard, & Norlin, 2006). The primary goal of the project was to improve surveillance and screening for ASD within medical homes located in Utah. A secondary goal was to improve ongoing care within the medical home following a diagnosis of an ASD. The specific aims of the project included 1) improve developmental surveillance by participating primary care providers by reviewing the early signs of autism and teaching age-specific probes that can be incorporated into everyday practice, 2) perform screening for ASD at all 18- and 24-month visits, 3) develop a registry of children identified as at risk for ASD, 4) implement a medical home approach for children with ASD and their families by implementing a parent-driven goal, and 5) increase provider knowledge of community resources for families of children with ASD.

Structure   The project will last 3 years and will include three separate 6-month LCs involving 32 primary care practices in Utah. Year 1 participants included eight pediatric practices located in the Salt Lake City area. Year 2 participant practices, located farther outside of Salt Lake City, are a mixture of eight pediatric and family medicine practices. Year three practices will target 12 family medicine practices located in rural and frontier areas of Utah. Each practice team includes a physician, a nurse or medical assistant, an office manager, and a parent partner. Each member of this team is crucial to the success of the LC. Physicians are necessary to perform the ASD surveillance and screening during health supervision visits and to provide leadership for the project. The office manager provides administrative support and linkage between UPIQ staff and the practice throughout the LC. The nurse or medical assistant might assume a number of roles such as distribution of screening tools and providing case management support. The parent partner is typically a parent of a child with an ASD within the practice. As users of "the system" parents keep the team focused on practical goals that are family-focused, provide passion to sustain effort, and provide the accountability for the team to deliver on promises. Each practice team maintains contact with the UPIQ staff throughout the LC during monthly site visits and conference calls.

During the LC, UPIQ staff provides the knowledge and experience of the process of quality improvement, expertise in the primary care of children with ASD, and the tools and incentives to help practices achieve the desired outcomes. The UPIQ Director is responsible for oversight of all aspects of the LC and UPIQ staff. The project coordinator (PC) is a quality improvement specialist with an MBA. The PC oversees planning and development of each LC and provides ongoing support to each practice team. The consultant physician (CP) is a general pediatrician with expertise in the evaluation and ongoing care of children with ASD. The CP provides technical advice in the planning, development, and implementation of the LC and works with the UPIQ Director to evaluate the LC. The family liaison (FL) is the director of the Utah Family-to-Family Network, housed within the Utah Department of Health. The FL ensures that the UPIQ team incorporates family-centered goals and practices into the LC, recruits family partners for practice teams, and supports family partners throughout the LC.

Potential participant practices were recruited via e-mail invitations to pediatric and family medicine providers located within the area of the upcoming LC. Pediatricians are offered Maintenance of Certification credit required by the recertification process of the American Board of Pediatrics. Parent partners were offered a small stipend to compensate for their time and travel/child care expenses. With these incentives in place, the recruitment process has been a success.

Intervention　Each practice team received training on medical home strategies, information about and the rationale for ASD surveillance and screening, and basic concepts of quality improvement at a daylong learning session. Presentations by UPIQ staff reviewed the rationale for ASD surveillance and screening and the system-level challenges in implementation of an ASD screening program. Instructive cases, video examples, and extensive input from parents of children with ASD about their experiences within primary care allowed detailed and meaningful exploration of each topic. The learning session also provided practice teams time to formulate specific plans on implementing the goals of the LC. The implementation phase of the LC began with completion of the daylong learning session The learning session was followed by ongoing support during monthly site visits and conference calls. The in-office medical home training provided by the PC places an emphasis on practice-level systems that support the care of CSHCN. Examples include longer appointment times and care coordination services for children with disabilities. Monthly site visits also allowed UPIQ staff to interact with practice team members to review progress toward goals and address any current system-level challenges in implementation. Monthly 30-minute conference calls throughout the LC between UPIQ staff and practices provided an opportunity for exploration of topics not addressed during the learning session and for practices to share "lessons learned" for the benefit of other participants. Topics addressed during conference calls included management of conditions commonly associated with ASD such as sleep difficulties, the use of medications for associated psychiatric conditions and maladaptive behavior, and the importance of interdisciplinary and family-centered care.

To encourage sustainability, physicians completing the year one LC have been recruited to serve as mentors to practices participating in the second year. During the year two learning session, physician mentors will offer advice in the planning process for new practice teams and provide ongoing support throughout the LC. Physician mentors benefit from additional training with the UPIQ physician consultant and the experience of academic detailing with their peers. Archived video presentations from previous LCs, and distance technology such as video and telephone conferencing, will be utilized to address the challenge of reaching practices in rural and frontier areas during year three.

Evaluation　In order to evaluate the impact of the LC, we developed an institutional review board (IRB)–approved study with the following objectives: 1) to evaluate participating primary care providers' effectiveness in implementation of ASD-specific screening during all 18- and 24-month visits and 2) to evaluate change in participating primary care providers' perceived self-efficacy in the areas of ASD surveillance, screening, and ongoing management. The specific aims of the study are 1) to perform monthly chart audits of five recent 18- or 24-month visits to ascertain whether there is physician documentation of screening for ASD and 2) to compare responses on pre- and post-LC questionnaires completed by participating physicians. The physician questionnaire consists of two sections: 1) demographics, such as years in practice and estimated number of patients with ASD, and 2) self-perceived efficacy in providing comprehensive care for children with ASD.

Impact　This project is currently in the second of 3 years. Eight practices and 13 physicians have completed the Year 1 LC. Preliminary analysis has shown a significant increase in practice-reported screening for ASD during 18- and 24-month visits (Figure 10.2).

The increased rate of screening for ASD reported by these 13 pediatricians increased the total estimated number of screenings performed by 1,365 during the 6-month period of the LC. Registry data was received from all of the 13 participating pediatricians. According to these registries, a total of 10 children failed the screening tool used during the LC, the Modified Checklist for Autism in Toddlers (M-CHAT) at either the 18- or 24-month visit. Six more children were found to be at risk based on parent or provider concerns. Based on a previous study of the M-CHAT (Kleinman et al., 2008) and the estimated 1,950 screenings performed, approximately 13 failed screens would be expected. Thus, pediatricians that participated in the 6-month LC successfully implemented autism screening and identified the number of children that would be expected from such a screening effort. These preliminary results suggest that with practice-level support, universal screening for ASD for toddlers can be implemented in community settings.

Participating practices also qualitatively described a number of system-level changes that were made as a result of the LC. Practices reported addressing the challenge of having parents complete a screening tool for ASD in the context of a health supervision visit using different approaches. Some practices reported success with parents completing the screener in the waiting room prior to the visit while others gave it to parents upon entering the exam room. Other practices preferred to mail the screener prior to the appointment, and one experimented with completing the screen over the phone prior to the appointment. Some practices found that conducting the screenings during sick visits of 18- to 24-month-old children helped to capture those patients who might miss well visits. Practice teams reported that the parent partners were helpful in making changes that increased family-centered care. One practice implemented a "get to know me" form in which parents of CSHCN could give providers helpful information about their child's needs during office visits. Another practice made changes to the check-in procedure to accommodate children who may have a difficult time waiting or making transitions from the waiting room to an exam room. Another practice is now contacting parents of CSHCN prior to visits to identify important issues that families wish to discuss during the visit. A focus group of parents of children with

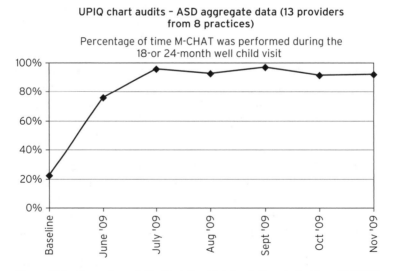

Figure 10.2. Percentage of Modified Checklist for Autism in Toddlers (M-CHAT) autism spectrum disorder (ASD) screening done at 18- and 24-month visits during the study period based on chart audits (*n* = 455). (*Key:* UPIQ, Utah Pediatric Partnership to Improve Healthcare Quality.)

ASD was conducted by another practice and found that it helped the staff better understand some of the challenges that are faced by families. Several practices formalized procedures to connect interested families of children with disabilities with each other. Another practice was able to develop the resources to hire a full-time care coordinator to work with families of CSHCN.

Barriers   Participating physicians in the Year 1 LC identified a number of barriers to universal surveillance and screening for ASD in the medical home. Some physicians questioned the utility of screening because they perceived a lack of adequate resources and qualified providers to evaluate children identified by screening. Some physicians perceived poor access to evidence-based treatments because of lack of insurance coverage and a shortage of trained treatment providers. Others believed that ASD is overdiagnosed by local evaluation clinics. The majority of physicians who participated in the year one LC report that lack of care coordination services, practice guidelines, time during visits, parental concerns about vaccine safety, and available community resources are barriers to providing comprehensive ongoing care to children with ASD.

Recommendations   This LC has addressed some important questions regarding the feasibility of universal screening for ASD within the medical home. A previous study of the M-CHAT predicted an approximate 1% failure rate in a primary care setting (Kleinman et al., 2008). Although our practices reported that screening for ASD had increased during the year one LC, the expected rate of failed screens and referrals for comprehensive evaluations was slightly less than expected. This suggests that there may be attitudinal barriers about the utility of screening on the part of primary care physicians (PCPs) and persistent system-level issues involved in properly implementing a two-step screening tool such as the M-CHAT. In speaking to pediatricians during conference calls and site visits it became clear that some either did not score the screen properly, modified the screen in ways that altered the validity, or simply did not refer children that failed screens. For future LCs, we have made changes in the content of the daylong learning session to address these issues and will more closely monitor the registry of practices during site visits so that we can give timely feedback about failed screens and referrals. We also believe that PCPs will have more enthusiasm about surveillance and screening if they perceive that a community system that offers more timely comprehensive evaluations and better access to evidence-based treatments is easily accessible.

Our experience indicates that an LC is an important step toward implementing recommended guidelines in evaluation and ongoing care of children with ASD within the medical home (Johnson & Myers, 2007; Myers & Johnson, 2007). The project illustrates the strengths of practice-level support and the meaningful changes that can occur over relatively short periods of time. By the end of the LC we hope to have created a large network of practices that are proactive in the approach to developmental concerns and are well equipped to offer comprehensive care to children diagnosed with ASD or other developmental disabilities.

The Children with Special Health Care Needs Satellite Clinics

The CSHCN satellite clinics provide comprehensive multidisciplinary evaluations of children from Utah's rural areas who are suspected of having an ASD. Although the 80% of Utah's 2,736,424 people who live along the Wasatch Front, an urban area of three counties centering on Salt Lake City, have easy access to specialists in Salt Lake City, the remaining 547,000 live in the vast expanses of the state's 84,889 square miles, much of which is designated as "frontier" (National Center for Frontier Communities, 2000). Approximately one third of Utah's residents are under 18, which is nearly 40% higher than the national average ("Utah Has Youngest Population in U.S.," 2010). It is estimated that there are approximately 180,000 children and youth in rural Utah (Utah's Indicator-Based Information System for Public Health, 2012). With a prevalence of 1 in 88 ("Prevalence of Autism Spectrum Disorders," 2012), there are approximately 2,000 children in rural Utah with an ASD. Because the number of children who identified as at risk on the basis of screening and surveillance is considerably higher, there is a substantial need to provide comprehensive, accessible diagnostic and management services for this population. The eight CSHCN satellite clinics are in place to meet this need.

For children identified at risk for ASD the satellite clinics provide all components of the comprehensive evaluation that has been recommended by the AAP:

> 1) a health, developmental, and family history; 2) a physical exam; 3) a developmental or psychometric evaluation; 4) a laboratory investigation to search for known etiology or coexisting condition; 5) determination of the presence of a categorical *Diagnostic and Statistical Manual of Mental Disorders, Fourth Edition* (*DSM-IV; American Psychiatric Association, 1994*), diagnosis, with tools that operationalize the *DSM*–criteria; and 6) assessment of parental knowledge of ASD, coping skills, and available resources and supports (Johnson & Myers, 2007, p. 1183-1215).

These components are performed by the multidisciplinary team in each clinic that consists of a pediatrician, an audiologist, a speech therapist, a physical or occupational therapist, a child psychologist, and a social worker. In addition to this core team, a pediatric neurologist, geneticist, and a transition specialist rotate through the clinics at less frequent intervals.

Each clinic lasts 2 days, with most providers staying overnight between clinic days and others flying in for 1 day. Only one clinic location (Ogden) is within reasonable driving distance (1.5-hour drive each way) of Salt Lake City. For the other seven clinic sites, the CSHCN Bureau contracts with the Utah Division of Aeronautics to provide reliable air transportation over rugged terrain and frequently challenging weather conditions. Most sites hold between three and six clinics per year, depending on the needs of the community. Appointments with each provider are at least 1 hour, allowing adequate time to address the family's concerns. At the end of each CSHCN satellite clinic day, there is a staffing session attended by the local and clinic staff and the multidisciplinary team. These sessions allow team members to discuss findings from their individual evaluations and to formulate a coordinated treatment plan from the entire team. Efforts have been made to include local medical home and educational representatives at the staffing sessions.

During the time between clinics, the local staff remains at the clinic site to provide case management for enrolled patients. Most of the CSHCN satellite clinics are housed within the local public health department with local public health employees serving as the case managers. Efforts have always been made to recruit local CSHCN satellite clinic staff from applicants that live within the communities they serve. Referrals to the CSHCN satellite clinics come from medical homes, early intervention programs, surrounding schools, and parents. The CSHCN clinic staff is responsible for performing an intake interview with the parent prior to scheduling appointments. Based on the needs identified during the intake interview, appointments are made with appropriate individual team members. Attempts are made to obtain medical and educational records prior to the patient's visit.

Support of local medical homes is an integral part of the CSHCN satellite clinics. Presently, only half of the communities served by CSHCN satellite clinics have a local pediatrician. The other communities are served by family medicine physicians and mid-level providers. Continued efforts have been made to make all medical homes in rural Utah aware of the satellite clinics and to request input from them for quality improvement efforts.

For example, in 2009 an outreach program was initiated to increase the involvement of primary care providers in the referral process. A referral form was sent to all medical homes and was made available on the CSHCN web site (Utah Department of Health, 2010). This referral form allows the PCP to provide pertinent information and to specify the concerns to the CSHCN staff, such as a failed screening test for ASD. If the referral to the CSHCN satellite clinic comes from an outside provider the form is sent to the medical home to inform the PCP that the child will be seen. Once the child has been evaluated at the satellite clinic, the form is sent back to the medical home within 48 hours, offering a brief description of findings and recommendations. A more thorough summary report is sent to the medical home and the family once transcribed, in 2–3 weeks. This process was instituted based on input from medical homes requesting more involvement and timely feedback from the satellite clinics. For the child with a newly diagnosed ASD, the transcribed reports provide a thorough description of the entire visit to the clinic and contain detailed recommendations for the local treatment team.

The CSHCN satellite clinics serve the primary purpose of providing an interdisciplinary diagnostic evaluation for children who have been identified as at risk. Once a diagnosis has been made, attempts are made to comanage issues involved in ongoing care with the medical home. More than occasionally, however, medical homes in rural Utah express that they do not have the training or experience to provide the ongoing treatment recommended from the CSHCN satellite clinic. This is particularly true in the case of utilizing medications to manage certain associated conditions in children with ASD such as sleep problems, attention-deficit/hyperactivity disorder (ADHD), anxiety, or other maladaptive behaviors. To compound this need, access to mental health providers in rural Utah is extremely limited. In these cases, children with ASD are frequently seen in follow-up at the CSHCN satellite clinics for treatment as well as to provide ongoing support for the family and the medical home. There are ongoing attempts, such as the learning collaborative described earlier, to provide education and support for providers in rural Utah that have interest in increasing self-efficacy in the long-term management of children with ASD and other developmental disabilities.

The funding for the CSHCN satellite clinics is a blend of federal, state, and private sources. The total annual budget is $1.3 million, with roughly one third of this funding coming from state government. Nonstate funding comes from the Maternal and Child Health Bureau Title V block grant and reimbursement from public and private insurance. The CSHCN satellite clinics offer a sliding scale to those being seen who show financial need and every effort is made to overcome any financial barriers that may exist for a particular family. Currently, the physicians providing services in the CSHCN satellite clinics are contracted through the University of Utah and the clinic bills insurers directly. Ancillary services such as speech and occupational therapy are provided by CSHCN Bureau employees. There are a number of ongoing challenges to providing services through the CSHCN satellite clinics. As noted earlier, a significant financial investment is necessary to maintain the quality of the clinics and funding streams can fluctuate from year to year. Due to the recent economic downturn, the CSHCN Bureau has incurred significant cuts in state funding over the last 3 years (Figure 10.1), prompting the closure of one of the CSHCN satellite clinic sites. Additionally, an ongoing commitment is required from Salt Lake City–based providers to temporarily leave work and family responsibilities to travel for 2 days to serve rural communities. Telehealth is one example of an emerging technology that is being piloted within the CSHCN satellite clinics to address the need for more cost- and time-efficient care. Despite the challenges, the CSHCN satellite clinics have been serving families in rural communities for more than 25 years. The providers who make the commitment to staff the clinic are well aware of the benefit of improved access to services that might not otherwise exist. Families receive high-quality, interdisciplinary evaluations within their community, eliminating a long drive (from 4–8 hours) and often an overnight away from family and work. The coordinators of the clinics receive multiple phone calls after each clinic from families who are thankful that they found needed support for their children without traveling long distances to find it.

REFERENCES

American Psychiatric Association. (1994). *Diagnostic and Statistical Manual of Mental Disorders* (4th ed.). Washington, DC: Author.

Brachlow, A.E., Ness, K.K., McPheeters, M.L., & Gurney, J.G. (2007). Comparison of indicators for a primary care medical home between children with autism or asthma and other special health care needs: National Survey of Children's Health. *Archives of Pediatric and Adolescent Medicine, 161*(4), 399–405.

Carbone, P.S., Behl, D.D., Azor, V., & Murphy, N.A. (2010). The medical home for children with autism spectrum disorders: Parent and pediatrician perspectives. *Journal of Autism and Developmental Disorders, 40*(3), 317–324.

Centers for Disease Control and Prevention. (2010). *The Autism and Developmental Diseases Monitoring Network.* Retrieved from http://www.cdc.gov/ncbddd/autism/addm.html

Dawson, G., Rogers, S., Munson, J., et al. (2010). Randomized, controlled trial of an intervention for toddlers with autism: The Early Start Denver Model. *Pediatrics, 125*(1), e17–e23.

Health Resources and Services Administration. (2010). National Survey of Children with Special Health Care Needs 2005–2006: Utah CSHCN data. Retrieved from http://mchb.hrsa.gov/cshcn05/SD/utah.htm

Institute for Healthcare Improvement. (2010). Testing changes. Retrieved from http://www.ihi.org/IHI/Topics/Improvement/ImprovementMethods/HowToImprove/testingchanges.htm

Johnson, C.P., & Myers, S.M. (2007). Identification and evaluation of children with autism spectrum disorders. *Pediatrics, 120*(5), 1183–1215.

Kleinman, J.M., Robins, D.L., Ventola, P.E., et al. (2008). The modified checklist for autism in toddlers: A follow-up study investigating the early detection of autism spectrum disorders. *Journal of Autism and Developmental Disorders, 38*(5), 827–839.

Lord, C., Rutter, M., Goode, S., Heemsbergen, J., Jordan, H., Mawhood, L., & Schopler, E. (1989). Autism diagnostic observation schedule: A standardized observation of communicative and social behavior. (Research Support, Non-U.S. Gov't.) *Journal of Autism and Developmental Disorders, 19*(2), 185–212.

The medical home. (2002). *Pediatrics, 110*(1 Pt. 1), 184–186.

The Medical Home Portal. (2010). Retrieved from http://www.medicalhomeportal.org/

Myers, S.M., & Johnson, C.P. (2007). Management of children with autism spectrum disorders. *Pediatrics, 120*(5), 1162–1182.

National Center for Frontier Communities. (2000). 2000 update: Frontier counties of the United States. Retrieved from http://www.frontierus.org/2000update.htm

Prevalence of autism spectrum disorders—Autism and Developmental Disabilities Monitoring Network, 14 sites, United States, 2008. (2012). *Morbidity and Mortality Weekly Report. Surveillance Summaries, 61*(3), 1–19.

Prevalence of autism spectrum disorders—Autism and Developmental Disabilities Monitoring Network, United States, 2006. (2009). *Morbidity and Mortality Weekly Report. Surveillance Summaries, 58*(10), 1–20.

University of Utah Department of Pediatrics. (2010). *Utah Pediatric Partnership to Improve Healthcare Quality.* Retrieved from http://medicine.utah.edu/upiq/

Utah Department of Health. (2010). *Children with special health care needs.* Retrieved from http://www.health.utah.gov/cshcn/index.html

Utah Has Youngest Population in U.S. (2010, June 13). *Deseret News.*

Utah Regional Leadership Education in Neurodevelopmental Disabilities. Retrieved from http://urlend.org/

Utah's Indicator-Based Information System for Public Health (IBIS-PH). (2012). Retrieved from http://ibis.health.utah.gov

Young, P.C., DeBry, S., Jackson, W.D., et al. (2010). Improving the prevention, early recognition, and treatment of pediatric obesity by primary care physicians. *Clinical Pediatrics, 49*(10), 964–969.

Young, P.C., Glade, G.B., Stoddard, G.J., & Norlin, C. (2006). Evaluation of a learning collaborative to improve the delivery of preventive services by pediatric practices. *Pediatrics, 117*(5), 1469–1476.

11

Autism and Tertiary Behavior Support Through the Kansas State Department of Education

Developing Collaborative Teams for Identification and Consultation

Lee Stickle and Sarah Hoffmeier

The Technical Assistance Statewide Network Autism and Tertiary Behavior Support (TASN/ATBS) operates with funding provided by a Title VI-B grant administered by the Kansas State Department of Education's Special Education Services Division. TASN/ATBS, formerly known as the Neurologic Disabilities Support Project, was funded in 1987 to provide training and technical assistance in the area of traumatic brain injury (TBI) and attention-deficit/hyperactivity disorder (ADHD). In 2000, autism spectrum disorder (ASD) was added to the project's areas of emphasis. Currently, TASN/ATBS is part of the TASN. TASN/ATBS is a statewide network that serves public and private schools by providing training and technical assistance to educators, related service providers, parents, and community service providers. Since 2000, TASN/ATBS has been charged with extending these services to providers of school-age (3–21 years old) children; however, in 2009 a concerted effort was made to increase the collaboration of school-age services and services provided to children birth to 3 years old. In Kansas, services to the birth to 3-year-old populations are under the direction of the Kansas Department of Health and Environment rather than the Kansas State Department of Education. Through this collaboration significant strides have been made in the development and implementation of a statewide plan with regard to the training of providers who serve children with ASD and those who are suspected of having ASD by implementing evidence-based practices (EBP) as defined by the National Professional Development Center on Autism Spectrum Disorders (National Professional Development Center on Autism Spectrum Disorders, 2012).

Kansas is the 17th-largest state in the nation with a population of 2,818,747—the 33rd-largest based on population. Kansas has 290 school districts covering 105 counties, and 94 of the 105 are classified as either rural or frontier counties. Most of its population—93%—lives in 10% of the counties. Kansas has more rural and frontier counties now than it did 100 years ago. The rural nature of the state creates some challenges in service delivery

(Kansas Department of Health and Environment, Bureau of Community Health Systems Kansas Primary Care Office, 2012).

TASN/ATBS offers a number of services: training, consultation, program review, and diagnostic services for Part C networks and both public and private schools. The training offered encompasses a variety of formats (e.g., face to face, Interactive Television Network, webinars). Consultative services take a variety of forms as well (e.g., on-site visit, telephone, e-mail, or video conferencing). Program review is provided upon request and involves both the review of records and on-site visits to assess the implementation of EBP.

There is significant variation in delivery models throughout the state. In many cases delivery models are dictated by population; however, since TASN/ATBS has been providing training and consultation, the number of districts using EBP has increased significantly (Stickle, 2011). Students with ASD in Kansas are served in a multitude of settings, including the general education classroom, class within a class, special education resource classrooms, self-contained programs, special day schools, and in residential placements. The IEP team, based upon the needs of the student, determines programming needs and services, which are then to be delivered in the least restrictive environment. All of TASN/ATBS's services are available to staff, families, and students regardless of the setting.

Training is an essential component of TASN/ATBS. It is our task to develop an infrastructure of statewide support for teachers who instruct students with ASD and ensure sustainability of that system. To that end, we have developed a variety of training opportunities and we divide our trainings geographically. We provide statewide training for our autism interdisciplinary teams (AIT) and autism diagnostic teams (ADT). These trainings occur two times per year at locations that are chosen to ease the travel burden for participants. The AIT model that is used is based upon the model developed and described by Tyler in the article "Improving Educational Services for Students with ABI Through Statewide Consulting Teams" (Glang, Tyler, Pearson, Todis, & Morvant, 2004). The ADT Model is one developed by TASN/ATBS and the University of Kansas Medical Center's Center for Child Health and Development (KUMC-CCHD). TASN/ATBS provides regionally based trainings eight times per year in the area of transition, assessment, and communication supports. District-level training is developed through a district improvement plan (DIP). The DIP includes a survey of needs, an inventory of local resources, and the identification of resources beyond the local district. Once that information is gathered, an annual plan is developed to provide high-quality professional development in EBP. In addition, TASN/ATBS also offers a 1-week Summer Institute each year designed to introduce educators to the principles of structured teaching. The Summer Institute is unique because in addition to the 1 week "hands on" experience educators have with students, TASN/ATBS also provides three follow-up visits in participant's classrooms.

Training offered by TASN/ATBS incorporates the principles of implementation research described by Fixsen in *Implementation Research: A Synthesis of the Literature* (Fixsen, Naoom, Blase, Friedman, & Wallace, 2005). Training is essential in improving outcomes for children with ASD. The 2006 Kansas Legislative Post Audit Report indicated that 60% of teachers in Kansas were 40 years or older; given the recent surge in the number of students with ASD, it is logical to assume those educators beginning their career prior to the surge seen between 1997 and 2010 have little preservice training in the area of ASD.

Kansas, like many rural states, has had a difficult time extending diagnostic services to rural and medically underserved communities. In February 2008, the Association of University Centers on Disabilities (AUCD) in conjunction with the Centers for Disease Control and Prevention (CDC) began holding regional summits to bring key state leaders from the early intervention and the early childhood community together for the purpose of enhancing relationships and collaborations among key stakeholders and providing a forum to share information and insights on the opportunities, challenges, and barriers for families and children with ASD and related disabilities in the identification, assessment, diagnosis, and intervention areas. As a result of that summit, TASN/ATBS and the KUMC-CCHD collaborated to develop and pilot a system of screening and diagnostic services in medically underserved areas. The prevalence rate of ASD in Kansas lags behind those that have been seen nationwide. Between the years of 1992 and 2008 the number of children (6–22 years of age) identified and reported to the Kansas Department of Education as having an ASD increased 2,312%, yet the prevalence rate for public schools in Kansas is 1 in 219, significantly behind the national prevalence rate of 1 in 110 children (Kansas State Department of Education, Special Education Services, 2010).

Consultation is another service provided by TASN/ATBS. The majority of requests for consultation come from smaller school districts that do not have autism specialists on staff. TASN/ATBS responds to approximately 700 requests for consultation each year. Each request for consultation is addressed based on five guiding questions:

1.   What is the desired outcome?

2.   What are the strengths and needs of the student?

3.   How does the ASD present in the student?

4.   What resources can be brought to bear?

5.   What are the capacities of the systems involved to change and adapt?

When we identify answers to these questions we are much more likely to develop a plan that will be successful. TASN/ATBS based these questions upon the information presented by the State Implementation and Scaling-up Evidence-based Practices Project (SISEP). The intensity of support provided is determined based upon the needs of the student, staff, and care providers, and is provided in the school setting.

TRAINING: IMPROVING OUTCOMES THROUGH APPLYING THE EVIDENCE-BASED PRACTICE WITH FIDELITY

The Kansas State Department of Education (KSDE) has been focusing on the development of capacity to serve students with ASD at the local level for 10 years. During that time, training models have been tested; many have failed. In early 2008, KSDE required all projects to read and discuss *Implementation Research: A Synthesis of the Literature* (Fixsen et al., 2005). Given the information presented, TASN/ATBS developed an entirely different approach to training and evaluation of training. We had stumbled into a common pitfall; we were training beyond our capacity to support and evaluate. Since that time we have divided our training into two categories: knowledge and skill. The majority of our knowledge-based training involves the use of online training modules from a variety of sources or from narrated PowerPoint presentations provided to participants. The acquisition of knowledge is determined through pre- and posttests that the participants take. Knowledge, unlike skill, has little to do with the change of practice; traditionally, one-time training can be effective in the dissemination of information but has shown to be ineffective in changing practice. In order to change outcomes for students, it is imperative that we change the practice of service providers. To that end, we have changed our evaluation of the effectiveness of training to focus on how participants have implemented the training that they have received rather than what they "thought" of the training. We gather that information using an online survey and we survey our participants at the 4-, 12-, and 24-week intervals following training. We are looking for the extent to which participants have implemented the information and the sustainability of the change. We engage in the most rigorous follow-up on the trainings that provide the greatest opportunity for skill building.

TASN/ATBS provides a weeklong, hands-on training for educators in the area of Structured Teaching. In order to attend the training, participants must complete the application process, which includes a portion that must be filled out by the applicant's administrator. In order to be considered for the training, the applicant's administrator must agree to support the classroom with materials necessary to implement the principles of structured teaching, and the administrator must allow other educators from their region to visit the classroom. In addition, both the administrator and the applicant must agree to a minimum of three follow-up visits by TASN/ATBS staff and to attending three1-hour follow-up webinars. Once all applications are received, they are divided into the eight educational regions from which they are located. TASN/ATBS has guaranteed that each region who applies will have an applicant chosen. Once the applicants are divided into regions, each application is scored on a rubric. Those applicants with the top scores are notified of their acceptance pending the completion of four online modules (ASD Characteristics, Communication, Person Centered Planning, and Assessment), submission of photographs of their current classroom, and a copy of their school calendar. Once all prerequisites have been met, participants are provided with the logistical information they need to make hotel reservations, and arrive at the training site.

The training site actually has two simultaneous events occurring. One is the training for the participants; the other is a classroom for the children staffed by master teachers. Each of the master teachers is someone who has had extensive training in structured teaching and has been observed implementing the principles of structured teaching by TASN/ATBS staff.

Once on-site, participants are provided information in a lecture format, followed by activities designed to put that information to use immediately with students with ASD. For example, the first day of training includes a quick review of the characteristics of ASD, followed by an activity in which the participants go into the classroom, observe a student for 15 minutes, and record the characteristics of autism that the individual displays. Once they return to the lecture hall, a guided group discussion takes place. At the end of the first day, each of the participants is divided into groups of five; each group is assigned a student for the week and provided with information about that student. Group members have roles to fulfill and each day the roles are rotated. The roles include

- The Facilitator who is to work with the student directly and to make sure that group members are involved in the decision-making process

- The Note Taker, who is to record the discussion and decisions of the group

- The Reporter, who is to share the group's decisions

- The Follow-up Person, who makes sure that any products that are to be made are completed and that the home communication notebook is ready to go home with the student

- The Time Keeper, whose job has proven to be the most challenging, keeps the group on schedule

In addition, group members observe the student during lunch time. Each group is assigned a TASN/ATBS staff member, who is available to answer questions, provide feedback and coaching, and fill in missing information about the student. Throughout the week, physical structure, individual schedules, independent work systems, visual structure, communication, and leisure/social skills are addressed. Each lecture is followed by an activity designed to provide the participant with the opportunity to observe the classroom and the opportunity to restructure and/or develop the component covered in the lecture. Once the group has completed the activity, the master teacher provides feedback and coaching. Each group meets with the master teacher who is working with the student to which they are assigned two times each day in addition to the time that they spend with them in the demonstration classroom. The meetings take place during lunch and at the conclusion of the day.

Once the participants have completed the training, they meet with the TASN/ATBS staff member who is assigned to them to complete the follow-up visits. Prior to leaving the training site, the three follow-up visits are scheduled, the fidelity check document is shared and the criterion for each visit is discussed. TASN/ATBS staff has a timeline in which to complete the visits. The first visit must be completed by October 1, and, on that visit, the staff is determining the extent to which the participant has physically structured the classroom and has developed an overall classroom schedule. A copy of the completed fidelity checklist is then shared with the participant, building principal, and the district's special education director. Suggestions for improvement are made and progress toward the implementation of the principles of structured teaching is noted.

Once the first visits have been completed for all participants, the TASN/ATBS staff meets to determine what the follow-up training needs of the participants are to cover in the webinar. Each subsequent visit follows the same pattern; the participants know what the staff member is evaluating and is aware of what products, if any they need to make available. The follow-up trainings are related to any pattern of deficit that is noted by the TASN/ATBS staff; training information and activities are developed and presented in the webinar. This training model follows what the implementation research has shown; select the very best people you can find (application), make sure that they will be supported by their system (administrators' portion of the application), ensure that they are all arriving with a core of knowledge (prerequisite modules), provide them with information and activities, give them a chance to demonstrate the skill, provide feedback (coaching) in the classroom, and evaluate the outcome (feedback loop). The subsequent fidelity checks follow the same pattern, with the expectations clearly identified, the checklist is shared well before our visits, and administrators are kept in the loop. Our follow-up training is always designed based upon our findings during visits.

The commitment to the implementation research has proven to be worth the effort. A review of fidelity checklists provides the following data: 88% of those that attended the training implemented the principles of structured teaching with fidelity; 92% of participants stated that the training changed the way that they teach; 88% indicate that their classroom data show improvement in behavior and performance. For those teachers who have developed model classrooms and whose administrators identify as leaders in their schools, we extend an invitation to intern with a master teacher the following summer. Interns' responsibilities include differentiating lessons for the students, developing materials, and they have the opportunity to work with a variety of students with coaching from the master teacher. The intern program allows us to provide advanced training to the very best of the previous training year's participants. We then have a larger pool from which to select our master teachers.

TRAINING/DIAGNOSTICS: BUILDING COLLABORATIVE TEAMS BETWEEN THE EDUCATION AND MEDICAL COMMUNITY

In late 2008, TASN/ATBS and KUMC-CCHD began a joint venture to extend diagnostic services to medically underserved areas. These areas present with a common set of barriers to quality diagnostic services. First, there is a significant lack of developmental pediatricians. Second, diagnosticians are not equipped to provide a multidisciplinary approach to diagnostics. Third, Kansas law does not require insurance to cover the costs associated with diagnostic/intervention services for people with ASD (Golnik et al., 2009).

In most rural and frontier areas of Kansas, medical services are provided by family practice physicians and/or physician assistants. At this time, the American Academy of Family Physicians has not adopted the American Academy of Pediatricians Recommendations with regard to autism spectrum disorders. These guidelines include the following.

American Academy of Neurology and the Child Neurology Society, Clinical Practice Recommendations

1. Developmental surveillance should be performed at all well-child visits from infancy through school age, and at any age thereafter if concerns are raised about social acceptance, learning, or behavior.

2. Recommended developmental screening tools include the Ages & Stages Questionnaires, the BRIGANCE Screens, the Child Development Inventories, and the Parents' Evaluations of Developmental Status.

3. Because of the lack of sensitivity and specificity, the Denver-II (DDST-II) and the Revised Denver Pre-Screening Developmental Questionnaire (R-DPDQ) are not recommended for appropriate primary-care developmental surveillance.

4. Further developmental evaluation is required whenever a child fails to meet any of the following milestones: babbling by 12 months, gesturing (e.g., pointing, waving bye-bye) by 12 months, single words by 16 months, two-word spontaneous (not just echolalic) phrases by 24 months, or loss of any language or social skills at any age.

5. Siblings of children with autism should be monitored carefully for acquisition of social, communication, and play skills and the occurrence of maladaptive behaviors. Screening should be performed not only for autism-related symptoms but also for language delays, learning difficulties, social problems, and anxiety or depressive symptoms.

6. For all children failing routine developmental surveillance procedures, screening specifically for autism should be performed using one of the validated instruments.

7. Laboratory investigations, including audiologic assessment and lead screening, are recommended for any child with developmental delay and/or autism. Early referral for a formal audiologic assessment should include behavioral audiometric measures, assessment of middle ear function, and electrophysiologic procedures using experienced pediatric audiologists with current audiologic testing methods and technologies. Lead screening should be performed in any child with developmental delay and pica. Additional periodic screening should be considered if the pica persists.

(Centers for Disease Control and Prevention [CDC], 2006)

As a result, they have not incorporated into their practice the same rigorous standards for developmental surveillance that are recommended and practiced by developmental pediatricians. Without adequate surveillance and screening, many children with developmental delays are late in being identified as having special needs. In May 2009 Shattuck reported that most children diagnosed with an ASD are not diagnosed until they are nearly 6 years old. Current research would indicate that that is more than 3 years later than the children who could reliably be identified. In 2005, Mandell, Novack, and Zubrisky found that children living in rural areas received a diagnosis of an ASD on average 0.4 years later than children in urban areas. In addition, the same researchers found that "near-poor" children were diagnosed 0.9 years later than children who were 100% above the poverty line (Mandell & Novak, 2005). The conclusions the researchers drew from their findings include the following: "many physicians have limited knowledge of the presentation, prognosis, and treatment of ASD." The conclusions that Mandell, Novack, and Zubrisky reached seem to have merit in Kansas as well.

The partnership between TASN/ATBS and KUMC-CCHD is a multifaceted initiative. We needed to identify the specialties that constitute a multidisciplinary team and determine who in communities are seeing children that may be on the autism spectrum. A review of referrals to KUMC-CCHD revealed that physicians, Infant and Toddler Service Providers (Part C), community mental health, local education agencies, and Community Developmental Disabilities Organization constituted the majority of agencies that referred children for ASD evaluations. Given that information, it became clear that we needed to target those agencies for training in both screening and diagnostic measures. Although there is a significant need statewide for diagnostic services, TASN/ATBS and KUMC-CCHD's limited resources helped us to focus our training efforts in medically underserved areas of the state. Once we had determined our geographic area of emphasis, we needed to find agencies that were likely to come in contact with infants, toddlers, and children and extend the invitation to apply to attend the training. Next, we needed to create a bridge between the team and the local physician. In order to create that bridge, teams applying to attend the training must secure a letter of support from a local physician. Securing the letter from the physician is the first step in building the bridge between the service providers and the physician. In addition to making contact with a local physician, applicants must have the support of their employing agency to act as a diagnostic team once training has been completed and complete online training modules to ensure that all teams arriving at the training have a solid foundation of knowledge in ASD. Once we had those elements in place, we were ready to train the teams in the diagnostic measures that they will use to gather the information needed to present to the physician in order to make a determination of an ASD.

In accordance with the ASD protocol used at KUMC-CCHD, teams are trained by TASN/ATBS staff to administer screening tools (Childhood Autism Rating Scale, Second Edition [CARS-2] and the Modified Checklist of Autism in Toddlers [M-CHAT] and follow-up interview). KUMC-CCHD staff trains the teams in the use of a structured caregiver interview (Autism Diagnostic Interview–Revised [ADI-R]) and a structured observation (Autism Diagnostic Observation Schedule [ADOS]). Each team trained is provided with a copy of the *Caring for Children with Autism Spectrum Disorders: A Resource Toolkit for Clinicians* published by the American Academy of Pediatrics to share with the physician that provided the letter of support for the team. In addition, the Learn the Signs. Act Early. campaign materials for health care providers, early childhood educators, and parents are provided to the teams to distribute in their communities. The training notebook that teams receive includes copies of the PowerPoint slides used by presenters, example protocols to use during and after the training, report examples, consent form examples, and resources. During the training, teams are provided with case studies, including video vignettes to practice scoring the items within the assessments. Both TASN/ATBS and KUMC-CCHD staff provide feedback before and after the training. Teams are then trained on how to write the report that shares their findings with the local physician, or in the case of some of the teams, the physicians at KUMC-CCHD who will be seeing the children and their families via Telemedicine, our interactive television system. Telemedicine (Telehealth) began in 1991 with a single connection between the University of Kansas Medical Center in Kansas City, Kansas, to a community in western Kansas; the Kansas Telehealth network now has access to more than 100 sites throughout the state.

TASN/ATBS and KUMC-CCHD had developed a strict protocol regarding receiving services through the Telemedicine system. First, the child *must* be screened using an approved screening tool and the results of that screen must be positive for an ASD before being seen by the entire team. If the screening tool used is the M-CHAT, the follow-up interview must be completed prior to the team seeing the child. Once the child has been referred to the team, TASN/ATBS is to be contacted in order to track the time between positive screen, evaluation, and appointment with a physician. That data are important in that not only is the project designed to extend diagnostic services, it is also designed to reduce the time between positive screen and diagnostic services. Currently, the wait time for families to gain access to traditional diagnostic centers in the region is in excess of 6 months. Data collected since the beginning of the project reveal that the average wait time using the extended system is less than 45 days. In the first full year of the project 38 teams have been trained that cover 62 of the 105 counties in the state. The teams, referred to as ADTs, receive support from both the TASN/ATBS and KUMC-CCHD staff. Supports include provision of protocols and testing materials, letters of collaboration between the ADT and the physicians at KUMC-CCHD, and on-site coaching by highly experienced TASN/ATBS staff when administering the assessments. TASN/ATBS is responsible for securing Telemedicine appointments and finding local sites capable of providing the interactive television network connection necessary to carry out the appointment. All costs associated with the training of the teams and the Telemed appointments are covered through a grant secured from the Children's Cabinet and Trust Fund. The 1999 Kansas Legislative session created the Kansas Children's Cabinet to oversee the expenditures from the Master Tobacco Settlement. Almost all, 95%, of the funds from the Master Tobacco Settlement in Kansas are dedicated to improving the lives of children. The funding provides protocols, manuals, and training materials for each team. Test kits for the ADOS are separated by modules and sent to teams on an as-needed basis. Costs for shipping are covered by the grant as well.

This entire initiative was put together using existing resources; the teams comprise psychologists, speech and language pathologists, social workers, educators, occupational therapists, and physical therapists that are employed through various agencies that have local presence on a statewide basis. Physicians, both in the community and at KUMC-CCHD, were already in place as is the Telemed system that was established more than 10 years ago. The missing element was training and expanding the skills of the professionals in the community. The dissemination of the Learn the Signs. Act Early. materials is expedited through this project, thereby raising awareness of the cognitive developmental milestones for children and increasing the awareness of autism in rural and frontier areas within the state.

TECHNICAL SUPPORT: INTENSE SUPPORT TEAMS

During the 2009–2010 academic year, TASN/ATBS developed and implemented a new type of consultative model for public school districts in the state. According to the New Jersey Council on Developmental Disabilities, families and students may pay a high cost for special day schools or out-of-district placements. Frequently, few, if any opportunities for integration with nondisabled peers are available in such placements; in addition, access to the core curriculum is very limited. Private schools are not required to have the same professional credentials as are public schools and frequently, there is a sense of the child becoming "invisible" within his or her community because of the lack of social opportunities that neighborhood schools provide. School districts costs are measured in dollars. Based on data from the IDEAdata.org in 2000, it cost on average an additional $10,463 to educate a child in a private setting than in the public school setting. In 2003, Kansas had 229 students in private placements. On average 9% of students in private placements during the 2003 school year were diagnosed with an ASD; thus, approximately 21 students with ASD were educated outside of the public school systems. In an effort to serve students in their home schools and to build the capacity of local education agencies to serve students with significant needs, TASN/ATBS developed the concept of intense support teams (IST). School districts who have exhausted their local resources in the development of an educational program for students with ASD and as a result are considering out-of-district placement or placement of the student in a district-run special day school are encouraged to contact TASN/ATBS to access the support of an IST. Unlike other teams developed by TASN/ATBS, the IST is not standing teams; in fact, each team is developed based upon the unique and individual needs of the student and the district. An initial assessment of the child, setting, and local resources is completed by a TASN/ATBS staff member. Once the relevant information has been gathered, a team of experts is pulled together from existing statewide projects and/or higher education. Experts have included behavior analysts, speech and language pathologists, vision specialists, and so forth. The makeup of the team is driven entirely by the needs of the student and district. The focus of the team is the child; however, in order to focus on the child, training of local education agency (LEA) staff must occur. A capacity-building plan is developed and shared with the district administrative team; once they agree to the provisions within the plan, the team is scheduled to arrive on-site, complete an in-depth evaluation of the child, develop and deliver the program, and provide on-site coaching of the LEA staff to deliver the program.

The evaluation piece is critical to the success of the child. TASN/ATBS has come to rely on the Ziggurat Model developed by Ruth Aspy and Barry Grossman (2007). The Ziggurat Model offers a sequential process for addressing the complex needs of individuals on the autism spectrum. The model incorporates assessment tools designed to identify the deficits and strengths of an individual and to better understand behaviors. Interventions are then developed to target the challenges by building on strengths and established skills. A key premise of the model is that autism is a *pervasive* developmental disorder. By using the model, we are able to develop a comprehensive plan. The tiers of the model provide a framework for practitioners to utilize; each tier addresses a key component that must be considered as we plan interventions. Each student seen through the IST has a Ziggurat completed; other assessment pieces (e.g., academic, adaptive behavior) are determined based on the cognitive ability, age, and needs of the student. The gathering of this information, while time-consuming, is the foundation for the intervention team's plan. As the assessment is being completed, LEA staff is trained in the use of the assessment tools selected, thereby building their capacity to complete the process independently in the future.

Once the assessment is complete and the information is analyzed by the IST and the child IEP team, a program is developed. The program is developed exclusively using interventions identified as "Best Practices" by the National Professional Development Center on Autism Spectrum Disorders, thereby exposing LEA staff to research-based practices. Once the program is developed, IST members deliver the program for a minimum of 2 days with LEA staff observing and taking data. At the conclusion of the second day, data is reviewed and adjustments are made if necessary. The third and fourth day of intervention with the student includes the LEA staff delivering the program with coaching from the IST members. The fifth day of the intervention has the LEA team delivering the program with a minimum of one member of the IST on-site to help with troubleshooting. Progress is monitored closely for the next 12 weeks. On a daily basis, data collected by the LEA team are shared with the IST and the parent/caregiver via e-mail; adjustments are made as necessary. On-site follow-up occurs on a weekly basis for the first 6 weeks and then on a semimonthly basis for the duration of the follow-up period.

The success of the IST Model has been remarkable: 75% of the students seen have been able to remain in their public school setting, and 50% of those who remained have moved to lesser restrictive settings within their school. The resources that such intense intervention requires are significant; however, the success rate would support the use of the system.

Clearly, the IST Model does not have a 100% success rate, and the 75% rate does not take into account those districts that once presented with the plan and the Commitment Contract decided to opt for the out-of-district placement. The commitment on the part of the IST and the LEA is significant. Each Commitment Contract includes provisions for ongoing staff development and a resource list for that staff development. The involvement of the parents/caregivers is essential in the development of a comprehensive plan and a sound educational program. The unique aspect of the IST Model is that expertise is drawn from all areas of the state in order to meet the needs of not only the student, but the professionals as well.

REFERENCES

Aspy, R., & Grossman, B.G. (2007). *The Ziggurat model: A framework for designing comprehensive interventions for individuals with high-functioning autism and Asperger Syndrome.* Shawnee Mission, KS: Autism Asperger Publishing Company.

Centers for Disease Control and Prevention. (2006). *Developmental surveillance and screening.* American Academy of Pediatrics (AAP), July 2007. Retrieved from http://www.cdc.gov/ncbddd/autism/hcp-recommendations.html

Fixsen, D.L., Naoom, S.F., Blase, K.A., Friedman, R.M., & Wallace, F. (2005). *Implementation research: A synthesis of the literature.* (FMHI Publication #231.) Tampa: University of South Florida, Louis de la Parte Florida Mental Health Institute, The National Implementation Research Network.

Glang, A., Tyler, J., Pearson, S., Todis, B., & Morvant, M. (2004). Improving educational services for students with TBI through statewide consulting teams. *NeuroRehabilitation, 19*(3), 219–231.

Golnik et al. (2009). Medical homes for children with autism: A physician survey. *Pediatrics. 123*(3), 966–971.

Kansas Department of Health and Environment, Bureau of Community Health Systems Kansas Primary Care Office. (2012). *Primary care health professional underserved areas report Kansas 2012.* Retrieved from http://www.kdheks.gov/olrh/download/PCUARpt.pdf

Kansas State Department of Education, Special Education Services (2010). *FY10 prevalence.* Retrieved from http://www.ksde.org/Default.aspx?tabid=2836

Mandell, D., & Novak, M. (2005). The role of culture in families' treatment decisions for children with autism spectrum disorders. *Mental Retardation and Developmental Disabilities Research Reviews, 11,* 110–115.

National Professional Development Center on Autism Spectrum Disorders. (2012). *What are evidenced-based practices (EBP)?* Retrieved from http://autismpdc.fpg.unc.edu/content/evidence-based-practices

Stickle, L.A. (2011). Annual report of the TASN Autism and Tertiary Behavior Support Project, submitted to the Kansas State Department of Education, Grant Review Team. Unpublished manuscript.

III

Exemplary National Initiatives

12

Learn the Signs. Act Early.

The Public Health Approach to the Early Identification of Children at Risk for Autism Spectrum Disorder and Other Developmental Disabilities

Georgina Peacock, Sue Lin, Jennifer Bogin, Cheryl Rhodes, and Rebecca B. Wolf

When residents of Brick Township, New Jersey, were concerned that a seemingly large number of children in their town had an autism spectrum disorder (ASD), the Centers for Disease Control and Prevention (CDC) undertook an epidemiologic investigation of ASD prevalence there. The resulting study, published in 2001, represented an early step toward CDC's current role in ASD surveillance, epidemiology, health communication, and system enhancement.

The Brick Township study showed a prevalence of 6.7 cases of ASD per 1,000 children—a rate that fell within the range found by other studies at the time that used equally rigorous case-finding methods (Bertrand et al., 2001). Although the rate was not unusually high, the residents' concerns and the study itself focused attention on ASD and the need for reliable prevalence estimates. CDC responded by developing the Autism and Developmental Disabilities Monitoring (ADDM) Network. This network of grantees measures prevalence of ASD in a state or a part of a state, such as the five-county metropolitan Atlanta area. Each site determines ASD prevalence through assessing medical, and, in some sites, educational records, to determine the number of 8-year-old children in their catchment area with an ASD. The most recent ADDM estimate (2006) of ASD prevalence in the United States is about 1 in 110 children, or 1% (Prevalence of Autism Spectrum Disorders, 2009).

With extensive reporting of these results in the news media, CDC's pivotal role in ASD has become much more visible than it was in the days of the Brick Township study. Along with the growth of the ADDM Network, CDC's public health efforts to reduce the impact of ASD on children, families, and communities have grown to include epidemiologic research, health education and communication, and enhancing collaboration among

The findings and conclusions in this report are those of the authors and do not necessarily represent the official position of the Centers for Disease Control and Prevention/the Agency for Toxic Substances and Disease Registry.

We would like to acknowledge the contributions to the Act Early Initiative from the following people: Joseph Sniezek the Centers for Disease Control and Prevention (CDC), Bonnie Strickland and Laura Kavanagh Health Resources and Services Administration (HRSA), George Jesien, Adriane Griffen Association of University Centers on Disabilities (AUCD), all of the Act Early teams and in particular teams and leaders from the four featured states: Lee Stickle (Kansas); Regina Guarneri, Patrice Yasuda, and Patricia Schetter (California); Stephen Hooper (North Carolina); and Mary Theresa (Terri) Urbano and Frederick Palmer (Tennessee).

state-level programs and systems that serve children and families affected by ASD. This chapter will first touch briefly on each of those roles and then describe more thoroughly an example of how CDC sought to improve health communication and increase system capacity through the Act Early Initiative, with regional summit meetings and subsequent work with the Act Early state teams.

CENTERS FOR DISEASE CONTROL AND PREVENTION: THE EXAMPLE OF POPULATION-BASED HEALTH

CDC is a public health agency; as such, it focuses on improving the health of populations through communitywide health promotion efforts to prevent disease, injury, and disability. Many models of public health have been developed. The ASD work of the CDC focuses on the following three areas of public health:

- Surveillance (define the problem)

- Epidemiology and preventive research (identify causes of and ways to prevent or control the problem)

- Intervention through health communication and education (develop, test, and implement prevention strategies to encourage widespread adoption)

Surveillance

Beginning in 1996, ASD surveillance was added to the Metropolitan Atlanta Developmental Disabilities Surveillance Program. This program has monitored the occurrence of intellectual disability, cerebral palsy, hearing loss, and vision impairment among children ages 3–10 years in the five-county metropolitan Atlanta area since 1991 (Yeargin-Allsopp et al., 1992). The current ADDM network, built on this earlier effort, now funds 11 sites around the country. At each site, abstractors review 8-year-old children's medical and education records for a diagnosis of an ASD or other developmental disability as well as for mention of behavioral or educational problems that could reflect the presence of an ASD. All abstracted evaluations are reviewed by a clinician trained in diagnosis of ASD. From these records, prevalence estimates of ASD among 8-year-old children in a defined geographic area are developed. The Early ADDM network is using similar methods of data collection to determine prevalence in 4-year-old children (see www.cdc.gov/addm).

Epidemiology

Not long after CDC's National Center on Birth Defects and Developmental Disabilities was created by the Children's Health Act of 2000 (PL 106-310), Congress funded CDC to conduct research to identify potential causes of ASD and other developmental disabilities (DD). This epidemiologic research, the Study to Explore Early Development (SEED), currently conducted at six centers across the United States, is looking at factors associated with a child's risk for developing ASD, health conditions among children with and without ASD, and physical and behavioral characteristics of children with ASD, children with DD, and children without a developmental delay or disability. SEED researchers in six sites are gathering information about the prenatal and early childhood periods, blood and hair samples, and clinical information from about 3,300 children ages 2–5 years to identify risk factors associated with the development of ASD (see www.cdc.gov/seed).

Intervention

Until the causes of ASD are fully understood and can be directly addressed, the best approach to improving the lives of children with ASD and their families is to identify developmental delays as early as possible so children and families can get the services they need.

Early intervention, before age 3, can have a significant impact on a child's ability to learn new skills (Dawson, 2008; Dawson et al., 2010; Lord & McGee, 2001). However, many children with a developmental disability are not identified until after they enter school (Prevalence of Autism Spectrum Disorders, 2009). Recognizing this, and with direction from Congress, in 2003 CDC began development of a health education and communication campaign with the goal of improving early identification and referral to services for children with ASD and DD across the United States. Based on research with parents, members of advocacy groups, and health care providers, the campaign was named Learn the Signs. Act Early. (see www.cdc.gov/actearly). We now describe this campaign in more detail as an example of a health education intervention and the resulting Act Early Initiative as a potential model of systems change.

LEARN THE SIGNS. ACT EARLY.: A HEALTH EDUCATION AND COMMUNICATION CAMPAIGN

As researchers spoke with parents in focus groups across the country to understand their information needs for the new campaign, they learned that parents were hungry to know more about child development beyond the common milestones of height, weight, first steps, and first words. As part of the formative research for the campaign, focus groups with parents suggested that parents were unaware of developmental milestones—how a child plays, learns, speaks, and acts—children should reach at certain ages. Parents also said that a campaign that highlighted the term *autism* and focused primarily on warning signs of DD would be less likely to be effective than one that focused on the positive signs of development and the importance of acting on concerns. Parents of children with an ASD stated that messages explicitly about autism could be so distressing as to lead to avoidance or inaction when their child was exhibiting delay.

Thus the campaign Learn the Signs. Act Early. was born. The campaign has three goals: increase awareness of developmental milestones and early warning signs of developmental delay, increase dialogue among parents and providers about child development, and spur early action on developmental concerns. Campaign messages were developed and tested through formative research.

The campaign has three target audiences—parents of young children, early educators, and health care providers. Parents of young children are the primary audience of the Learn the Signs. Act Early. campaign. They know their children best, are in the best position to notice a delay in reaching milestones, and are motivated to both obtain further evaluation and advocate for their child to get the services he or she needs. Health care providers who serve young children and early educators (early childhood teachers and child care providers) are secondary audiences that can both help reach parents with campaign messages and materials as well as benefit from campaign information themselves. Early educators are in a unique position to monitor development because they routinely care for very young children and have regular contact with parents.

Partnering with autism advocacy groups, professional organizations, and other federal agencies was essential in developing the Learn the Signs. Act Early. health education messages and materials. CDC worked with the American Academy of Pediatrics (AAP), the Association of University Centers on Disabilities (AUCD), the Autism Society of America (ASA), Autism Speaks, First Signs, the Health Resources and Services Administration (HRSA), the National Association for the Education of Young Children, and the Organization for Autism Research. CDC worked with partners and marketing experts to design a campaign that conveyed the importance of knowing that there are developmental milestones and acting on concerns about developmental delay.

Campaign Messages and Materials

The legend, "It's time to change how we view a child's growth" (see Figure 12.1), appears on materials for parents, health care providers, and early educators to remind them that there are important ways to measure growth and development besides height and weight. Campaign materials display important developmental milestones for the social/emotional, language/communication, cognitive, and physical/motor development domains for each of the ages of well-child pediatric visits. The follow-on message, "The good news is, the earlier a delay is recognized the more you can do to help your child reach her full potential," encourages parents, health care providers, and early educators to take action if a delay is recognized.

A prominent message for health care providers is "CDC has free information to help educate parents about childhood development." A prominent message for early educators is "Every day you see them reach milestones. There are free resources to help you spot a few more."

Campaign Channels

CDC and its partners disseminate campaign messages and materials widely via traditional and nontraditional communication strategies. The campaign has appeared in mass-media vehicles such as on a billboard in Times Square, New York City, on the side of the Goodyear Blimp, and in popular television shows. CDC staff have promoted the campaign's messages and materials at myriad professional conferences through talks and exhibits. Campaign ads have appeared in popular magazines for parents and in articles for health care providers and early educators. In addition, the campaign provides widgets, buttons, and e-cards for partners to link to on their web sites. Parents of young children understanding the importance of monitoring milestones and acting early on concerns have been featured in radio, print, and television public service announcements in media markets across the country. The "Baby Steps" video, stressing the importance of these messages, is also used to educate parents about talking with their child's doctor about potential developmental delay.

To further enhance the reach of the campaign and its messages, CDC works to integrate campaign materials with other national programs that serve parents of young children and that have a mandate to or interest in providing information about child development to the communities they serve, such as Head Start, home visiting programs, and others.

Campaign Results

Since Learn the Signs. Act Early. launched in October 2004, campaign resources have been made available to more than 11 million health care professionals, parents, partners, campaign champions, and child care providers. CDC has fulfilled requests for more than 300,000 resource kits, and online materials have been downloaded from the campaign web site more than 400,000 times. The campaign web site averages more than 20,000 visits per

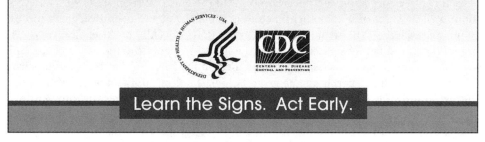

Figure 12.1. This flyer from Center for Disease Control's Learn the Signs. Act Early. health education campaign delivers the message that how a child plays, learns, speaks, and acts offers important clues about his or her development.

month and enjoys one of the highest consumer satisfaction ratings seen across government agencies. In addition, survey results show that pediatricians who have heard of the campaign are more confident discussing cognitive development with parents; more likely to be aware of resources available for referral, treatment; and more likely to have resources to educate parents (Daniel et al., 2009).

THE ACT EARLY INITIATIVE: ACT EARLY SUMMITS–A MODEL OF SYSTEM CHANGE

As the Learn the Signs. Act Early. campaign reached parents, health care providers, and early educators, CDC found that increased public awareness revealed system-related challenges among programs serving children and their families at the state level that warranted engagement of additional partners from federal agencies and national-level support. In addition, increased public awareness created additional demand on early intervention systems and state infrastructure serving children with special health care needs (Title V programs). CDC, HRSA, and AUCD partnered to address the barriers, convening key stakeholders in regional Act Early summits to work on issues related to access and coordination of services for young children identified with developmental delays, including those at risk for an ASD, and their families.

HRSA's Maternal and Child Health Bureau (MCHB) served as an ideal federal partner with its mission to increase the number of children receiving health assessments, ensure access to health care services, and support family-centered, community-based state systems of care for children with special health care needs. The AUCD network, which is a national network of university-based, interdisciplinary programs focused on serving individuals with disabilities through education, research, and service, provided a platform to engage state-level stakeholders, representing advocacy, early intervention, education, medical, and other systems. Members of the AUCD network, including University Centers for Excellence in Developmental Disabilities (UCEDDs) and Leadership Education in Neurodevelopmental and Related Disabilities programs (LENDs), located in all 50 states and territories, served as anchors to facilitate development and coordination of state teams in an effort to identify and overcome barriers to the provision of services and support needed by children with ASD and DD and their families through increased awareness and collaboration among stakeholders.

Another integral partner is the birth-to-3 system in each state. Depending on the state, education or public health systems serve young children identified with developmental delay. The birth-to-3 system in each state is required through a federal mandate under the Individuals with Disabilities Education Act (IDEA). Part C of this law covers children birth to 3 years old who have certain disabilities and also children who exhibit a certain level of developmental delay. Entry into the Part C system starts with an evaluation in all domains of development including social, language, cognitive, gross and fine motor, and adaptive skills. Following these evaluations, if a child meets eligibility criteria, an individualized family service plan is developed, incorporating the needs of the child based on the developmental assessment and the family's goals for the child. Services from therapists, including speech/language pathologists, physical therapists, occupational therapists, and early educators, work with a child's family to provide early intervention.

Despite the existence of education and public health systems that serve young children identified with developmental delay in every state, parents and providers reported difficulties in gaining access to the services they needed. In many cases, parents and their health care providers reported difficulty knowing how to gain access to the Part C program, medical and other health care providers for diagnostic workup, and other social service, education, and public health agencies that might support their child with delays.

Act Early Initiative Framework

The Act Early summits were designed to enhance the collaboration among state service systems to improve earlier identification, earlier diagnoses, and access to systems of care for children at risk for ASD and DD. The summits offered a unique opportunity to foster dialogue and to support state-level coordination among key state leaders from the early detection and intervention community, including parents, state agencies, provider groups, autism and other related disability organizations, and relevant university personnel. Continued work within states postsummit was supported through grant opportunities, technical assistance, and dissemination of national resource materials.

The desired outcomes of the Act Early Regional Summit project were to

- Increase awareness and use of the CDC's Learn the Signs. Act Early. campaign and its reach and impact in the target regions

- Develop a common understanding among state stakeholders of the opportunities and challenges to address the needs of families and children with ASD and other DD

- Develop sustainable state teams to enhance the coordination of statewide service provision for families and children with ASD and other DD

Regional summit attendees were invited to attend based on their expertise in ASD and roles and knowledge in their state. Individuals identified from each state included representatives of state and local government, provider organizations, and public health advocacy groups. Parents of children with disabilities were also represented, sometimes from both the parent perspective and as a representative of one of the organizations given in the following list. Participants included but were not limited to

- Part C of IDEA State Services

- State Preschool Special Education—Section 619 of IDEA

- State Children with Special Health Care Needs—Title V

- State Developmental Disabilities Office (MRDD)

- State Public Health

- State Child Care Resource and Referral

- Child Foster Care Bureau

- State Head Start and Early Head Start

- AAP State Chapters

- UCEDDs

- LENDs

- State Autism Organizations—Autism Society of America, Autism Speaks, Easter Seals, Network of Autism Training and Technical Assistance Providers

- State Parent Organizations—Parent Training Center, Family Support, or Parent Health Information Center

- State Medicaid and Health Insurance Programs

- State Legislature members or staff

Presummit Work

Approximately 4–6 weeks prior to the summit, the state teams had one or two teleconferences with state team members mediated by an AUCD facilitator. Sometimes team members had not worked together before, despite having common goals of serving young children with developmental delay. These early meetings served as an opportunity for team members to understand each other's roles. States were encouraged to broaden their thinking of groups and individuals who work to improve identification of these children, thereby including representation of a broad variety of organizations. In addition, during these discussions, the teams began to talk about resources in their state. Each team created a "State of the State" presentation, which outlined the most important aspects of activities related to early awareness and identification of and intervention for ASD and other DD in their state. Each presentation included an overview of state systems, a list of the barriers and gaps, and the team's overall vision for the summit.

Summit Work

State team members came prepared to work together to improve identification of children with developmental delay and those at risk for ASD, as well as improve access to services and improve awareness of developmental milestones. These teams were brought together in one of 11 Act Early regional summits, organized according to the 10 Department of Health and Human Services Regions; Region IV was split into two meetings due to the large number of states in that region. An earlier summit, held prior to the onset of the first Act Early summit in early 2008, and sponsored by the MCHB-funded National Autism Medical Home initiative, served as the basis for the framework of the subsequent Act Early summits.

During the summit, state team members had opportunities to network with others in similar roles from different states, listen to presentations on national and federal initiatives focused on early childhood and disability, and work together in their state teams to create a state plan.

Summit discussions were structured using the Kellogg Foundation logic model format (Logic Model Development Guide, 2011) to guide the identification of resources and to help agree upon outcomes and related activities to achieve outcomes for the team to undertake after the summit. Each state developed a plan to improve the system of services for children with ASD and other DD. Many plans highlight the following themes:

1. Early and continuous screening for ASD and other DD.

2. Partnerships among public service systems, professionals, and families of children with an ASD.

3. Access to a culturally competent care for clinical practice, pediatric subspecialties, and community-based services.

4. Increased overall public awareness of ASD and DD.

Postsummit Work

Following the summit, each state team had the opportunity to apply for a 1-year Act Early minigrant. These minigrants provided support for state teams to continue to meet and address high-priority activities in their state plan. These minigrant funds were used to carry out activities such as statewide dissemination of Learn the Signs. Act Early. campaign materials, additional team meetings, and engagement of broader audiences within their state. Additional technical assistance from both CDC and AUCD assisted state teams in maintaining the momentum in addressing relevant, state-level ASD and other DD issues.

Information sharing occurred in various ways. Materials and information were disseminated through dedicated webpages archiving presentations and handouts from all of the summits (www.aucd.org/actearly). State team collaboration was further fostered through a shared online workspace designed to support and facilitate work among summit participants and state teams. In addition, an Act Early Forum e-mail discussion list provided a way to further disseminate information of interest.

A database for ASD-related state legislation was developed in collaboration with the National Conference of State Legislatures (NCSL) (Autism Legislation Database, 2011). NCSL provides research, technical assistance, and opportunities for policy makers at state legislatures in the United States (states, commonwealths, and territories) to exchange ideas on the most pressing state issues. NCSL is an effective and respected advocate for interests at the state level. Since 2008, there have been more than 1,000 pieces of state legislation related to ASD in the areas of awareness, criminal justice, education, employment, financing, infrastructure, pilot programs, professional training, screening, task force formation, and appropriation. State teams had indicated the importance and the need to learn about legislation in other states to assist in their efforts to develop innovative and effective policies for the early identification, assessment, and service coordination for young children with ASD and other DD in their states. The database is currently available to the public through the NCSL web site, www.ncsl.org. In addition, NCSL produced and distributed an information card that illustrated and highlighted important ASD issues. The information cards contained a concise narrative that explained the issue and the challenges of developing a coordinated system for the early identification, diagnosis, and provision of services for young children with an ASD and other DD.

Subsequently, with the development of another partnership with the Association of Maternal Child Health Programs (AMCHP), CDC and AMCHP have offered grants to 10 Act Early teams to continue activities described in their state plans. The areas of activity include dissemination and customization of Learn the Signs. Act Early. materials, development of resource guides and ASD diagnostic guidelines, training clinicians and community providers to understand the importance of early identification, developmental screening and screening for ASD in multicultural community and medical settings, creating guides or road maps for families and for professionals to navigate the systems that serve children with developmental delay, and continued collaboration through Act Early team meetings, forums, summits, and webinars.

Evaluation of Act Early Activities

State Plans   Key themes from the state plans were reviewed to better understand areas of focus and facilitators and barriers to success. Common barriers included few well-trained professionals, disparities among ethnic groups in access to services, use of non–evidence-based services, and diminished funding. In order to address these concerns, states proposed to increase public awareness about ASD and other DD, improve seamless transition among service systems, provide statewide training for families and practitioners, and address disparities by increasing services for the underserved.

Surveys and Interviews   In order to determine the impact of summit activities, we surveyed and/or interviewed states about the outcomes of having participated in an Act Early summit. The postsummit interview process made it possible to identify themes and similarities among states in their work after the summit. The interview protocol asked past state team leaders questions in three areas. First, the team leaders were asked whether or not they felt that the summit itself was helpful in increasing early identification of ASD and other DD in their states. Second, they were asked about their postsummit activities including additional meetings, product development, dissemination initiatives, and so forth. Finally, team leaders were asked about the needs they had for future technical assistance and the next steps that they thought would help continue the efforts that were started at the summit. The direct outcomes of the Act Early summit varied considerably by state.

ACT EARLY STATE TEAMS: EXAMPLES OF SYSTEM CHANGE

Since the Act Early initiative began in 2008, states teams have returned to their states to implement parts of their state plans. States have conducted activities to increase awareness of the importance of early identification of children with developmental delays. Some have done this by customizing CDC's Learn the Signs. Act Early. materials with state or local information, and conducting targeted awareness activities through the use of health fairs and public service announcement campaigns. A number of states have attempted to help families and professionals navigate the many systems serving young children with delays through the creation of a variety of navigation tools. In addition, many teams have sought to increase collaboration among state stakeholders and awareness in their states through continued meeting and expansion of state Act Early teams. Other states have focused on professional training to increase screening for ASD and other DD.

We have highlighted examples of state successes in the next sections, although we should note that many more states have also achieved success through the continued work of their Act Early state teams. These successes focus on three anticipated outcomes:

- Increase awareness and use of the CDC's Learn the Signs. Act Early. campaign and its impact in the target regions through local collaboration that sometimes include information on local resources.

- Develop a common understanding among state stakeholders of the opportunities, challenges, and barriers to address the needs of families and children with ASD and other DD.

- Develop state teams to enhance the coordination of statewide service provision for families and children with ASD and other DD.

Throughout these interview processes, several factors seemed to be directly associated with the amount of positive change reported by states. These include strong consistent leadership, availability of funds (either through CDC or another source), existing structure to support dedicated staff time, support from the state, county, and local level for ASD activities, and buy-in from at least three of the major state agencies, namely, departments of public health, education, and developmental services.

Kansas

The Kansas state team participated in the first Act Early summit in Kansas City, Missouri, in February 2008. The team consisted of 18 members from several sectors in the state including Kansas Director of Children with Special Health Care Needs (CSHCN) services, Director of the Kansas Children's Developmental Services, Medicaid, University Centers, Kansas Instructional Support Network, Kansas Coalition for Autism Legislation, Part C, Director of Community Supports and Services, and several pediatricians, provider groups, and higher education. Approximately half of the Kansas team members were involved in the Kansas Autism Task Force, which had been created by the Kansas state legislature in 2007.

The Kansas team members stated that their biggest challenges were lack of training, long wait times for diagnosis, too few qualified personnel, inadequate funding, inconsistent health insurance coverage, and geographic and socioeconomic diversity around the state. During the summit the team identified 10 short- and long-term outcomes that would lead to successful achievement of its vision. These outcomes included

- All children will receive screening for developmental delays within the first year of life.

- All children with a positive ASD screen are enrolled in a program of evidence-based early intervention.

- There is an adequate number of qualified personnel.

- Funding is not a barrier.

- All Kansans will have access to a centralized source of information regarding ASD.

The first outcome that the team chose to target was to establish "regional centers across Kansas to provide diagnosis, treatment, follow-up and support for providers, individuals, and families of Kansans with ASD."

One year after the summit the team members reported that they had developed a pilot program to establish "autism diagnostic teams" around the state. Their strategy was to provide training to practicing professionals in their local communities in the latest methods and tools for screening and diagnosing children with ASD. Locally trained autism teams currently exist in 65 of the state's 105 counties; the team plans to continue their efforts and eventually reach every county. After teams are trained, they have access to ongoing technical assistance, available through an autism training network and the state department of education.

One of the main charges of the teams is to screen and identify children in child care centers, medical clinics, and schools in their local community. After receiving a positive screen a child is immediately referred for a diagnostic evaluation. Through the use of their existing telehealth technology, they are able to set up diagnostic assessments with developmental behavioral pediatricians in the urban areas. Currently 10–15 children are seen per month through this technology. As evidence of the success of this program, the Kansas team has been able to reduce the wait time from a positive screen to a diagnostic assessment from more than 7 months to 45 days. The team leader reports that without the summit they would not have had the necessary relationships with the physicians at the large medical schools, the local doctors, the department of education, and the university centers to set up the diagnostic teams.

The Kansas team has also been able to increase their training efforts by utilizing the Kansas Instructional Support Network and the Kansas Center for Autism Training and Research. They have developed an autism certificate program with Pittsburg State University via their Interactive Television Network. A state team leader from the Kansas Act Early state team, Lee Stickle, reports that the program initiated by the summit is "an absolute success." She goes on to describe how the process of getting everyone to "sit down and agree on common goals and common activities" was what allowed the collaboration enabling achievement of their goals. "We are nowhere near done with our work," she reports, "but we are heading in the right direction."

California

The California state team participated in an Act Early summit in June 2009. The California team was large, with 43 participants. Individuals from many sectors were represented on the team, including those from the health, education, early intervention/Part C, social services, California state legislature, and Head Start. This team was unique in the large number of parent representatives as well as those from higher education institutions who participated.

The majority of members on the California state team had been meeting as a group for almost 2 years when they came to the summit. The team had formed in anticipation of applying to be one of the state partners to receive technical assistance from the National Professional Development Center on Autism Spectrum Disorders (NPDC on ASD) cooperative agreement funded through the U.S. Office of Special Education and Rehabilitative Services within the Department of Education. NPDC on ASD is a national technical assistance and development project focused on promoting the use of educational evidence-based practice for children and adolescents with autism spectrum disorders. Many of the same team members were also involved in drafting the California Legislative Blue Ribbon Commission Report on Autism highlighting specific issues that impose barriers and challenges to the health and well-being of individuals with an ASD, the Superintendent's Autism Advisory Committee recommendations, and the Department of Developmental Services Best Practice Guidelines for Screening, Diagnosis and Assessment. The knowledge and history that these team members brought to the summit added significantly to the discussions and provided a framework for next steps.

Because the California team was very large, they created three active workgroups to address their priority short- and long-term goals. These workgroups focused on screening, training, and transition.

The goal of the screening workgroup was to decrease the average age of diagnosis. The benchmarks toward reaching that goal included more parents report that their developmental concerns were heard, parents have accessible information about how to determine where to get their needs addressed, diagnostic accuracy is improved, and all children will receive the services they need regardless of whether their diagnosis is medical or educational.

The long-term goal of the training team was that professionals and families would receive training in evidence-based practices including assessment, treatment/interventions, inclusive of cultural competencies, and family support. This goal would be evidenced by an overall decrease in staff turnover and burnout and a greater number of highly qualified professionals working with children with an ASD.

Finally, the subcommittee on transition focused their efforts on coordination as they learned that gaps in services most often occurred when a child moved from one agency to another. The goal of the transition subcommittee was that in all regional centers and schools, roles would be identified, language would be unified, and any overlapping mandates between IDEA and early intervention would be discussed. The outcome would lead to better coordination of transition services at age 3 across agencies and there would be common approaches across regional centers and school districts.

Immediately following the summit, the California state team worked with AUCD to create an online collaboration through a SharePoint site that was open to all of their team members. The team met in the fall of 2009 to discuss their next steps and to train all of their members in the use of the SharePoint site. Through the use of the site, the team was able to share all of the materials from the summit as well as resources from other sites with all of the team. The team was also able to utilize the site successfully for receiving technical assistance from NPDC on ASD. California was successful at being awarded funding through NPDC on ASD and their subcommittees continue to meet and move their agenda forward.

When reflecting on the summit process the California team leaders talk about how helpful the summit was in breaking down the silos that exist in the state. They comment that before the summit people were not aware of some of the activities and initiatives in the state. Having the representation from education, public health, and the current state-wide screening initiative gave the team a forum for discussing joint projects. The leaders of the California state team call the summit a "win-win" situation in that it allowed them to establish new partnerships and find new opportunities for collaboration. The team hopes that the partnerships and new joint projects coming from the summit will positivity impact the state's capacity to screen, diagnose, and serve young children with an ASD and other developmental disabilities.

North Carolina

The North Carolina Act Early team brought 15 members to the Region IVa Act Early summit in January 2009. The team included members of the pediatric community, Part C/early intervention, public health, and academic communities, as well as several members from the Autism Society of North Carolina, which has several very active chapters. As part of their activities leading up to and following the summit, the members of the North Carolina state team assembled a critical group of stakeholders in North Carolina called the North Carolina State Autism Alliance. Its priority was to increase coordination of clinical services and training initiatives across the state and identify targeted initiatives. The group intentionally included active researchers to provide ongoing input into promising practices and new knowledge, which would guide the committee's evidence-based policies and practices. These teams have now blended.

The challenges and gaps that the team identified were in the areas of interagency communication, ensuring an adequate workforce to serve the needs of children with ASD, increasing public awareness, and maintaining stable funding given the possibility of large budget deficits. The high-priority activities identified on the North Carolina state plan were around service coordination, resources, research to practice, alliance/policy coordination, evaluation, and training. The team identified several short- and long-term impacts related to these activities, which included improving access to screening through a child's medical home, earlier intervention, and earlier referral for community-based supports. Their premise was that early surveillance leads to earlier referral to early intervention, which in turn leads to earlier referral for other community-based supports. In addition, they expected that assessments and treatments should be evidence-based, timely, and could be provided through academic centers.

The North Carolina Autism Alliance continues to grow and expand; what started as a group of 15 people is now a group of more than 50. The alliance has broken into task forces focused on specific goals. Three task forces focus on inventorying resources, legislative advocacy and policy, and access to health care. The task force structure has led to greater accountability, as there is regular reporting to the larger group. The first task force is to create an inventory of training initiatives across the state and consolidate them into a training calendar for the state. The second task force advocates for ASD-related legislation as well as advises staff on policy initiatives. The alliance continues to invite state senators and staffers to their meetings. The third task force is planning to continue working on a brochure that outlines how and where families can gain access to diagnostic and other clinical services in the state. The connection between the Autism Alliance and other legislative task forces has also proven to be helpful in bringing a focus on children with an ASD into rural health initiatives. The North Carolina team leader lists this as a perfect example of how strong linkages can effect change.

The North Carolina team leader fully attributes the expansion of the North Carolina Autism Alliance to the Act Early regional summit. He talks about how the summit came at a "perfect time" in North Carolina and how the state plan, which came from the logic model at the summit, continues to provide them with a blueprint and a method for evaluation. The team leader also stresses how important it was to have all of the people in the state come together to discuss what they are doing so they could all stop "reinventing the wheel." Almost 2 years after the Region IVa summit, the North Carolina Autism Alliance is still strong. The linkages that were started at the summit have continued to grow and develop into new partnerships, and in turn, new possibilities.

Tennessee

Tennessee was the host site for the Region IVa summit in Nashville in January 2009. The team had 23 members who represented a wide range of agencies, families, and two LEND training programs. Moreover, the Tennessee Act Early team included five individuals engaged in policy representing either the Governor's Office of Children's Care Coordination or the Tennessee Commission on Children and Youth. During the summit, the Tennessee state team identified several resources such as the Tennessee early intervention system, active Autism Society chapters, committed parent-to-parent support programs, the two LEND programs, and the Governor's Office on Children's Care and Coordination as assets. The main challenge that the team identified was that there was "no system of care for children with ASD in Tennessee." They also cited inconsistent access to services and diagnostic assessments, geographic disparities, long waiting lists, and lack of up-to-date standards for quality ASD services as other challenges.

The team identified priorities at the summit. The first priority was to coordinate an Act Early group that would include representatives from all of the summit team participants. Their second priority was in the area of media/awareness. Some of the benchmarks included developing a social marketing approach to increase awareness, utilizing existing materials, providing materials to the Home Visiting Coalition, identifying and reaching out to underserved groups, and reaching out to existing early intervention initiatives. Their third priority was to promote family involvement and supports. The activities for this priority included providing an orientation for families of newly diagnosed children, developing a resource guide, involving families in all planning, and developing statewide ASD family and professional networks. The fourth priority of their state plan was to build capacity by providing training, improving existing services, and building infrastructure and legislative activities.

In the 2 years since the summit, the Tennessee Act Early summit team has continued to meet three to four times per year as a whole group and more frequently as smaller workgroups. The workgroups, which mirror the goals in the state plan, are public awareness, training, family support, and state agency collaborations. The team leaders from the Tennessee state team report that breaking into the smaller workgroups allows them to achieve more "concrete operational planning" while the greater group provides system-level vision.

One reported outcome of the summit is that the three Autism Society of America chapters in the state have been able to build more cohesive partnerships and jointly take on projects. The team has used an Act Early minigrant to provide travel reimbursement to parents and ASA chapter representatives who live in different parts of the state so they can participate in Act Early activities. The public awareness workgroup has been able to collaborate with people at the UCEDD and LEND to put together a resource guide and tip sheet for parents of newly diagnosed children. These tip sheets can be adapted to any part of the state as they are disseminated. This workgroup has also done some Spanish-language radio broadcasts with the help of the UCEDDs. Through the collaboration with the UCEDDs the workgroup has been able to send out packets with both the Learn the Signs. Act Early. materials as well as the tip sheets to every child care center in the state as well as the state Part C early intervention system.

Since the summit, the training workgroup has also collaborated with the state chapter of the AAP. Through its partnership with the AAP, the team has been able to identify people throughout the state that can train primary care providers, including pediatricians and family physicians, to conduct ASD-specific assessments. The group has been able to identify practitioners in all five areas of the state with the hopes that they will be able to circumvent bottlenecks to getting a diagnosis. The work of the state team has also connected with some current legislative initiatives through the governor's office. One of the leaders from the state team has been able to attend the Governor's Office of Children's Care Coordination meetings and provide information about ASD and a list of resources to the council members.

When asked about the effectiveness of the Act Early summit, both team leaders agree that the summit was a worthwhile venture for their state team. They report that the collaborations that have come out of the summit have been integral to their progress. Their dissemination efforts and plans have been much more coordinated. They also report that they are able to reach a wider population of children and families across the state due to their connections with the parent and advocacy agencies. Although the team leaders state that they "still have a ways to go," they both agree that the summit was "the perfect kick-off" to reaching the goals developed at the summit.

LESSONS LEARNED

The Act Early Initiative has enabled CDC to systematically promote public awareness of the importance of early identification of developmental delays and on acting on these concerns through referral for evaluation and intervention through the strategic dissemination of Learn the Signs. Act Early. materials in states. In addition, CDC has been able to gain a pulse on local and state activities related to the early identification of children with developmental delay. This connection to states has been invaluable.

CONCLUSION

CDC's role in addressing the urgent public health concerns related to ASD encompasses a number of segments of the public health model, including surveillance, epidemiology, and intervention through development of prevention strategies and encouragement of widespread adoption through health education and communication.

The ADDM network has monitored prevalence of ASD in 8-year-olds since 2000 and now will be providing additional information about prevalence rates of 4-year-olds through the Early ADDM project. Epidemiological work through the SEED study will help to identify risk and protective factors for ASD.

The Learn the Signs. Act Early. program provides the framework for intervention and prevention strategies. This health communication campaign provides messaging to parents of young children, early educators, and health care providers and serves as the basis for the early identification efforts at the CDC. The Act Early summit initiative was conceived and implemented to coordinate and catalyze action among state key stakeholders focused on the early identification of children with delays, including those at risk for ASD. As demonstrated by these state examples and many others not reported previously, states have been able to form Act Early teams and sustain collaboration to increase action focused on the early identification of children. These states have worked hard to increase awareness using the Learn the Signs. Act Early. messages, developing teams to coordinate state service provision and developing a common understanding among team members of opportunities and barriers.

Continued support of these Act Early initiatives with blended federal funding from both CDC and HRSA in partnership with national organization such as AUCD and AMCHP will strengthen partnerships and keep attention focused on this important public health issue. Early identification of children with delay, including those at risk for ASD, is an important step in helping to support families to help their children reach their full potential.

FUTURE DIRECTIONS

The summits were held regionally to address geographic and demographic similarities among states. Initial discussions considered arranging summits based instead on special populations who experience specific barriers to early identification through language barriers or poverty. As the Act Early Initiative continues, holding summits to highlight and aid populations with significant barriers to identification may be considered. These issues, however, have been addressed to varying degrees already by Act Early teams through their postsummit work.

The Act Early Initiative has catalyzed action in states to improve early identification of ASD and other developmental disabilities. Community awareness about the Learn the Signs. Act Early. campaign has increased through the development and continued support of the Act Early teams. To sustain and further improve this awareness, a new program is being launched. The Act Early Ambassador project will identify local points of contact for the Act Early Initiative and the Learn the Signs. Act Early. campaign. These ambassadors will train local professionals on the importance of acting early on concerns about a developmental delay. They will be strengthening the connection between their state's Act Early team and Act Early's national (AUCD and AMCHP) and federal (CDC and HRSA) partners.

REFERENCES

Autism Legislation Database. (2011). *National Conference of State Legislatures web site*. Retrieved from http://www.ncsl.org/default.aspx?tabid14109

Bertrand, J., et al. (2001). Prevalence of autism in a United States population: The Brick Township, New Jersey, investigation. *Pediatrics, 108*, 1155–1161.

Daniel, K.L., et al. (2009). Learn the signs. Act early: A campaign to help every child reach his or her full potential. *Public Health, 123*, e11–e16.

Dawson, G. (2008). Early behavioral intervention, brain plasticity, and the prevention of autism spectrum disorder. *Developmental Psychopathology, 20,* 775–803.

Dawson, G., et al. (2010). Randomized, controlled trial of an intervention for toddlers with autism: The Early Start Denver Model. *Pediatrics, 125,* e17–e23.

Logic Model Development Guide. (2004). *W.K. Kellogg Foundation web site.* Retrieved from http://www.uwsa.edu/edi/grants/Kellogg_Logic_Model.pdf

Lord, C., & McGee, J.P. (Eds.). (2001). *Educating children with autism.* Washington, DC: National Academy Press.

Prevalence of Autism Spectrum Disorders–Autism and Developmental Disabilities Monitoring Network, United States, 2006. (2009). *Morbidity and Mortality Weekly Report, 58*(SS-10).

Yeargin-Allsopp, M., et al. (1992). A multiple-source METHOD for studying the prevalence of developmental disabilities in children: The Metropolitan Atlanta Developmental Disabilities Study. *Pediatrics, 89,* 624–630.

13

National Professional Development Center on Autism Spectrum Disorders

An Emerging National Educational Strategy

Ann W. Cox, Matthew E. Brock, Samuel L. Odom, Sally J. Rogers, Lisa H. Sullivan, Linda Tuchman-Ginsberg, Ellen L. Franzone, Katherine Szidon, and Lana Collet-Klingenberg

The National Professional Development Center on Autism Spectrum Disorders (NPDC) was conceived from the concern and frustration that its authors and primary investigators experienced in trying to help motivated and committed professionals in the public schools apply best practices for children with autism spectrum disorder (ASD) in their classrooms. Before helping professionals to apply best practices for working with children with ASD, the NPDC had to answer numerous questions: What were the best practices? Who decides what they are? How would general education public school teachers, or other school-based professionals, learn to use the practices? How would they know if they were using them correctly? How would they measure their effectiveness? How would they apply a practice to the individualized education program (IEP) goals as written? What might a high-quality program look like?

These concerns were less about the teaching staff and more about the large amount of disparate information scattered throughout the educational literature. First, the information lacked integration and synthesis; the research was not organized into a coherent body of information. Second, there was a lack of consensus in the field about definitions of an evidence-based practice (EBP) in ASD. Finally, the research on ASD was published in many different journals, in language inaccessible to most, and with too little information in the articles for a teacher to be able to replicate the practice in a classroom.

When the U.S. Department of Education issued a request for proposals in the fall of 2006 for the creation of a national professional development center to support educators

Funding for preparation of this chapter was provided by Grant No. H325G070004 from the Office of Special Education Programs, U.S. Department of Education.

who work with students with autism, a team of individuals from the Frank Porter Graham Child Development Institute at the University of North Carolina at Chapel Hill, the Waisman Center at the University of Wisconsin, and the Medical Investigation of Neurodevelopmental Disorders (MIND). Institute at the University of California at Davis Medical School saw an opportunity to address these concerns. They conceptualized a possible approach to these problems by developing a professional development/coaching model for states that would

1. Support local school districts to provide high-quality education and early intervention to children and youth with ASD based on empirically tested and supported educational practices

2. Support teamwork between families and school personnel in educational planning and programming for children;

3. Develop needed assessment tools and self-instructional materials from the highest-quality educational approaches in ASD, package them in multiple formats (print, Internet, video), and encourage school adoption of these practices and procedures for ongoing evaluation of student progress

4. Develop a high level of training and implementation expertise combined with NPDC resources so that state-level training teams could continue to train and support new sites in their state

The proposal was submitted in January 2007 and funding was awarded that summer. Teams were assembled at each of three coordinating university sites—Wisconsin, California, and North Carolina. These were headed by a co-principal investigator, managed on a daily basis by a project coordinator, and staffed with a number of ASD experts from various disciplines. These individuals had expertise in using empirically supported practices for children with ASD, teaching and training other professionals, developing training materials, and working with parents. Administrative support staff rounded out the teams.

Now, more than 5 years later, hundreds of people have participated across 12 states, and training materials are being placed on the Internet regularly. More than 700 participants have attended summer workshops, several of which are being carried out independently by state teams who have participated with the NPDC. Seventy-six programs are serving as model or expansion sites and new sites are added yearly. And more than 189 preschoolers, elementary students, and teenagers with ASD have directly benefited from training and coaching provided by NPDC team members in classroom sites.

The developers of the NPDC sought to address their original concerns in practical and sustainable ways but found that some information was not readily available or needed to be developed. The model that has emerged is based on working with entire states, and programs within the states, for 2 years. Attention has centered on engaging the state through a strategic planning process before focusing on work in sites and classrooms. A great deal of time has been devoted to developing training and technical assistance resources that are used and remain with a state after their work with the NPDC ends. Much of this work is presented in the next three sections. The chapter concludes by sharing lessons that have been learned during this process and a concluding "state success story" that illustrates how capacity is built and sustainability assured.

Note that the work of the NPDC on ASD also addresses the needs of children younger than 3 years of age; however, in this chapter, we focus on our work with individuals 3–21 years of age.

IDENTIFYING AND CREATING NEEDED RESOURCES

Our first work as a center focused on identifying the instructional or intervention practices that had been demonstrated in the scientific literature as effective with children with ASD and tools to help practitioners better understand the elements of quality programs for children with ASD. These resources were not already available for us to use, so NPDC researchers set about addressing these areas in a systematic way.

What Are the Best Practices for Learners with Autism Spectrum Disorder? How Were These Identified?

A key feature of the NPDC work has been to identify from the research literature instructional and intervention practices that are effective and could be translated into practices that teachers and other service providers may use in programs for learners with ASD. The NPDC investigators and staff followed a systematic process for identifying EBPs from the research literature. Initially, researchers from the NPDC conducted computer-based literature reviews. Specific procedures are provided in Odom, Collet-Klingenberg, Rogers, and Hatton (2010).

The NPDC researchers and staff then sorted intervention articles by important outcome areas (e.g., social, communication, interfering behavior) and age groups and grouped the articles by intervention practices. After articles were identified and grouped, two NPDC researchers reviewed the methodology of each article to determine that essential methodological quality criteria for group and single case experimental designs were met (Gersten et al., 2005; Horner et al., 2005). Acceptable articles were then grouped by practice type. For a practice to be classified as evidence-based, there had to be 1) at least two acceptable experimental or quasi-experimental design studies, 2) five single case design studies conducted by a minimum of three different researchers, or 3) a combination of group (a minimum of one study) and single case design studies (a minimum of three studies).

From this review, NPDC investigators identified 24 practices that had sufficient research studies to be classified as evidence-based. The practices are listed in Figure 13.1 by domains of instruction that were targeted in the research making up the evidence base for each practice.

Many of these practices are based on applied behavior analysis principles. There are basic behavioral interventions, such as reinforcement or prompting, as well as more complex practices such as peer-mediated intervention or self-management, that include these basic behavioral features as part of the overall practice. Also, there is a cluster of practices (i.e., functional behavior assessment, redirection, extinction, antecedent-based interventions, differential-reinforcement of other behavior, functional communication training) that focuses on building more adaptive skills while decelerating or reducing challenging behavior and can provide the foundation for a system of positive behavior management. In addition, some practices come from frameworks other than applied behavior analysis (i.e., social narratives, speech generating devices, visual supports) and have sufficient research to qualify as being evidence based.

To be useful, the practices had to be translated into procedural guides that practitioners could use in classrooms and programs. For each of the 24 practices, staff has created clear descriptions of the features of the practice, steps for implementation, and an implementation checklist. Together these components are called *practice briefs*. The NPDC is also developing Internet-based modules, with video examples. Both the briefs and online modules are core training resources and are described later in the chapter.

EBP	Academics and Cognition			Behavior			Commun- ication			Play			Social			Transition		
	EC	EL	MH	EC	EL	MH	EC	EL	MH	EC	EL	MH	EC	EL	MH	EC	EL	MH
Antecedent-based interventions	■	■		■	■													
Computer assisted instruction	■	■	■															
Differential reinforcement				■	■	■							■	■				
Discrete trial training	■	■	■			■	■			■	■							
Extinction				■	■		■											
Functional behavioral assessment				■	■	■												
Functional communication training				■	■		■	■										
Naturalistic interventions					■		■	■		■			■					
Parent-implemented interventions				■	■			■		■	■							
Peer-mediated instruction/intervention							■	■					■	■	■			
Picture Exchange Communication System							■	■					■					
Pivotal Response Training	■	■					■			■			■					
Prompting	■	■		■	■		■	■		■	■		■	■				
Reinforcement	■	■		■	■		■	■		■	■		■	■				
Response interruption and redirection				■	■		■											
Self-management	■	■		■	■		■	■					■	■		■	■	■
Social narratives	■	■		■	■		■	■					■	■				
Social skills groups							■	■					■	■				
Speech generating devices (VOCA)							■	■										
Structured work systems	■	■								■	■		■			■	■	■
Task analysis	■	■											■	■		■	■	
Time delay	■	■					■	■		■	■		■	■				
Video modeling	■	■		■	■		■	■		■	■		■	■				
Visual supports	■	■		■	■		■	■		■	■		■	■				

Figure 13.1. Evidence-based practices (EBP) by instructional domains and age. Shading indicates that research was found to support the use of the practice in a given instructional domain and with a specific age range. (Key: Age Groupings: EC, early childhood (2–5 years); EL, elementary age; MH, middle/high school age; EBP, evidence-based practices (Disclaimer: The review completed by the National Professional Development Center on Autism Spectrum Disorder was not exhaustive. It is possible that yet unidentified evidence exists for practices and ages not indicated above or that have been published since the time of the last review.)

What Do Quality Classrooms for Students with Autism Spectrum Disorder Look Like? Can This Be Assessed?

Increasing quality of instruction in a classroom, a major goal of the NPDC project, assumes there is a procedure for evaluating quality of instruction. However, there were no such procedures available to teachers when the NPDC began. An instrument developed for this purpose, the Autism Program Environment Rating Scale (APERS), measures features of programs that reflect program quality, such as program structure, social climate, team functioning, communication, and family involvement (Autism Program Environment Rating Scale Development Group, 2012).

The development of the APERS was systematic and iterative. The selection of items and the format began with a review of the literature on assessment of program and learning environments for children and youth who are typically developing and for individuals with ASD. Based on a review of approximately 35 articles and 13 other environmental scales, a list of pertinent items was assembled. These items were sorted into categories representing features of learning environments and programs. NPDC team members reviewed items and provided feedback that was used to revise the items, which were finally assembled into domains. A scaling process was chosen and anchors were written and reviewed.

The items and domains were then assembled into the APERS Preschool/Elementary form (APERS-PE). This version was shared with practitioners in middle and high school programs for learners with ASD to create the middle-high school version (APERS-MHS). Items were revised to represent the different quality features of these programs, and one domain was added to include a focus on transition.

Research members then pilot tested the APERS in preschool, elementary, middle, and high school programs for learners with ASD. This pilot information was used to revise observation and data-collection procedures as well as individual items. Both forms were used at the initial state model sites of the NPDC in fall 2008 and spring 2009. Investigators provided detailed feedback about items and data collection procedures, which has been incorporated into the current versions of the APERS.

The current versions of the instrument include 64 and 68 items, respectively, for the APERS-PE and the APERS-MHS. Individual items are organized into subdomains, and each item has a five-point Likert scale format. Individuals completing the APERS observe in the program (a minimum of 3 hours of observation is required) and conduct interviews with the teachers, team members, and parents of children with ASD in the classroom. Both versions are suitable for self-contained classrooms and inclusive programs.

The instrument is still in its pilot phase. Validity studies have not been conducted and psychometric properties have not yet been established through research, although the research team hopes to begin such a process within a year. In the meantime, the APERS is being used to assist teachers and technical assistance providers to evaluate current classroom practices and identify goals for increasing program quality at our model and expansion sites.

As the EBPs were being identified and the program quality assessment was being developed, the NPDC began implementing strategies to identify states with sufficient infrastructure and commitment with which to partner.

DEVELOPING PARTNERSHIPS WITH STATES

Commitment from a team of state leaders is the most important first step in a state's involvement with the NPDC. State commitment coupled with a systematic approach that engages state partners through multiple opportunities for communication, clarification of roles, and review of commitments, has ensured that there is a good fit between NPDC priorities and state NPDC partners. The process leading toward the development of the partnership starts with a successful state application, is followed by completion of the state's 2-year strategic plan, and then the initial development of model sites.

How Are States Selected?

The NPDC developed a process to assist potential states in deciding if an application for a 2-year partnership with NPDC is feasible. The application packet, which is posted on the NPDC web site 9 months before the application is due, includes a comprehensive list of professional development and other responsibilities that are entailed in the partnership. Descriptions of the training, technical assistance/coaching, and financial resources that the NPDC will provide as well as the states' requirements to commit resources, including a state liaison, time of other state leaders and stakeholders, and financial resources associated with NPDC activities are described. In each state, a collaborative leadership team is formed that includes representatives from the department of education, the state's Part C office, and the University Center for Excellence in Developmental Disabilities (UCEDD). Representatives from other groups including parents, advocacy organizations, parent training centers, higher education faculty, and health care professionals may serve as members of the state's leadership team. This team decides if the state has the infrastructure needed to meet the participation requirements of partnership with the NPDC. The leadership team then develops the application.

Upon receipt, each application is reviewed by a team external to the NPDC and rated along criteria developed by the center. These ratings and comments are reviewed by the principal investigators of the NPDC, and three highly rated applications are selected and invited to work with the NPDC for 2 years.

How Is a State's Strategic Plan Developed and Who Needs to Be at the Table?

A state's interagency planning group (IAPG), whose primary task is to identify how the requirements of the NPDC will be meaningfully integrated into the existing infrastructure and activities of each state, is critical to shaping the NPDC partnership. Initial IAPG meetings occur within 6 months of the state's acceptance of the offer to participate. In some states this IAPG has been integrated or grown out of an already existing group. In other states, the IAPG has created the opportunity to bring together a group of key stakeholders for the first time around their common interests in improving their state's capacity for serving children with ASD and their families. Typically, members of the state leadership team, members of the state's training and technical assistance autism network, and representatives from local school districts are included. Parents and individuals with ASD contribute to the IAPG work.

In most states, the NPDC convenes the IAPG for a 1- or 2-day, face-to-face meeting to create a strategic plan, solidify members of the autism training team, and identify priorities for model sites if they have not already been selected. The strategic plan becomes the work plan for how the NPDC and the state will engage over the 2-year partnership. The plan details how the NPDC activities will be implemented within each state, including timelines and who will work on the planned activities. Although each state started this process in its written application, the IAPG meeting provides a forum for bringing participants to a common understanding of the commitments entailed in an NPDC partnership. These discussions often result in the identification of many strengths, but also gaps.

An important consideration within each strategic plan is the sustainability of activities that are undertaken through the NPDC partnership. Some states have a clear idea of how the NPDC will contribute to the professional development system in their state whereas others let that emerge. States establish priorities to strengthen their autism training and technical assistance networks that may include 1) embedding EBPs into the state's ongoing professional development, including summer institutes; 2) developing more networking opportunities among training and technical assistance providers; 3) using more coaching and consultation processes; and 4) increasing partnerships between training and technical assistance providers and higher education faculty.

Strategies for ongoing communication to help a state stay on target with the IAPG commitments in the strategic plan include periodic meetings, tele- and web conferences, and e-mail updates between the NPDC and state leadership staff. Each state's initial strategic plan is reviewed by the IAPG in 1 year and may be modified.

What Are Model Sites and How Are They Developed?

Selected sites (model, then expansion sites) within each state implement the NPDC model. The purpose of these sites is to select and implement EBP based on the needs of children and youth with ASD, implement these practices with fidelity, and monitor progress, all within a quality program. Model sites are developed during the first year of work with the NPDC. They become resources within states that implement EBP for children and youth with ASD within quality programs. These sites are places where practitioners from other programs and classrooms can spend time with skilled practitioners to learn how to implement EBP with students in self-contained and inclusive environments. All this begins by selecting sites, putting technical assistance and coaching structures in place, and completing an initial program of professional development.

What Is Expected of Model Sites and What Do They Agree to Do?   Minimum criteria are established for model sites. Each model site must have administrative support from the school's principal and district superintendent and must have a team of four to six practitioners and teachers who work with students with ASD. In addition, model site team members must

- Be willing to receive and act upon monthly on-site coaching

- Join in regular telephone conferences to focus on changes being implemented

- Be willing to be learning sites and be observed by visitors

- Collect data on student, teacher, and family outcomes

- Complete an array of professional development activities (online course, summer institute, EBP modules)

- Implement EBP that address priority goals of at least three students with ASD in self-contained and/or inclusive educational programs

By clearly defining these expectations, potential sites are informed about the specifics of their roles and responsibilities before agreeing to become a model site. These guidelines have become a useful resource in each state as model sites are identified.

How Is Technical Assistance/Coaching Organized and Who Does It?   Once model sites are selected, state and local technical assistance providers are identified. The decision to have both a local and a state/regional technical assistance (TA) provider for each site, if possible, allows each model site to have a local coach who is frequently available to the site during the year and into the future. The state/regional TA provider is available during the school year to visit each site for at least 1 day a month for training and coaching.

Both TA providers participate in professional development activities along with their model sites and learn to implement the NPDC model. After the year of work with the model site, each TA provider/coach is able to continue the coaching process and use the NPDC model with other sites with NPDC support during the second year of involvement, then on their own once state participation with NPDC ends.

What Initial Statewide Professional Development Is Completed by Model Site Teams and How Is It Delivered?

Professional development begins for all model site and technical assistance personnel in each state with the completion of an online course titled Foundations for Autism Spectrum Disorders and attendance in a weeklong summer institute.

Foundations for Autism Spectrum Disorders   This eight-session online course was developed as an up-to-date source of information about ASD. The sessions cover content on characteristics of ASD, screening and assessment of ASD, factors affecting learning and development, and promoting positive and reducing interfering behaviors among others. All model site team members and technical assistance providers are required to complete the course prior to initiating work with the NPDC in classroom settings. Both text-based and PowerPoint versions of the course content are available for downloading at the NPDC web site.

Summer institutes   The first-year summer institute is a 4- to 5-day training that is developed by the NPDC with the state leadership and hosted in the partner state by the NPDC. The summer institute brings together all model site team members, local and state TA providers, and state leadership to learn about the NPDC model and to plan specific activities for model sites and target students in the fall. An additional benefit is that all attendees have the opportunity to plan and learn together, meeting other model site team members and TA providers, often for the first time. During the second year, the state leadership takes the lead in planning and coordinating the summer institute with support from the NPDC.

The time, energy, and resources invested in developing relationships, identifying the components of the partnership with the NPDC, and providing professional development have been critical. This investment has set the stage for an ongoing collaboration that requires significant commitments from all partners. Then, how does this state-level work translate to the work in specific model sites and classrooms?

IMPLEMENTING THE NATIONAL PROFESSIONAL DEVELOPMENT CENTER ON AUTISM SPECTRUM DISORDERS MODEL

The NPDC model for working with teachers and practitioners in model sites emphasizes 1) measuring and targeting improvement in program and student outcomes, 2) selecting and matching EBP to student need, and 3) implementing EBP with fidelity through training and coaching.

Measuring and Targeting Improvement in Program and Student Outcomes

In order to support the implementation of EBP in school programs serving learners with ASD, the NPDC model focuses on measuring and targeting improvement for two interrelated outcomes: overall program quality and individual learner performance. These two outcomes are not easily separated. High overall program quality provides an optimal environment to implement EBPs that will effect change in individual learner performance, while at the same time the very implementation of EBP results in improvement of overall program quality. The NPDC model uses pre- and posttest measures of both of these outcomes to measure the impact of the implementation of EBP for learners with ASD. Together, these two complementary measures capture change at both the overall program and individual learner levels.

How Are Program Quality Measures Used by Model Site Personnel?   Overall program quality is measured using the APERS. As described in the previous section, the APERS is an environmental rating tool that can be used to rate both inclusive and self-contained programs for learners with ASD at the preschool, elementary, middle, and high school levels. The NPDC uses the APERS to measure baseline program quality at the beginning of the academic year (early in the fall) or toward the end of the previous academic year (late in the spring). The APERS is used again in the spring as a postmeasure to measure change in program quality.

After the APERS is administered, an APERS report is generated that communicates the overall results. This report has two major features: a graphic summary of the results that illustrates the relative strengths and weaknesses in a given program and a narrative highlighting the qualitative nature of program strengths and specific suggestions for improving weaknesses. Two different graphic summaries are used by the NPDC to convey results. One displays domain scores (Figure 13.2), whereas the other provides a more detailed graphic display of individual item scores by domains. With the help of technical assistance providers, teachers and team members work to build on strengths and address weaknesses using the suggestions from the report.

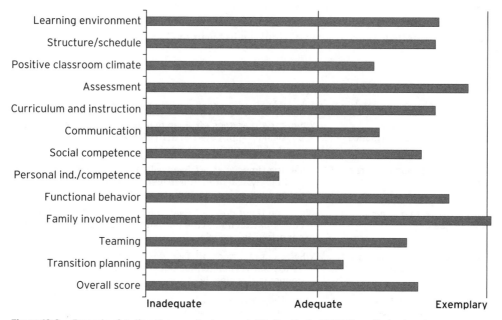

Figure 13.2.   Example of Autism Program Environmental Rating Scale (APERS) profile by domain.

What About Learner Performance? How Is that Monitored?   Individual learner performance is measured using goal attainment scaling (GAS). Although initially developed in the field of mental health (Kiresuk & Sherman, 1968), GAS has a history of use in special education for monitoring individualized goals for learners with disabilities (Balfour & Harris, 1979; Howe & Fitzgerald, 1976; McCarthy & Keener, 1976; Miller, 1975; Schuster, 1984). As used by the NPDC, GAS is a system for assessing the amount of progress that learners with ASD make on select goals over an academic year.

First, teachers, related service professionals, and family members work together to select three priority goals from the learner's IEP. It is critical to the scaling process that the selected goals are observable and measurable. Next, a five-point scale is developed to quantify progress on each selected goal. The lowest point on this scale, "much less than expected," describes the learner's present level of performance at the beginning of the academic year. The second point, "somewhat less than expected," describes a benchmark in between the present level of performance and the annual goal described in the IEP. The third point, "expected level of outcome," describes the progress expected to be made by the end of the academic year, as described by the selected annual goal from the IEP. The fourth and fifth points on the scale, "somewhat more than expected" and "much more than expected" describe learner performance that goes above and beyond the level of performance described in the IEP goal. Although traditional GAS uses a numerical scale (−2, −1, 0, +1, +2) to quantify each of the five points of the scale (Kiresuk & Sherman, 1968), some NPDC? staff found that these numbers were more confusing than helpful to special education practitioners and parents. Therefore, some NPDC coordinating sites have elected to use only descriptive labels and omit the numerical scale in discussions with parents and service providers, although the numeric scale is used in program evaluation. An example of a GAS developed for a learner with an ASD in collaboration with the NPDC is shown in Table 13.1.

At regular points throughout the academic year, learner progress is gauged using the GAS, and a point is selected at the end of the academic year that best describes the learner's level of performance for a given goal. This final rating summarizes the learner's progress relative to the expected annual outcome. Thinking in terms of GAS gives educational teams a

Table 13.1.   Sample goal attainment scaling (GAS) for preschoolers with autism spectrum disorder (ASD)

Much less than expected (Present level of performance)	When the timer goes off, Evan makes a transition with a full physical prompt between activities within the classroom 4 out of 5 opportunities weekly.
Somewhat less than expected (Benchmark)	When the timer goes off, Evan will make a transition with a partial physical prompt between activities within the classroom 4 out of 5 opportunities weekly.
Expected level of outcome (Annual goal)	When the timer goes off, Evan will make a transition independently between activities within the classroom 4 out of 5 opportunities weekly.
Somewhat more than expected (Exceeds annual goal)	When the timer goes off, Evan will make a transition independently between activities outside the classroom 4 out of 5 opportunities weekly.
Much more than expected (Far exceeds annual goal)	When the timer goes off, Evan will make a transition independently between both the classroom and the playground and the classroom and the lunchroom 4 out of 5 opportunities weekly.

framework to work with families to select priority goals (Kiresuk & Choate, 1994), identify appropriate expectations for a learner, and to closely monitor learner outcomes (Oren & Ogletree, 2000).

Once a learner's goals are clearly defined using goal attainment scaling, the next step is to determine which EBPs will be used to support the learner in meeting his or her goals.

Selecting Evidence-Based Practices to Address Student Goals

Identifying and selecting the most appropriate EBP for the learning goals of an individual learner is an important step in the instructional process. This decision is based on a number of factors including the EBP available, consideration of the individual learner, and preferences of the team of professionals who will be implementing the practices.

Where Should I Begin When Selecting Evidence-Based Practices?   Figure 13.1, presented earlier in this chapter, provides a listing of 24 EBPs identified by the NPDC by domains of instruction and age groups targeted in the research. Although this format provides professionals with information on what practices may be most useful in targeting certain skills, it is not meant to be restrictive.

The NPDC has sometimes encouraged teams to identify a single EBP to use with an individual goal. This has been especially helpful for teams who are hesitant about the process and/or less confident in their teaching skills. However, few practices are ever really used in isolation. Prompting and reinforcement, for example, are used in almost all of the other practices. Task analysis, too, is used prior to teaching skills through video modeling, visual supports, and so forth. Teams are encouraged, through coaching and mentoring, to explore the *overlap of practices*. For example, video modeling can be used to teach a self-management system. A social narrative can be written to explain the routine of a social skills training group. A speech-generating device may be used by a learner in the context of a peer-mediated intervention. The understanding required to use practices concurrently, while still being mindful of fidelity of implementation, is an important component in the development of skillful teachers and practitioners.

Consideration of the Individual Learner   Not all students are alike, which is why experienced educators know that no single teaching practice will work for all students. The value in having a list of identified EBPs is that the characteristics of individual learners can be the foremost consideration when selecting practices for instruction. There are four areas for consideration when identifying EBP for individual students, including 1) learning style, 2) temperament, 3) interest and motivators, and 4) history of what has and has not worked.

Team Preferences and Strengths   Combining scientific understanding with professional wisdom has always been considered best instructional practice. Teachers and other practitioners are encouraged to look at their own strengths and interests in the selection of EBP. Technology-minded professionals may be interested in exploring the use of video modeling; other professionals may be more inclined to initiate a parent-implemented intervention. Environmental factors may also influence the selection of EBP. For example, if a classroom is already set up as a structured teaching environment, then structured work systems may be an obvious place to start. If a student is to be served in an inclusive preschool setting, naturalistic interventions may be most appropriate. The NPDC encourages practitioners to build on strengths and interests but also cautions that not every EBP will work for every learner. Thus, just because a professional has had intensive training on Picture Exchange Communication Systems (PECS) does not mean that it will be the appropriate intervention for all students in that setting.

A case example illustrates how consideration of these factors contributes to an appropriate EBP match with student goals.

✳ Nate

Nate was a fifth-grade student with a diagnosis of autism. He was included in a general education classroom for most of his school day. He was academically on target but struggled with small-group work during science and social studies. He loved basketball and video games, and he had some good friends at school who had known him since kindergarten. His mother reported that he was having some trouble with kids in the neighborhood when they would all gather outside after school. His team wanted Nate to improve his social skills in order for him to be more successful during small group work and then generalize these skills to his neighborhood. The team identified the following annual IEP goal, which was further delineated using goal attainment scaling:

> Given a visual prompt, Nate will complete 5 reciprocal turns (listening and verbally responding) in a peer-initiated conversation, within a daily small-group session, in 4/5 opportunities across 5 school days.

Nate's team considered its options by consulting the list of EBP presented in Figure 13.1. They saw that many practices targeted social skills, including discrete trial training, PECS, social narratives, social skills training groups, and video modeling. Next, the team considered Nate. They knew that he really loved interacting with his peers. They knew that he was motivated by topics that are typically of interest to fifth-grade boys-basketball and video games. However, he tended to monopolize conversations around these topics and was at a loss when some other topic was initiated. Finally, the team considered themselves and the setting. Nate was clustered in his regular education setting with two other boys, one with Asperger syndrome and another with attention-deficit/hyperactivity disorder (ADHD). He liked these boys, and they all struggled with many of the same challenges. The special education teacher and the speech-language pathologist (SLP) had a strong collaborative relationship. Taking all of these factors into consideration, Nate's team eventually decided to implement a social skills training group with Nate and the two other boys from his class. The special education teacher and the SLP took turns running the group, and they focused on topic maintenance. They paid attention to their prompting practices as they ran the group and used visual supports. As the group progressed in their skills, the team turned its attention to generalization of these skills to the classroom. They realized that a self-management strategy might help Nate understand his responsibility in the group, and they worked to implement this strategy to fidelity.

Implementing Evidence-Based Practices with Fidelity Through Training and Coaching

The third component of the NPDC model for working with teachers and practitioners describes the resources that are available to learn about implementing EBP with fidelity and the technical assistance and coaching practices that are followed.

What Training Resources Are Available for Practitioners to Use?   In order to assist teams to implement with fidelity the practices they select, the NPDC team has created professional development resources in the form of briefs and modules. These briefs and modules provide the information and tools necessary for professionals to use the EBP with fidelity.

Evidence-Based Practice Briefs   EBP briefs have been developed for all 24 identified practices. These briefs provide concise, text-only documents introducing practitioners to the practices and describing how to effectively implement them. Within the brief, the practice is described in four main documents (Table 13.2). The EBP briefs are available at no cost on the NPDC web site at http://autismpdc.fpg.unc.edu.

Evidence-Based Practice Internet Learning Modules   The NPDC is developing online modules for all 24 EBP. The modules are a more dynamic instructional tool for educators to learn about each of the practices. Each module contains the resources from the briefs as well as more specific guidelines for using the practice, video and case study examples, frequently asked questions, a glossary of terms, discussion questions, suggested activities, and a pre- and postmodule assessment.

State partners are encouraged to use the online modules as part of the training process for implementing EBP. Once school site teams select the EBP that they intend to implement with target students in their program, specific online modules and briefs for the practice are reviewed and used as an integral part of the implementation process. The online modules have been developed in collaboration with the Ohio Center for Autism and Low Incidence Disabilities (OCALI), are posted in its Autism Internet Modules web site (www.autisminternetmodules.org), and are free to the public.

Who Will Help Me Learn to Use These Materials in the Classroom and How?   In addition to the training resources, the NPDC has developed a *coaching model* to address learning needs for participating team members and NPDC partners providing technical assistance/coaching. The NPDC coaching philosophy and guidelines for effective coaching practices are described in a coaching manual. A coaching log has been designed to be used by technical assistance providers to guide coaching practices with participating

Table 13.2.   Evidence-based practice (EBP) brief documents

EBP brief documents	Description of document contents
Overview of the practice	Gives a brief description of the practice and general guidelines for most effective uses of the practice.
Steps for implementing the practice	Provides step-by-step and detailed instructions for implementing the practice. This document also may include sample data collection sheets.
Implementation checklist	Contains all of the steps for implementation in a checklist format. It is designed to be utilized by technical assistance providers and practitioners to monitor fidelity of implementation of the EBP.
Evidence base for the practice	Allows practitioners to have access to the studies that demonstrate the effectiveness of the practice with students who have an autism spectrum disorder.
Optional data sheets	Sample and blank data collection sheets may be provided in a separate document in the brief.

model sites throughout the year. The coaching materials provide a framework for actively working with practitioners during the process of implementation and program improvement.

NPDC personnel also provide *technical assistance* to collaborating partners. The NPDC works with states intensively for 2 years to provide technical assistance in program development, the selection and implementation of EBP, target student progress monitoring, and monthly assistance to teams. This technical assistance has several components including coaching/training, classroom feedback through the use of the APERS findings, monthly site visits by state TA providers, and monthly check-ins from NPDC staff (by phone or in person) for problem-solving and planning.

Coaching Training

A coaching training component, offered during the NPDC annual summer institute, has been designed to instruct technical assistance. The NPDC coaching philosophy and guidelines for effective coaching practices are covered. Video examples and professional development activities are included to demonstrate and practice effective coaching. Materials to plan for and record coaching activities during the year are included.

APERS Feedback

Model sites receive program quality feedback from NPDC staff following administration of the APERS. The recommendations and observations from the APERS guide programwide improvement efforts during the intensive year of work with each model site.

Monthly Site Visits

Technical assistance to model site programs is provided during monthly on-site visits by state and local autism trainers. These technical assistance providers or coaches work with model site teams to implement an agreed-upon plan for each model site. The plan draws upon recommendations from the APERS report (program quality), the GAS developed for each target student (learner outcomes), and context-specific factors (e.g., type of program, age of students, resources available onsite). During monthly site visits, coaching practices outlined in the coaching manual are followed.

During monthly site visits the coaches work with teachers and team members to 1) monitor progress toward reaching student's targeted goals, 2) select EBP that support goal attainment, 3) coach teachers and others in the appropriate use of EBP and to establish fidelity of practice implementation, 4) assist in defining other classroom issues and plan actions, and 5) provide support with data collection. Implementation fidelity of EBP is monitored by completing the practice implementation checklist, which is contained within the brief and module for each practice. This checklist is completed at baseline prior to implementation and then in an ongoing fashion throughout the year. Also, technical assistance providers use the coaching log to plan monthly visits and guide the discussion around EBP use in the classroom.

Monthly Phone Calls

Following monthly site visits, NPDC team members have a conference call with the technical assistance providers and model site team members to discuss outcomes associated with each on-site visit. Topics covered in the monthly calls include an update on implementation of EBP, a progress report on the goal attainment for target students, the completion of the coaching log, and updates on NPDC resources and materials. In addition, priorities and plans for the upcoming month are outlined.

WHAT LESSONS CAN WE SHARE FROM OUR WORK?

The NPDC has learned a great deal about the implementation of EBP and other factors that influence the success of a program through work with model site teams and coaches. Likewise, lessons have been learned about state-level implementation. Some of these are described next.

Measurable and Attainable Goals Are Essential   In developing GAS for multiple students with multiple teams, it has been essential to step back and revisit the process of writing functional, observable, and measurable goals. Although goal writing is a skill that is taught in all special education training programs, the practice of goal writing sometimes deteriorates as a teacher works in real classrooms with real caseloads of students. Often teachers and staff lose sight of what the "target act" of a lesson or set of instructions is; they forget what it is they actually want to accomplish during this circle time or that science lesson. Refocusing the team on selecting a target act that is discrete and observable, measurable, and attainable helps to increase the precision of teaching.

Start with the Fundamentals   Certain EBP seem to attract teachers more than others. The effective implementation of video modeling, social skills training groups, and computer aided instruction are but a few examples. It is rare that teachers show enthusiasm for improving their skills in the areas of prompting, visual supports, or functional behavior assessment. Yet, the results of our APERS often point to these practices as the elements of programming that would have the most beneficial effect on the classroom. Refining the prompting practices of, for example, five staff members that work together in a classroom can have a profound effect on day-to-day behavior and learning. Improving the visual supports can instantly change the way a classroom operates. Fundamental practices are strongly encouraged as part of our technical assistance suggestions.

Make Evidence Based Practices Work for You   Some of the practices that have been identified by the NPDC as evidence-based are individualized and labor intensive. Implementing these with large class sizes and limited resources is challenging. PECS and discrete trial training (DTT), for example, require one or two adults to work with a single student, at least during the critical early phases. One of our model site teachers wanted to use both practices in her classroom. She quickly realized that she needed to teach her other students how to work more independently in order to create a time in the day where two adults could implement PECS and/or DTT. This realization led her to improve her classroom structure (with the help of the structured work systems module) to make it possible for other students to learn to be on-task, independent workers. By initially focusing on one EBP (structured work systems), she was able to scale up to address the more complex and labor-intensive practices of DTT and PECS.

Administrative Support Is Crucial   Administrative support is imperative in order to implement innovation. NPDC staff has been fortunate to experience some model site environments where the administrative support has clearly helped teachers make changes to their teaching. In one location, districtwide professional learning communities have supported opportunities for teams to come together to collaborate and plan for change. In another district, an administrator with personal and professional passion for working with children who have ASD has led the team to use peer-mediated interventions to make the school a positive and more socially successful environment for their learners with ASD. Teams in both settings have made ASD program improvement a schoolwide goal for the educational community.

Everyone Needs a Coach   Because every district has a slightly different infrastructure, it can be hard to identify someone to act as a coach or mentor for a teacher or team working with learners with ASD. The same job title can have a very different job description depending on where you work and what individual district and community needs are present. However, it is important that *all* teachers have someone to go to for brainstorming, guidance, resources, and general support.

Turnover Happens   One of the reasons infrastructure is so important—whether it is formal through a state network or informal through a strong team process and peer-to-peer coaching—is that turnover happens. People leave the district for one reason or another; teachers are transferred to different buildings. If a program relies on one great teacher, it really is a house of cards. When that teacher has questions or wants guidance, there is no one for her to turn to. If that teacher were to take a position elsewhere, where does that leave the program? Having a team who takes advantage of—and learns from—each other's expertise leads to a program that is sustainable and that can withstand the inevitable turnover.

You Don't Have to Do It All At Once   The NPDC uses the technique of starting small, and then scaling up. Although our partnership is with an entire state, three model sites are initially identified, a minimum of three target students are selected from each site, and three priority goals are selected for each target student from his or her IEP. The belief is that, by focusing on and increasing proficiency in one area with success, more areas of improvement, more learners, more programs, and more schools can be added. Our teams are encouraged to approach change in this manner. If school teams take smaller steps, change is much more manageable.

Practice Makes Perfect   A lot of great teaching for students with ASD happens in schools. Many teachers already use some of the practices that the NPDC has identified as having an evidence base. Teachers in our project looked at NPDC materials and did, in fact, improve their use of the practice. In one school, a teacher working with social narratives looked at the implementation checklists and improved her use of data collection practices so that she had documentation of the increased understanding these students gained. She was already a fine, skillful teacher, but by taking a closer look at her teaching and making sure she was following all the steps of the implementation checklist, she brought her use of the practice closer to fidelity. She reported that using tools like the implementation checklist increased her own confidence in her teaching and made her more consistent in her use of social narratives.

Don't Throw the Baby Out with the Bath Water   Some professionals fear operationalized, step-by-step directions, thinking they suggest cookie-cutter teaching. Teaching is never simply a matter of checking items off a to-do list. Teachers are encouraged to retain the positive things they are doing such as building rapport with a student, developing relationships with families, having fun with their students, and laughing and joking with colleagues. All of these things are integral to good teaching, and no step-by-step guide will replace their value. It has been a privilege to spend time in so many different schools, and that untouchable quality of school climate—that feeling of positivism and respect—is real.

NPDC staff encourage teachers to hold onto that "art" of good teaching while working to implement scientifically based practices with fidelity.

No Program Is an Island   Sometimes, individual classrooms stand as almost their own miniprograms—the teachers within each classroom meet and collaborate, but opportunities for cross-classroom teaching are few. For example, one classroom may become very skilled at the use of functional behavioral assessment, and another at social skills training groups. But without the chance to share their knowledge with one another, there is no expansion of these successful practices. Another "island" example is a classroom that many educators are familiar with: special education students in a basement, in a corner. The out-of-sight-out-of-mind-mentality has a negative impact for staff, typically developing learners, and those with special needs. A shared environment leads to a shared set of expectations for behavior, a common understanding of community, and mutual respect.

Recruit the Right People for the Interagency Autism Planning Group and Leadership Team   Without leaders with the vision for how the system should look across the state, commitment to building capacity, ability to think of better ways to proceed, and authority to commit resources, very little will happen after the initial 2 years. The entire state partnership is built by having the right people at the table, owning the process, and implementing the expansion in subsequent years.

Talk About and Plan for Sustainability from the Beginning   Sustainability is discussed from the beginning of the planning process with states and continues with each site and the state leadership throughout the 2 years. There is a deliberate process in which the NPDC engages with states that transfers increasing responsibility for planning and implementation to states while reducing responsibility for the NPDC. By the end of the 2 years of collaborative work between the state and NPDC, the state is equipped to continue implementing the model. Briefs, online modules, coaching processes, APERS, strategic planning procedures, online course, forms, and other items are available for use by the states during the time they actively partner with the NPDC and after.

ONE STATE'S SUCCESSES

Although all of our state partners look for ways to translate their partnerships with the NPDC into sustainable infrastructure and capacity building, one state in particular has demonstrated an exceptional level of commitment in using the NPDC model as a catalyst for statewide change.

From the moment that they partnered with the NPDC, this state's representatives focused heavily on sustainability, taking a number of steps to promote rapid dissemination of knowledge, materials, and technical assistance. One year into the partnership, they took ownership of the NPDC online course at a state university to allow additional practitioners to be able to complete it sooner and registered an additional 700 participants in only the second year of the NPDC partnership. During the second year of the partnership, this state tripled their number of model sites (from 4 to 12) and regional summer institutes (from 1 to 3) on EBP, supporting them with state and local personnel following the NPDC model. Training cadres have been formed in every school district across the state, consisting of at least two professionals able to implement and model EBP with fidelity. Members of the cadres not yet involved in the project are invited to shadow and learn from currently participating districts, so that everyone will be trained and prepared to implement the model at the conclusion of the NPDC partnership. State leaders and technical assistance providers worked closely together, always considering what the next step would be in scaling up the model.

With an ambitious vision, a strategic plan, and a high level of commitment, this state has used the NPDC partnership as a springboard for statewide training and coaching in the effective implementation of EBP for students with ASD. Although states plan to sustain their work in different ways, all states that have partnered with the NPDC have taken steps to ensure that a sustainable infrastructure for improving education services for students with ASD continues in place long after the NPDC partnership concludes.

REFERENCES

Autism Program Environment Rating Scale Development Group. (2012). Chapel Hill: Frank Porter Graham Child Development Institute, University of North Carolina at Chapel Hill.

Balfour, M.J., & Harris, L.H. (1979). *Sail, an innovative mainstream special education project for drop-out prone students: Validation report* (Research Report). Hopkins, MN: Author.

Gersten, R., Fuchs, L.S., Compton, D., Coyne, M., Greenwood, C., & Innocenti, M. (2005). Quality indicators for group experimental and quasi-experimental research in special education. *Exceptional Children, 71,* 149–164.

Horner, R., Carr, E., Halle, J., McGee, G., Odom, S., & Wolery, M. (2005). The use of single subject research to identify evidence-based practice in special education. *Exceptional Children, 71,* 165–180.

Howe, C.E., & Fitzgerald, M.E. (1976). *A model for evaluation of special education programs in Iowa area education agencies.* Des Moines: Iowa State Department of Public Instruction, Division of Special Education.

Kiresuk, T., & Choate, R. (1994). Applications of goal setting. In T. Kiresuk, A. Smith, & J. Cardillo (Eds.), *Goal attainment scaling: Applications, theory, and measurement* (pp. 61–104). Mahwah, NJ: Lawrence Erlbaum Associates.

Kiresuk, T.J., & Sherman, R.E. (1968). Goal attainment scaling: A general method for evaluation of community mental health programs. *Community Mental Health Journal, 4,* 443–453.

McCarthy, R., & Keener, N. (1976). *Goal attainment follow-up at a preschool diagnostic center.* Minneapolis, MN: Program Evaluation Resource Center.

Miller, G.H. (1975). Problem and goal-oriented evaluation system. In B. Willer, G.H. Miller, & L. Cantrell (Eds.), *Information and feedback for evaluation* (Vol. 1, pp. 34–43). Toronto, Ontario, Canada: York University.

Odom, S., Collet-Klingenberg, L., Rogers, S., & Hatton, D. (2010). Evidence-based practices in interventions for children and youth with autism spectrum disorders. *Preventing School Failure, 54*(4), 275–282.

Oren, T., & Ogletree, B. (2000). Program evaluation in classrooms for students with autism: Student outcomes and program processes. *Focus on Autism and Other Developmental Disabilities, 15*(3), 170–175.

Schuster, S. (1984). Goal attainment scaling with moderately and severely handicapped preschool children. *Journal of the Division of Early Childhood, 8*(1), 26–37.

IV

Facing Autism Nationally

How to Improve Services Through Training, Research, and Policy

14

What We Have Learned

How to Create Integrated Networks that Improve Access, Increase Capacity, Develop Expertise, and Address Meaningful Outcomes

Peter Doehring

The final section of this book seeks to draw conclusions from the overview chapters and those describing regional, statewide, and national programs for services, training, research, and policy surrounding autism spectrum disorder (ASD). This chapter begins by returning to the question of outcomes: Does the spectrum and lifelong trajectory of ASD suggest new ways to design regional, statewide, and national programs for services, training, research, and policy to improve outcomes? It then evaluates patterns in the other elements of the network for ASD—the domains addressed, level and type of agency, and the type of population served. Next, it revisits the components—the service, training, research, and policy—and the natural relationships between them that appear to emerge at the local, state, and national level. The chapter concludes by offering some principles for understanding how different kinds of services for ASD draw from training, research, and policy at the local, state, and national level. Throughout, the chapter draws from the descriptions in the overview chapters in Section I and those of the specific programs described in Sections II and III. It frames the discussion as specific lessons or principles that program leaders should consider. This sets the stage for the final chapter, which puts forth recommended specific strategies for regions just beginning to develop and organize their networks, as well as strategies for those regions that already have key networks established and are seeking to grow. These strategies draw on the key services, training, research, and policy described next and are linked back to examples described in the program chapters whenever applicable.

Throughout this final section, the emphasis is on how the potential interrelationships between services, training, research, and policy at the local, state, and national level may support the development of a truly integrated network. As outlined in Section I, the network of local, state, and national agencies and organizations was not built logically, from the ground up, to better understand and support people living with ASD through services, training, research, and policy. Therefore, the current network can be characterized as ad hoc, emerging through informal relationships between public and private agencies and organizations, with often complementary (but sometimes competing) mandates. In some cases, this ad hoc network has successfully adapted to the growing needs of these children and families, but in too many other cases it has failed. In many respects, the goal for this book is to provide the information needed to redefine and reinvigorate this network and promote a seamless integration of services, training, research, and policy addressing ASD at the local, state, and national level that takes full advantage of the growing awareness, understanding, and commitment to help people living with ASD fulfill their potential.

INITIATIVES MUST DEMONSTRATE PROGRESS TOWARD OUTCOMES FOR INDIVIDUALS WITH AUTISM SPECTRUM DISORDER, THEIR CAREGIVERS, AND THE SYSTEM OF SERVICES

Each of the programs in Sections II and III described innovative programs for addressing specific elements of services, training, research, and policy addressing ASD. To draw conclusions from these initiatives, the question of outcomes must be revisited. What do the programs reviewed here tell us about how local, state, and national initiatives related to services, training, research, and policy addressing ASD might improve outcomes? What lessons can be learned and what solutions can be suggested that will help design a more effective and integrated network? Whenever possible, the outcomes must be discussed at both the individual level (e.g., improving the quality of life for people living with ASD) and at the network level (e.g., improving the efficiency with which services and supports can be delivered). All services, training, and research initiatives should require demonstration of measurable progress toward outcomes related to improved quality of life for individuals and improved delivery of services and associated training.

There are several reasons outcomes must be revisited. First, the tremendous challenge of developing services, training, research, and policy at the local, state, and national level has caused professionals to lose sight of the very outcomes most agencies pursue: improving the lives of people living with ASD. Many agencies and organizations adopt ambitious mission statements professing the desire to improve such outcomes, but they neither gather data to clearly demonstrate progress toward these outcomes, nor are they held accountable for a lack of progress: A treatment center may describe the number of individuals or caregivers served but provide little data on satisfaction with services; a university center focused on training will define impact in terms of the number of professionals trained, not whether services improved as a result; researchers are more likely to be evaluated in terms of the number of peer-reviewed publications produced and not on the translation of research into practice; policy makers focus on the passage of legislation and often lose focus with developing the regulations that define how the legislation takes life. Many agencies inevitably err toward more narrow definitions of desired outcomes when reconsidering their mandates during times of fiscal restraint.

My colleagues and I believe that other problems contribute to these gaps. For example, many agencies and organizations either never fully grasp, or simply lose sight of, the full range of needs and outcomes for individuals with ASD and their caregivers across the life span. They may struggle to achieve narrowly defined outcomes while missing easier opportunities to address a broader outcome that is more meaningful to families. In addition, important decisions are more often based in opinion and tradition instead of data, and settings sometimes pursue the prestige of a highly specialized program instead of ensuring an essential level of access or competence across the network. One of the most compelling themes in the emerging research findings since 2000—that ASD varies tremendously from one person to another and across the life span—further complicates the task of translating research findings into practice. Together, these problems may also help to explain how some of the gaps in services, training, and policy have widened despite growing awareness of the broad impact of ASD.

There is a real opportunity for a new kind of research that can inform policy, training, and practice by considering the full spectrum of outcomes across the life span for both the individual and the network and barriers to translating research finding into practice. Translational research can foster better integration of services, training, and research across local, state, and national networks by emphasizing the transfer of practices from the research laboratory to the community. Setting-specific goals that address the quality of life of people living with ASD may help reenergize parents, practitioners, and policy makers who have become disillusioned with the disconnection between traditional academic research and the plight of people living with ASD (Burgess & Gutstein, 2007). In many respects, the power of these research designs to uncover subtle differences in the characteristics of ASD—how these change with development, as a function of other skills, and in relation to other neurological features—has far outpaced the ability of practitioners to translate these discoveries into real and meaningful improvements in outcomes.

The Ability to Gain Access to Critical Services Is a Key System Outcome

Empirical research offers the greatest potential to improve the lives of people living with ASD, and the next chapter describes some of the steps professionals need to take to fully realize the promise of evidence-based practices (EBP). Before any of the benefits of EBP can be realized, however, the fundamental problems of access must be tackled. Can people living with ASD gain access to the services already available and already recognized as key to successful outcomes? How do professionals identify barriers to gaining access to services? How do they test strategies to push through these barriers? Data from the 2005 Pennsylvania Autism Census (Lawer & Mandel, 2009) summarized earlier (see Chapter 3) and data now beginning to emerge from the 2011 Pennsylvania Autism Needs Assessment (see Chapter 6) begin to illustrate some of the challenges of identifying and addressing fundamental problems of access. Why are 60%–90% of people with a possible diagnosis of ASD in Pennsylvania not receiving health and/or education services under this label, and what does this mean for outcomes?

- *Some individuals with ASD may not need, or may no longer need, services from any of these agencies.* By studying this group, those in the field may discover important characteristics of the individual or the network contributing to positive outcomes.

- *They have not yet been identified with ASD.* Some of the barriers to identification include the failure to universally adopt recommended methods for screening for ASD and the lack of a cost-effective diagnostic protocol for community-based practitioners (see Chapter 3). Other barriers suggested by the results of the needs assessment include the long wait for a diagnostic assessment, the initial misdiagnosis of ASD, and the lack of qualified diagnosticians (Bureau of Autism Services, 2011c).

- *They may not be referred to appropriate services.* Results of the needs assessment indicated that, even among preschool children recently identified with ASD, less than one half were referred to specific treatment or follow-up appointments, and more than one quarter were not referred to early intervention services (Bureau of Autism Services, 2011c).

- *They may need services but cannot gain access to providers.* Barriers suggested by the needs assessment include the limited availability of trained providers, the lack of providers who accept Medicaid, the challenging behavior of the person with an ASD, and the lack of transportation to services (Bureau of Autism Services, 2011a). Thus, identifying effective services is only one of many steps needed to improve outcomes.

- *They may need services but cannot afford them.* Respondents to the needs assessment reported that the cost of services or the lack of insurance prevented them from gaining access to care (Bureau of Autism Services, 2011a). In addition, more than 60% of caregivers or their partners reported a significant change in employment that had direct impact on their ability to pay for services (Bureau of Autism Services, 2011b).

The problem of access can be framed in terms of both the individual living with ASD and the network seeking to improve the services, training, research, and policy. It is clear that until these fundamental problems of identification and access are addressed, the potential for positive outcomes for individuals living with ASD will be limited. At best, there may be isolated pockets of success, but the majority of people with ASD continue to be underidentified and underserved. These fundamental problems of identification and access also suggest potential goals for local state and national initiatives related to services, training, research, and policy. Relative to the goals most often identified by agencies—for example, to identify core features of ASD, causes of ASD, and evidence-based interventions for ASD—goals related to improved identification may be more realistic in the short term (given the many initiatives described herein). Similarly, goals related to access may be more meaningful in the intermediate term, to the extent that problems of access will ultimately limit the speed with which new policies and practices can be implemented.

All Service, Training, Research, and Policy Initiatives Should Adopt Broader Goals that Address Quality of Life

The spectrum of potential outcomes considered should include a balance between the traditional, narrowly defined outcomes (e.g., that address specific, individual goals) and those defined more broadly to address the quality of life (see Figure 14.1). This might require a realignment of resources to better assess the range of needs and to better document impact, but such a broadening the range of goals for programs related to services, training, and policy may be the only way to prevent this drift away from improving the quality of life of people living with ASD. This realignment is consistent with a growing interest in quality-of-life issues for people with ASD (Burgess & Gutstein, 2007).

Working from the top down—that is, thinking in terms of broad outcomes framed as issues of quality of life—may be important for several reasons. First, it may help to recalibrate goals and resources in important ways when designing individual treatment plans. On the one hand, the professional may adopt a narrow goal to improve a child's requesting and thus may be content with evidence of increased requesting in a weekly session with a speech pathologist in his or her office. On the other hand, the professional may adopt a broad goal to improve the child's quality of life by ensuring that the person can independently communicate his or her essential wants, needs, and interests across settings. The latter goal may compel the service professional to adopt more functional goals (e.g., to identify all of the toys the child likes to play with before moving on to more abstract language functions and concepts), shift resources to promote generalization (e.g., to include opportunities for

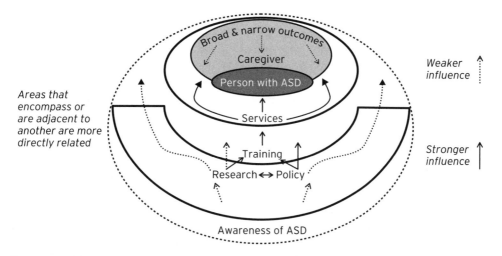

Figure 14.1. Interrelationship of awarenes, services, training, research, policy, and outcomes for people living with autism spectrum disorder (ASD).

parent training), and realign the schedule and curriculum (e.g., to maximize communication opportunities outside of the session with the speech language pathologist).

Working from the top down may help to counteract the tendency of agencies to function in silos and instead pushes them toward a common goal, as long as there are opportunities for collaboration. My colleagues and I were privileged to observe a number of different Act Early state teams (see Chapter 12) working to develop state plans to improve early identification. We found that teams who came to frame these goals more broadly (e.g., to increase access to timely and accurate diagnostic services) seemed more likely to look beyond their traditional roles, to recognize barriers to gaining access to services, and identify potential partnerships to overcome these barriers. Working from the top down may also prevent professionals from overlooking easier opportunities to have a more meaningful impact. As discussed next, the failure to provide training and support to caregivers appears to be one of the more persistent gaps in the ad hoc network. But one simple solution to improve the quality of life of caregivers is to facilitate the provision of before- and after-school care, respite, and summer programs.

Consider Needs Across the Life Span When Allocating Resources

Whether one considers the availability of specialized services and associated training, the amount of research, or the types of policies enacted, the focus appears exclusive to children with ASD. Yet when one considers that many people with ASD can live into their old age and that many continue to require intensive levels of support if they and their caregivers are to achieve and maintain a reasonable quality of life, adults with ASD merit at least equivalent if not a greater focus relative to children. It is difficult to dispute the long-term potential for early identification and intervention to change the trajectory of outcomes for people with ASD and perhaps decrease or even largely eliminate the need for such a focus on adults with ASD. This potential is far, however, from being fully realized; tremendous strides have been made in many aspects of intervention but have certainly not achieved a cure or significant recovery in the majority of children. Moreover, recent findings suggesting that ASD may have multiple and complex genetic bases (Glessner et al., 2009; Wang et al.,

2009) makes the discovery of a cure or a single powerful intervention even less likely. Thus, there is no scientific basis for the almost exclusive focus on children with ASD. Instead, this focus probably reflects the concerns of each new generation of advocates from among the thousands of caregivers struggling to cope with the recent diagnosis of a young child with an ASD, together with a new generation of researchers, clinicians, and policy makers eager to make a difference and hopeful for a cure. Although each new generation brings new energy to these endeavors, failure to rely on the available scientific evidence when deciding where to focus efforts and resources has led to the neglect of tens of thousands of adults living with ASD across the country.

Over the past decade, advocates have begun to draw attention to the tremendous lack of services and supports for adults with ASD. In part, this may reflect that the generation of advocates, originally mobilized when their children were first identified with ASD in the 1990s, has been preparing for the transition out of education services. Most now face an abrupt decrease in services that accompanies the transition into adulthood, and this situation is unlikely to improve without significant injection of new resources because the number of individuals with ASD entering adulthood will increase dramatically going forward.

These stark realities are reflected in some of the other recent findings in Pennsylvania. The 2005 Pennsylvania Autism Census projected that the number of adults with ASD will increase from 1,421 in 2005 to 3,825 by 2010, and 10,140 by 2015, for an overall increase of more than 600% in 10 years (Lawer & Mandel, 2009). The 2011 Pennsylvania Autism Needs Assessment indicates that the adults with ASD face many unmet needs once they leave the education system in the areas of health, employment, behavior support, and other services (Bureau of Autism Services, 2011d). Caregivers of adults with autism reported that 55% of individuals were unemployed and that more than 50% had unmet needs related to employment (e.g., transitional planning, career counseling, vocational training, and/or supported employment) and social skills training. These gaps extend into research, training, and policy related to adult outcomes. For example, when my colleagues and I reviewed the outcome research published in three prominent journals (*Journal of Applied Behavior Analysis, Journal of Autism and Developmental Disorders,* and *Journal of Positive Behavior Interventions*) between 2000 and 2006, we found that less that 8% of articles describing outcome research (and less than 2% of all articles) described outcome research involving adults (Doehring et al., 2008).

Identify Outcomes for Caregivers

One of the most significant changes over the past decade is the increasing involvement of caregivers not only in the treatment and care of their children but also in the broader network of training, research, and policy. Although research and policy may generally acknowledge the importance of the caregiver and family, most programs providing services or training focus on the individual with an ASD. Individual education plans are written for the student; health care is directed to an individual patient. There is now a watershed in the evolution of the role of caregivers; a shift from participant to true partner, and potentially the manager if not the direct recipient of key services, supports, and associated training. Caregivers can—and sometimes do—fulfill a role that professionals will never be able to assume, stepping into the breech to compensate for an inadequate system of services and supports and sometimes amassing more knowledge and providing more intervention in key areas than the professionals around them. There is a need to go far beyond providing compassionate understanding and consider training and supporting caregivers directly. This is reflected in Figure 14.1, in which the caregiver plays many different roles in mediating the impact of services and support on the person with an ASD. This is not to discount the important and often overlooked role played by other family members (e.g., siblings, grandparents), but the focus here is on the caregiver's involvement and responsibility because it is broad and lifelong.

• *Service provider:* There are many instances in which caregivers play a direct and unique role in service delivery. This goes far beyond traditional parental responsibilities, and, when expressed as hours of intervention, is far greater than that of professionals. When adequately trained educators, physicians, behavior analysts, speech pathologists, and case managers are not available, parents do their best to teach, treat, and track down resources. Caregivers essentially function as the most important of service providers because the intense, complex, and ever-evolving needs of their offspring, combined with the many gaps in service and support that already exist, mean that the traditional system of services and supports fall far short of meeting the needs of people with ASD. Caregivers are sometimes the only ones generalizing specific skills and plans to more natural settings. The most meaningful difference between the majority of caregivers and the professionals with whom they work is that the latter chose to assume that role, are more likely to have received formal training in that role, and can set that role aside at the end of the work day.

• *Case coordinator:* For most people with ASD, a well-supported and well-informed caregiver will provide lifelong, person-centered, cross-agency case coordination and management that is far superior to any provided by a professional (although this may be moot because there are few examples of cross-agency case management).

• *Advocate for the person in their care:* In additional to coordinating services, caregivers may provide the voice for the person in their care, if that person cannot assume that role. For a significant proportion of people with ASD, this is a lifelong responsibility. By extension, caregivers may also provide the voice for broader systems change.

Not all caregivers are able to assume all of these roles at all points throughout their lifetime; some may never be able to do so, even with improvements in training and support. Some caregivers may struggle with their own cultural, mental health, or family issues. Supporting families who can assume these roles does not, as a society, obviate our responsibility to support those families who cannot act as a service provider, case-coordinator, and/ or advocate.

The central role played by many caregivers in the lifelong care and support of people with ASD casts a new light on the potential impact of ASD on caregivers. Thus, as the role of the caregiver increases, the impact of ASD on caregivers is magnified: It affects the caregiver directly and affects the person with ASD via the effect it has on the ability of the caregiver to fulfill his or her multiple roles. As described earlier in this section, caregivers face many significant barriers to gaining access to services. The cumulative impact of these barriers can leave caregivers increasingly bitter and disillusioned; they can lose the patience to negotiate the service maze and nurture the alliances they so carefully built with different professionals, schools, and other agencies. And all of this is likely to happen when the person with the ASD approaches adolescence, after the caregiver may have already struggled for many years. Too often, caregivers are pulled into a maelstrom in which the deteriorating behavior of the person with an ASD increasingly limits the ability of the caregiver to adapt and respond. This leads to further deterioration, until the person is finally removed from the parent's care. In most cases, these tragic outcomes could have been avoided: They result not from a lack of knowledge but from a failure of implementation.

OTHER COMPONENTS OF AN INTEGRATED NETWORK

In Section I of this book, I described many of the components of the network: the elements (services, training, research, and policy); the sector (public, private); the domain (education, health, and community supports); and the level (local, regional, state, and national). These are summarized in Figure 14.2. All professionals should recognize that the distinctions between some of these elements may not always be clear; national agencies can (and in many cases, should) have mechanisms for influencing the action of local agencies and vice versa, and a given agency may address multiple components and/or domains. Nonetheless, most agencies and organizations can be generally categorized according to these components, and that these distinctions help to describe the most common boundaries, and to disentangle agencies with overlapping mandates. Before professionals can begin to grasp the true potential and the limitations of an integrated network, however, they also need to distinguish between other components not discussed thus far. These are indicated in Figure 14.2 in italics and discussed next.

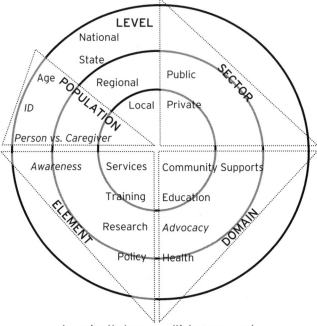

Agencies that span multiple components

Figure 14.2. Components of an integrated network of support for people living with autism spectrum disorder.
(*Key:* ID = intellectual disabilities.)

The Population(s) Served

Set Research-Based Priorities to Better Meet the Needs of the Entire Population It is generally acknowledged that ASD covers a broad spectrum. As exemplified by the programs described in this book, the range of components and domains addressing this spectrum appears to be equally broad. Yet professionals seem unable to precisely project the proportion of the population likely to benefit from specific interventions or programs, despite more stable estimates of the overall prevalence of ASD and the growing ability to characterize the many facets of ASD. There is little consensus on which types of programs must be developed first (at best, professionals can only agree that the services and supports needed by those living with ASD must be highly individualized). As a result, it is difficult to establish the priorities for overall program growth in a balanced and logical manner that takes the true extent of the needs of the overall population into account.

How do professionals draw on existing scientific data, or collect new data regarding the population of people living with ASD to more accurately project their future needs and more effectively and efficiently scale up services, training, research, and policy? In Chapter 3, I recommended that, in the long term, the focus must shift away from describing the causes and characteristics of people with ASD to more precisely describing their needs, their response to intervention, and the resources needed to implement these interventions effectively. In the short term, professionals might reconsider the potential value of broadly characterizing the range of needs according to general population categories. I understand why some might be skeptical of such a strategy, given that categorical distinctions between Asperger versus high-functioning autism do not seem to reliably predict response to treatment. Traditional, categorical distinctions between children, adolescents, and adults will continue to be useful—professionals can clearly justify offering some services exclusively to one group or another (e.g., early intervention, employment). Categorical distinctions based on presence or absence of significant intellectual disability may also have some use.

Build Bridges with the Community of Those Living with Very Significant Intellectual Disabilities Over the past decade, the focus on ASD as unique has been important to increasing awareness and mobilizing the energy for change. This focus has helped to uncover the characteristics common to people with ASD across the spectrum: that all people with ASD demonstrate a pattern of unusual interests or behaviors together with distinct deficits in social interaction, though the extent and specific manifestations of this pattern vary from individual to individual. Yet the emphasis on the unique characteristics of ASD has obscured the many areas of overlap between the needs of people with ASD and those with other disorders, most notably those with very significant intellectual disabilities (ID). (By very significant ID, I am broadly referring to those individuals with IQ scores clearly outside of the normal range on standardized measures of intelligence.) This is striking because, in many respects, the movement to improve the lives of people with ID sets the stage for advocates for ASD, bringing to light the deplorable treatment of people with ID and psychiatric disorders and leading to the passage of the landmark Individuals with Disabilities Education Act.

I believe that the determination to distinguish between those with and without ASD, within the overall population of people with very significant ID, may be misplaced and ineffective. On the one hand, there are clearly people with ASD who are also ostensibly identified with ID only because the right tests were not selected, reasonable accommodations were not offered, and/or the tester simply did not recognize specific and significant areas of potential that can be characteristic of ASD and that would render overall estimates of intelligence invalid. On the other hand, an argument can be made that the amount and types of services and associated training for people who truly present with very significant ID—with and without ASD—are more clearly determined by the level of ID than by the presence or absence of ASD. The emphasis on ASD and not ID has led to overlooking areas of common need and the potential for improvements in services, training, research, and policy that will ultimately benefit both groups. The emphasis on ASD to the exclusion of ID has also drawn attention away from the equally pressing need for lifelong services and supports for all people living with significant ID, not just those with ASD.

The functional irrelevance of the identification of ASD among those with very significant ID is evident in the challenge of differential diagnosis faced by community-based practitioners. In my experience, it is not uncommon for these practitioners to interpret significant deficits in communication and peer interaction, and the need for sameness or predominant focus on the sensory qualities of the world, in absolute terms, not in the context of the overall ID. Although these characteristics conform to the definition of ASD on face value, they are also entirely consistent with the person's overall development and functioning level. Even in more controlled laboratory contexts, assessment protocols are less effective in reliably diagnosing ASD as the level of ID increases (de Bildt et al., 2004). I argue that, in such cases, the additional diagnosis of ASD adds little to intervention planning, except to open the door to funding and intervention methods traditionally (and erroneously) designated solely for people with ASD.

There are several consequences of attempts to differentiate ASD among those with significant ID. First, interventions potentially beneficial to both populations do not always cross over readily from one to the other. One common area of need is behavior support informed by functional behavioral assessment (FBA) and driven by methods based in applied behavior analysis (ABA) generally and positive behavior supports (PBS) specifically. Practitioners may fail to recognize that some behavior interventions derived from research with people with ASD and ID apply equally well to those with ID but not ASD. In my experience, the intensity of obsessions/rituals and the reaction to certain sensory stimuli is perhaps more marked among some people with ASD, and the patterns of socially maintained behavior are perhaps more readily established among some without ASD, but otherwise the functions of behavior and response to other interventions are generally comparable: The expertise needed to successfully develop and implement behavior plans for people with ASD and ID translates readily to address the same needs in people with ID but without ASD.

Second, and perhaps more important, service systems developed for one population may be suited to all those with very significant ID, regardless of whether they also have ASD. This is particularly important in contexts when the limited number of people with a disorder precludes the efficient development of a service specialized for one population or another. For example, in a small rural school district, it may be impossible (and, as argued earlier, perhaps irrelevant) to develop a specialized classroom for those with very significant ID and ASD separate from a classroom with other children with similar needs but who lack the formal diagnosis of ASD. I discuss how to take advantage of these overlapping areas of need in the next chapter.

The Domain of Advocacy

Over the past decade, agencies and organizations focused primarily on advocacy have played an increasingly important role in shaping services, training, research, and policy at the local, state, and national level, and across a range of issues. Autism Society of America has continued to build on a strong network of state chapters to raise awareness and mobilize resources at the local, state, and national level. Autism Speaks has emerged as a new and powerful force for change, through its unprecedented contribution to research funding and the development of research networks, spearheading of state insurance reform to increase resources for services for ASD, and other initiatives. Other organizations have helped raise awareness and promote change in more specific areas, like early detection (First Signs), awareness of research (Organization for Autism Research), and participation in research studies (Interactive Autism Network). The increasingly articulate communities of care-givers and self-advocates put a face to ASD, ushering in a new era of accountability for program leaders. Together, these and other organizations have tipped the scales during the passage of the Combating Autism Act and other important legislation. I did not include more extensive discussion of programs primarily addressing advocacy because I wanted to demonstrate how to better utilize established government-, university-, hospital-, and school-based programs. Although advocacy will be key to mobilizing policy changes and helping to set priorities for these training programs, these other agencies and organizations will play a more direct role in actually scaling up services, training, research, and policy, at least in the short term.

The Component of Awareness

Anyone who is seeking to develop new programs or expand existing ones must first ensure that those concerned are at least generally aware of the condition. In this context, aware-ness is necessary to any effort to add elements or expand to domains served. I have not considered this component until now because initiatives addressing awareness of ASD have already been so successful that they may provide a unique study in how to increase the "name recognition" of a disorder. The Learn the Signs. Act Early. campaign described in Chapter 12 is an excellent example of a multifaceted and multilayered campaign in which the raising of awareness was tied to specific initiatives to increase and improve local ser-vices. As a result of these and many other campaigns, most organizations acknowledge the need to tailor their services, training, research, and/or policy to the needs of people living with ASD. Nonetheless, there are still some agencies and domains, at least at the local and regional level, for which increased awareness of ASD will be a necessary step in the develop-ment of a plan to increase services, training, research, and/or policy. Increased awareness is certainly necessary to germinate change in local, regional, and/or statewide networks but appears insufficient to sustain their continued evolution. Increased understanding and ac-ceptance of ASD, its characteristics, and its prevalence can help make others more open to research, training, and policy initiatives but will provide neither the guidance nor momen-tum needed for new and effective services to be developed to scale.

The Persistent Lack of Agencies that Span Multiple Components

The continued absence of agencies that clearly span traditional domains (e.g., education, health, and community-based services) or elements (services, training, research, policy) is striking, though not surprising. As acknowledged in earlier chapters, the distinctions between these domains function primarily to demarcate the responsibilities of different public agencies or categories of professionals. They do not mirror categorical differences in the needs of people living with ASD: More often, they create artificial boundaries that perpetuate service silos. They appear confusing or arbitrary to families simply trying to get help and become barriers when these families must seek supports that require co-ordination across domains. At the same time, I also believe that these distinctions are inevitable if not integral to the early evolution of agencies, disciplines, and even the careers of individual professionals. Without some degree of specialization, for example, individuals may never develop the expertise in a specific area needed to achieve important breakthroughs.

Significant increases in the degree of specialization appear inevitable whenever competition for resources increases. When there is pressure to shrink budgets specifically, or the role of government more generally, agencies work even more diligently to demarcate the boundaries of their responsibility in an attempt to better utilize dwindling resources. This increases the tendency to work in silos and may actively discourage cross-agency collaboration because of competition and distrust. A similar tendency can be seen in professionals: In an attempt to assure the maintenance if not the growth of their discipline, professional groups have devoted more resources to defining and defending unique responsibilities instead of promoting cross-discipline collaboration. Likewise, the pressure of publication and funding compels researchers to distinguish themselves from competitors by identifying increasingly specialized areas of expertise that bear less and less resemblance to the day-to-day challenges of ASD.

There are many instances in which the potential benefits of such specialization are far exceeded by the costs of lost opportunities to bridge gaps across traditional domains and the barriers created to the more effective and efficient care of people living with ASD. Consider the identification and treatment of problem behaviors using strategies based in ABA generally and FBA and PBS specifically.

- FBA for individual problem behaviors reveals a wide range of "fast" and "slow" triggers (e.g., reinforcement contingencies, teaching strategies, physical health, mood) that when understood together help in the development of more effective behavior support plans (Ingram, Lewis-Palmer, & Sugai, 2005). Data indicating that single-parent households are more likely to seek hospitalization for a behavioral crisis (Mandell, 2008) suggest that even social services and supports can play an important role in behavioral outcomes.

- To address these many different factors, people living with ASD may have to draw on the expertise of behavior analysts, educators, physicians (including pediatricians, psychiatrists, and neurologists), and other disciplines. In my professional experience, I have found that many of these professionals lack the training and experience to fully recognize the potential contribution of these other disciplines to comprehensive behavior management. As a result, interventions to decrease behavior can be narrow in their focus.

- These professionals listed earlier may be based in a wide range of settings, including private practice, hospitals, schools, and behavioral health agencies. As a parent and as a professional, I have found that it is often difficult or impossible to coordinate care across these different agencies, and that there is more likely to be parallel (and sometimes contradictory) plans for care across settings.

- Only in the past 3 years have both group and single case designs been recognized as contributing to standards for evidence-based practice (National Autism Center, 2009; Reichow, Doehring, Cicchetti, & Volkmar, 2011). Prior to this time, proponents of each type of design had stubbornly refused to acknowledge the potential contribution of the other. This has limited cross-fertilization between these two approaches, with the result that many journals and professional conferences tend to exclusively promote one or the other.

REEXAMINING THE ELEMENTS OF THE NETWORK AND THEIR INTERRELATIONSHIPS

What factors affect the growth of each of the four elements of services, training, research, and policy? What are the lessons beginning to emerge from some of the programs reviewed in Sections II and III, with respect to the potential relationships between different elements?

Services, Training, Research, and Policy Each Grow in Different Ways

Patterns in the Growth of Autism Spectrum Disorder Services During the course of my career, I have found that the growth in service providers seems to depend most directly on the pool of available talent and the means to pay and to train them. During lean economic times, when the pool of individuals seeking work is greater, I have found that it is easier to attract new people (and especially those with some college training) into the nonprofessional, direct service positions that are so important. I suspect that some of the same conditions may lead others into direct service careers as teachers, nurses, and social workers. Yet these are the same conditions under which training programs are more vulnerable to funding cuts.

My experience in developing new programs suggests that it takes 18 months to 5 years before a new program for ASD can begin to run smoothly. This is primarily because of the difficulty hiring professionals experienced in ASD, and because most new staff require a period of more intense training and supervision before they are comfortable independently developing and implementing more specialized education and treatment programs. The new professionals who benefited from more specialized training and internships in ASD at college may be ready in 1.5–2 years, while those who completed a generic training program may require 3–5 years. I have confirmed this time line with numerous discussions with colleagues.

Patterns in the Growth of Training in Autism Spectrum Disorder This is described in a separate section later in the chapter, because of the complexity of the issues and challenges associated with improved training.

Patterns in the Growth of Research in Autism Spectrum Disorder Many factors are likely to have contributed to the tremendous growth of research in ASD. This probably includes the growth in funding for research, the creation of peer-reviewed journals specific to ASD, the burgeoning market for books on ASD, and, most important, the tremendous increase in the number of parents and professionals desperate for guidance. Between 1990 and 2008, for example, the number of articles in autism in the OVID PsychINFO database increased sixfold, from about 200 to nearly 1,300 (Volkmar, Reichow, & Doehring, 2011). When speaking to the potential synergy among the four components, it is important to focus, however, on peer-reviewed publications describing the kind of outcome research needed to establish a practice as evidenced-based, or to evaluate other issues pertinent to the increase in overall service capacity (e.g., to establish the nature and extent of needs, assess access to services, evaluate effectiveness of training programs). In this context, it is interesting to note that the proportion of OVID PsychINFO database focused on treatment peaked at 28% in 2000 and then steadily decreased to 50% of that peak (to 14%) by 2008 (Volkmar et al., 2011). As discussed later in this chapter, I hope that this trend will be reversed, given that new approaches to establishing a practice as evidence-based (e.g., that acknowledge the contribution of single case designs) make it easier to conduct such research.

Patterns in the Growth of Policy Regarding Autism Spectrum Disorder
A somewhat different configuration of factors seems likely to affect the growth of policy regarding ASD. The most significant of these have been the organization and effectiveness of advocates, from the initial passage of the original Individuals with Disabilities Education Act in 1975 to the passage of the Combating Autism Act in 1996. Since the early 2000s this has begun to translate into action at the state level, most notably in efforts to pass autism insurance legislation. In many of these more recent cases, advocates have worked to create sustainable momentum, by supporting the development of subgroups of legislators keen to address a wide range of issues related to ASD (see Chapter 2).

The increasing impact of advocates on policy seems likely to result from the increased availability and quality of information about ASD and the effectiveness of campaigns to disseminate it. Rigorous, peer-reviewed research has repeatedly confirmed the high prevalence of ASD, and each new finding now is disseminated via the national and local media. In this context, it is interesting to note that funding for some of this research was itself the direct result of the lobbying of advocates, via their contribution to the passage of initiatives such as the Combating Autism Act.

Under the Right Conditions, Services, Training, Research, and Policy Can Grow Synergistically

One of the other reasons that the contributors and I sought to assemble this volume now is that we feel we are at a watershed—that services, training, research, and policy addressing ASD has matured to the point when each of these components can now contribute more meaningfully to the growth of the others. One lesson we have learned is that these elements are naturally interrelated when they are done well: Training and the research can inform the delivery of services, policy can provide funding and set broad parameters for services and training, and research on the needs of the population can drive policy. We would also argue that the particular nature of ASD—the fact that it draws on resources from different sectors, has captured the attention of policy makers, has benefited from the input of articulate advocates, and is riding a wave of new outcome research—makes it unique among disabilities and other mental health conditions and a model for how such growth may ideally work. As professionals, we must also recognize that new and coordinated service, training, research, and policy initiatives do not simply evolve naturally but that funding sources must be actively developed and the relationships between agencies providing various components must be actively pursued.

I have attempted to capture the degrees of interdependence among the different elements in the network of support systems in Figure 14.1 (with adjacent elements being more directly related) and expressed the potential for synergy in several principles outlined next. To exemplify this potential, I refer to the rise of early intensive behavior intervention (EIBI) programs in the 1990s, initially inspired by the work of Lovaas and his colleagues (Lovaas, 1987).

1. *In general, training, research, and policy do not directly determine outcomes.* With some isolated exceptions, the direct influence of training, research, and policy on real outcomes for individuals and caregivers is relatively weak; individuals and caregivers are more likely to benefit from the increase or improvement of services that are the direct result of training, research, and policy initiatives rather than the initiatives themselves. (As noted earlier, training provided to individuals with ASD or caregivers is defined here as a service.)

2. *The impact of training, research, and policy initiatives is almost always mediated by the availability and quality of services.* Thus, the goals set for training, research, and policy initiatives must always be defined and evaluated in reference to increases and improvements in specific services provided to people living with ASD. As support for EIBI increased, EIBI trainers effectively tapped underutilized but broadly available resources for direct care, undergraduate students and the broader population of community-based nonprofessionals working as one-to-one aides or assistants.

3. *Training mediates the impact of research on services.* In a similar fashion, it seems unlikely that research findings will contribute to improvements in services unless training programs are in place to translate these findings into improved practice. I believe that EIBI's explosive growth was due in part to the evolution of an informal network of trainers, initially drawn from research-based faculty and graduate students who then migrated into independent practice. These trainers drew on a common set of easily accessible teaching methods and curricula (Leaf & McEachin, 1999; Maurice, Green, & Luce, 1996).

4. *Policy changes are most likely to affect services directly by making funding available or by setting standards.* Decisions regarding who is eligible for services can release or deny funding to service providers. The availability of funding for research and training programs is highly dependent on policy decisions at the regional and the national level. Some policies puts people with ASD or their caregivers in direct control of where and how they gain access to services and therefore have a more direct and immediate impact on their lives. In the case of EIBI, advocates set a legal standard for the intensity of educational support needed to ensure reasonable progress. This standard was first applied in lawsuits filed against school districts and applied more recently to establish the level of funding for state autism insurance mandates.

5. *Training, research, and policy can also improve advocacy.* I recognize that training, research, and policy can help to make advocates more aware of the potential impact of services and thus have some effect on services by providing advocates with a more compelling argument for change. But even in this case, change will not occur unless services increase or improve. Advocates for EIBI drew heavily and effectively on the compelling outcome research findings (Lovaas, 1987; McEachin & Lovaas, 1993) and other data suggesting the potential medium- and long-term economic benefits (Jacobson & Mulick, 2000) when arguing for increased support of EIBI (see Chapter 3 for more discussion of this topic).

Developing a program that capitalizes on the synergy between services, training, research, and policy requires that professionals coordinate and balance the relative growth of the four components. Imagine each component as a horse, loosely hitched together in a team, pulling a fully loaded carriage, with Services and Training in the lead. The horses must pull in unison and in the same direction and must sustain this effort to gain momentum. The power and pace will ultimately be limited by the weakest animal and will never exceed the pace set by Services and Training. Thus, it is important to understand which factors affect the pace of each component, and how the pace of one affects the pace of the others, because the pace of total system change will be set by the component that is the slowest. In reality, there are few instances in which services, training, research, and policy are actually hitched together as a team: They sometimes appear to be, as it were, still wandering in the wilderness.

Several Factors Prevent the Synergistic Growth of Services, Training, Research, and Policy

The Lack of Training Resources Clearly Limits the Rate at Which Overall Service Capacity Can Be Scaled Up and the Likelihood that Research and Policy Initiatives Will Improve Outcomes I believe that, in the short to medium term, the availability of training resources (including trainers, training programs, and program leaders) is the lynchpin to the coordinated growth of the network of services, training, research, and policy. Even if overall system needs were clearly described, money was no object, rules and regulations were no longer a barrier to innovation, service providers were available, and evidence-based practices identified, little progress can be made until programs can effectively distill research findings into high-quality training for specific providers. In the case of ASD, there has been a general acknowledgment that there is a lack of individuals with sufficient expertise to provide the training needed (Committee on Educational Interventions for Children with Autism, 2001).

In my experience, several factors determine the speed with which a new training program can be developed. For example, increased specialization and intensity of training has particularly important implications for the training and experience required—and ultimately the availability—of trainers, and, by extension, the speed with which services can be scaled up. On the one hand, practices that can be mastered with less intense training can be scaled up much more quickly, because of the more limited commitment required of trainees and the greater availability of trainers. Services needed by many children and that require less intensive trainings thus have the greatest potential to benefit rapidly from a coordinated program of local and regional training. Given this potential, it is surprising that there has been relatively little interest in the development of less intensive but critical training programs. Perhaps funders, leaders, and policy makers are more attracted by the prestige of a more specialized training program? Program leaders need look no further than the EIBI programs described earlier in this chapter to appreciate the impact of a well-conceived training program that takes advantage of a widely available, nonprofessional workforce.

On the other hand, I anticipate that the lack of trainers will soon become the primary factor limiting the growth of new programs drawing on new research-based practices and entailing moderately to highly intense training, especially as the volume of trainees required increases. First, I have found that it can easily take 3–7 years between the emergence of a new, research-based practice that depends on postgraduate training and the availability of trainers to disseminate it; the findings must be peer reviewed (and often replicated); a program of training must be developed, and new trainers must themselves have completed formal training. Second, it takes a significant commitment of resources to develop a university-based training program: You must hire a lead faculty who may have extensive experience in relevant facets of intervention in ASD or in developing a training program, but rarely both. The faculty must develop syllabi and cultivate potential placement opportunities. In the case of postgraduate training programs, funding to support interns must also be identified. Thus, it is not surprising that there are relatively few well-established programs specifically designed to develop ASD trainers, though the number is growing each year. Programs for training behavior analysts are the exception, as these have drawn from a rapidly growing pool of professionals who are more likely to have extensive training in service delivery, who can more quickly identify community-based placements, and who themselves have already adopted a systematic approach to training that can prepare them for the challenge of developing a university-based program.

Given the shortage of more structured and comprehensive university-based training programs, I must remind readers here of the limitations relying in the interim on isolated, specific training workshops. As discussed in Chapter 3, the latter appear less likely to truly change practice. There are some specific workshops that can draw from evidence-based practices, provide some tools to support implementation and evaluate treatment fidelity, and can push an experienced professional to significantly change their practices. But in most cases, the workshops do not draw systematically on evidence-based practices and rarely include the follow-up coaching and consultation needed by a less experienced professional to establish the fidelity required to truly change practice. I have also observed that trainees returning from such workshops, energized by the promise of what they have learned, quickly confront barriers to implementation (e.g., colleagues unwilling to consider new approaches, snags in attempts to use the practice). Without opportunities for coaching and consultation, they revert almost immediately to their prior practices and can become disillusioned when considering other ways to change their practice.

Professionals must therefore be strategic in their use of available resources: They must situate new training programs in areas of documented need; they must recognize how specific opportunities vary greatly from one service to another, if they are to begin to build momentum; they must begin to look for areas of need that bridge traditional service domains (e.g., health, education, family support) and create a larger pool of potential trainees, and they must consider all of the time and resources involved. In the next chapter, I provide examples of programs and services that illustrate how a thoughtful consideration of intensity of services and training and the level of need may reveal barriers to, and opportunities for, program development. I also list examples of training programs I believe can be quickly and effectively implemented in regions beginning to develop a more integrated network and other examples for regions with already well-established services and related resources.

Increasing Specialization Will Interfere with the Relationships Between Individuals and Agencies Needed for Synergistic Growth Despite the natural relationships between services, training, research, and policy outlined earlier, I have found that few agencies devote significant resources to more than two of these components. Those providing services and/or training often are rarely involved in research or policy. Many institutions seeking to improve outcomes through research have a token involvement in direct services, training, or policy. It seems that agencies specialize in one component for the same reasons and under the same conditions that they specialize in one domain: Specialization demarcates the responsibilities of different kinds of agencies (e.g., those providing services vs. those conducting research), specialization helps both individuals and agencies to develop the expertise in a specific component and as such is inevitable if not integral to their evolution, and the pressure to specialize with respect to the components addressed also seems likely to increase whenever competition for resources increases.

I have found that agencies specializing in one component consistently underestimate the challenge of the remaining components. The failure to anticipate the complexities of developing and sustaining new services and their associated training activities is particularly problematic, because even the best funded research and policy initiatives are unlikely to have any meaningful impact on outcomes if they cannot be translated into services (see earlier discussion, and Figure 14.1). All too often, training, research, and policy initiatives fail take into consideration how funding for the new services will be sustained, how intensely services must be provided, and how service providers must see the value of a new program before investing in it. Similarly research and policy initiatives intended to increase or improve training rely on single workshops and fail to provide the ongoing coaching, consultation, and oversight needed for new concepts to truly change the practice of service providers. When competition for resources increases, training, research, and policy initiatives tend to become more specialized and likely to drift away from the services that should ultimately be provided. Under similar circumstances, the immediate pressure to provide services can prevent the development of a coherent strategy to increase training or gather data about services needs, even when this strategy clearly has the potential to improve services and even save money.

Many of the same solutions to domain-specific silos also hold here. For example, many of the Leadership Education in Neurodevelopmental and related Disbilities (LEND) and University Center for Excellence on Developmental Disabilities (UCEDD) (see Chapters 3 and 10) address multiple components, effectively leverage other faculty and related programs, and invest considerable energy in training new practitioners and researchers. Initiatives focused tightly on a specific need, like the Act Early summits (see Chapter 12) effectively merge services, training, research, and policy. Given how challenging it is for any individual to develop expertise in even one of these components, the solution will always require the creation of a multiagency team.

COORDINATING SERVICES, TRAINING, RESEARCH, AND POLICY ACROSS DOMAINS AND LEVELS: SOME PRINCIPLES AND EXAMPLES

In the previous section, I describe some of the relationships between the components of services, training, research, and policy and propose how these might grow more synergistically to constitute an integrated network. In this section, I add another dimension to this network, by discussing how the growth of these components can be balanced across local, state, and national level to most efficiently scale up and improve services for children with ASD. (I believe that the same rationale can be applied to programs for adults living with ASD but for the sake of brevity did not elaborate on these here.) Some of the principles describing the relative contribution of local, state, and national agencies, and the distribution of training and service needs across each of these levels, may appear self-evident to some readers but nonetheless have important implications for those seeking to increase capacity. In the absence of empirical data to address this question, I have drawn on my own experience to summarize some of the most common needs of children with ASD in Figure 14.4. Together, this information will help to identify immediate opportunities for emerging and established programs that I describe in detail in the final chapter.

Local, Regional, State, and National Resources Contribute in Predictable Ways to Services, Training, Research, and Policy

As suggested elsewhere in this book, and described next, there are consistent patterns in the relationship between the levels and components of the ASD network (see Figure 14.3).

The Majority of Services Are Provided at the Local and Regional Level   Except for some specialized services, most services are delivered at the local or the regional level. This is because many of the services must be accessible daily or weekly by children with ASD, and so must be available locally or regionally. The best example of this need would be early intervention and school-based services, needed by most people with ASD, and recognized as critical to long-term outcomes. In contrast, I know of no direct services provided at the national level.

Training Resources Are Distributed More Evenly Across Levels   As I argue later in the chapter, specific training needs vary as a function of many different factors. For some practices, training must be delivered more locally whereas for others, training is best delivered at the state or even the national level. Prior to the initiatives undertaken by the Centers for Disease Control and Prevention (CDC) and the National Professional Development Center (NPDC) (see Chapters 12 and 13), people would have been hard pressed to identify national training programs specific to ASD.

Research Resources Are More Concentrated at the State or National Level   Throughout this volume, I propose specific research questions that I believe can help to scale up services. Although many of these projects might be "local" to the extent that they take place at a specific university or focus on a specific region, I argue that such projects must be part of a multisite program or specific research competition organized at the state or national level.

Policy can Happen at Any Level at Which Decisions About Regulations, Funding, and Resources Are Made   Here I am defining policy broadly, to help recognize the potential to influence decisions at many levels: a local school district that

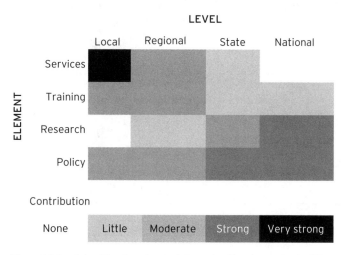

Figure 14.3.   Role of local, regional, state, and national agencies in different aspects of programming.

Intensity with which service is delivered

Intensity of training needed	Once or twice	Daily/weekly/bimonthly	2-6 Times/year	Time limited
Low	SCREENING (Asif)	PARAPROFESSIONAL SUPPORT* (Asif, Sophia); CHILD CARE*: *Inclusive and Specialized/respite* (Sophia); EDUCATION/EI: *Inclusive/in-home placement* (Asif, Joshua), *Special education program* (Sophia)	*Management of common comorbid conditions* (Sophia); DENTAL CARE: *Inclusive and Specialized* (Sophia); TRAINING IN RESOURCE UTILIZATION: CAREGIVERS *and Self-advocates* (Asif)	SUMMER CAMP: *Inclusive* (Joshua) and *Specialized*
Moderate	DIAGNOSIS and EVALUATION: Basic (Asif)	Specialized ASD school college support (Chloe); Outpatient therapies; Residential program (Sophia); CASE MANAGEMENT	Medication management (Chloe); Behavioral assessment and support (Sophia); POST-21 TRANSITION PLANNING (Liam)	
High	Specialized		Specialized medical management (Asif)	Behavioral stabilization (Sophia)

Level at which service is needed

Local	County/regional	State

Figure 14.4. Intensity of services and training by level, specialization, and type of intervention. Proportion of children with autism spectrum disorder needing the Service: **ALL/ALMOST ALL**; *Many*; *Some*; and *Few*. *All other services described here are delivered by professionals.

designates increased resources to students with ASD, a county Medicaid office that assembles a guidebook for parents seeking respite, a state chapter of a professional group that helps to promote new practice standards, a national agency that creates a grant competition to encourage outcome research.

The Intensity and Specialization of Services and Their Associated Training Together Determine the Overall Capacity and Growth of the Network at Each Level

As I began to envision how to efficiently scale up services by first describing some of the services and supports most often needed by children with ASD (see Figure 14.4), I realized that several different factors may differentiate services and supports that can or should be available locally (e.g., in most small- to medium-size towns or rural counties) and those that can or should be available regionally or statewide. These factors help to determine how many providers are needed, where they should be situated, and how difficult it might be to provide them with the necessary training and support. I also believe that these factors are themselves worthy of study, especially if professionals are seeking to scale up services as efficiently as possible, and so describe some specific research questions later in the section. In each of these cases, I draw from the subset of services reviewed in Chapter 2.

     The Prevalence of the Various Needs   The number of children potentially benefiting from the service is a critical factor determining how many providers must be trained and how many programs must be developed. Consequently, prevalence of a need will help determine whether the critical mass of potential trainees will be found at the local, regional, state, or national level. In the short term, one might crudely project these needs using a statewide needs assessment similar to that undertaken by Pennsylvania. For example, many people with ASD benefit from various forms of outpatient patient therapies (e.g., speech, occupational therapy, behavioral support, social skills training), which can be delivered in schools, homes, and in other community settings several times a week or month. All children will need dental care, provided either in community settings with guidance or support provided as needed, or in a hospital setting for those with more specialized needs.

     The Intensity of Services   By adding the intensity with which services are required, professionals can determine 1) the potential caseload for each provider, 2) how many providers are needed, and 3) whether these providers are most efficiently situated at the local, regional, or statewide level. For example, services needed daily or weekly (e.g., early intervention/education, paraprofessional support, child care) should be locally available to facilitate access. In contrast, it is more reasonable to expect families to travel outside of their town or county to receive services requiring only one or two visits (e.g., a specialized assessment, a one-day training session for caregivers), no more than bimonthly follow-up, or an intermittent, intensive service. More precise calculations of caseload are limited by the lack of research specifying the optimal level of treatment intensity. Such research will be needed to efficiently scale up services by determining the number and distribution of providers across a region.

     The Intensity of Training   To efficiently scale up services, professionals must know the type and intensity of training needed to achieve treatment fidelity, so that they can determine the number and distribution of training resources across a region or state. For purposes of the present discussion, I would define low-intensity training as requiring relatively little time (e.g., no more than the equivalent of a 6-credit college course), little or no need for ongoing coaching and consultation, and not requiring specialized skills. For example, this could include training that need only consist of 2- to 3-hour workshops that might be aimed at physicians (e.g., to educate them regarding screening for ASD or the management of common comorbid conditions such as sleep or gastrointestinal problems). I am excited by the potential for courses or certificates at smaller community and technical colleges to provide basic information about supporting children with ASD, targeting community-based providers of child care, after-school care, or respite care. I also acknowledge that many community-based organizations provide individual workshops seeking to educate and train caregivers about a broad range of services and supports, although in most cases these are too loosely organized to constitute a curriculum or course of study. I would also include training that is relatively more intense but that is not that specialized: a 3- or 6-credit introduction to teaching methods and curricula for ASD offered as a certification for regular education teachers or a community-college certificate for paraprofessionals.

I would consider other types of training to be more intense, for several different reasons. They may entail a specialized undergraduate degree or certificate (e.g., teacher certification in ASD) or be part of a graduate-level training program (e.g., speech pathology, behavior analysis). They may require the development of skills that are highly specialized (e.g., diagnosis, medication management) and/or multidisciplinary planning and case coordination that are often developed gradually over years of experience.

The most intense training requires a specialized postgraduate degree (e.g., neurologist, developmental pediatrician) or postgraduate placement (e.g., to provide experience in specialized diagnostic training or management). Other training may be highly intense because it includes program development (e.g., leading specialized, multidisciplinary education and treatment programs). In my experience, both moderately and highly intense training require coaching and consultation and opportunities to remain up to date with new developments, through collaboration with other programs and engagement in research (see Chapter 3). Thus, such intense training requires a greater commitment of time and effort from trainees.

To Efficiently Allocate Specific Services at the Right Level, Professionals Should Balance the Need to Ensure Reasonable Access with the Challenge of Scaling Up Training

Together, the factors described earlier help to establish some principles for determining the level at which different kinds of services should be optimally located. This level is selected so as to assure reasonable access to services, in the light of the difficulties developing and delivering the training needed by service providers, which is described next in greater detail.

1. If the service is needed by most children with ASD, and if the training required of providers is not intensive, services provided at least weekly should be available locally. Providers should expect, for example, to provide early intervention/educational programming, paraprofessional support, and child care locally. This ensures reasonable access to people living with ASD. Though screening need only occur once, its critical role in identification of ASD, and the fact that relatively little training is needed to screen effectively, suggests that screening for ASD should be available locally.

2. If the service is needed by most children with ASD, and if the training required of providers is not intensive, services provided at least biannually should be available regionally. Providers should expect, for example, to provide dental care, management of comorbid medical conditions, and training in resource utilization regionally. The less

frequent utilization of such services makes the additional travel more reasonable, except for those living in rural regions who do not own an automobile.

3. Services that require highly intensive training and that are not needed by the majority children with ASD may only be available at the state level: The relatively low number of children in need of the services makes it difficult to create the critical mass of trainees needed to justify a more significant investment in regional training capacity for services such as specialized diagnosis/evaluation, specialized medical management, behavioral stabilization, and more specialized residential programs.

4. Services that are needed by more than a few children with ASD, and that require at least moderately intensive training, may necessitate a longer-term investment in the development of regional training capacity in order to develop the necessary number of providers: The high number of children in need of services that require relatively more intense training (e.g., diagnosis of ASD, case management, outpatient therapies, medication management, behavioral support, post-21 transition planning) makes it necessary to develop regional training capacity, though the intensive nature of the training makes it difficult to develop such capacity quickly.

To Efficiently Allocate Training Resources at the Right Level in the Light of the Factors Listed Previously, Professionals Should Balance Training Need, Training Intensity, and Distribution of Service Providers The factors to be considered in the development of training capacity are somewhat more complex. Professionals must determine how many trainers are needed to scale up service capacity: 1) what kind of training is required (i.e., the intensity of the training), 2) how many providers must be trained (i.e., the prevalence of the need and intensity of the services), and 3) whether these providers must be dispersed locally or can be grouped at the regional or state level (i.e., the intensity of the services). The factors described earlier in the chapter also help to determine the number and types of programs that must be developed to train the trainers needed to scale up service capacity: 1) the prerequisite certification, training, and experience required of trainers, and 2) the specialization of the service required. Together, this information will help to determine the rate at which service capacity can be developed and the level at which training capacity should be developed—for example, at the local, regional, state, or national level. If professionals develop a plan that considers all of these factors, they can strategically scale up some services quickly as long as they can balance these limited resources. I describe next some other general principles for organizing training as a function of the other factors described earlier in the chapter.

1. In most cases, training is most efficiently delivered at the regional level when the training required is less intensive, and especially when trainees must be distributed evenly across a region to ensure access to services needed daily or weekly by most children with ASD. In general, it is easier to train trainers who are conducting a less intensive training, and so the development of local or regional training capacity is more feasible. The critical mass of trainees needed to justify the development of a training resource is more easily created when a service is needed by more people with ASD. When training can be completed relatively easily, it is more realistic to expect trainees to have to travel to a regional as opposed to a local training.

2. In most cases, training is most efficiently delivered at the state level when the training required is more specialized or when the services are needed by a small proportion of children with ASD. In general, it can be challenging to identify and train trainers for a

more specialized kind of service, and so it is more difficult to develop a local or regional training capacity. The critical mass of trainees needed to justify the development of a training resource may only be found at the state level for a given service that is needed by more people with ASD.

3. A critical mass of trainees may sometimes be created by identifying training needs that span traditional service delivery systems. Some service needs are largely comparable in different systems of service delivery, and so efficiencies of scale can be achieved by combining training for services utilized across multiple domains (e.g., education, behavioral health). For example, there is considerable overlap in the core understanding of ASD and core skills for monitoring behavior and implementing intervention for paraprofessionals working in a school, home, job site, residential program, or inpatient program. Regardless of whether they are working in a school, medical home, behavioral health agency, or other organization, all case managers must understand the range of services and service systems typically used by people with ASD and must facilitate the development of a plan that works for all parties.

Policy Initiatives at the State and the National Level Are Needed to Develop the Resources to Efficiently Scale Up Services Through Training

Earlier in this chapter, I emphasized that research and policy initiatives will only improve outcomes if they ultimately impact services and supports and this will only occur if these initiatives can be translated through training to service providers (see Figure 14.2). What other kinds of policy initiatives can help to scale up services and their associated training using the principles I described earlier? I believe that initiatives that specifically support the development of coordinated training programs (especially for more specialized training), and that demonstrate how to train and engage providers at the local level, will be particularly important.

More Specialized Training Programs Needed to Scale Up Services Will Likely Develop Only with State and Federal Support   Throughout this chapter and Chapter 3, I listed a number of challenges to the training needed to change practice on a regional, state, and national scale, especially as the intensity of the training required increases. In general, the need for state or federal support increases with the intensity and specialization of training required. Some of this support may be needed to simply offset some of the costs associated with such training. Moderately or highly intensive training often requires more extensive advance preparation and therefore an upfront investment in trainers and training time that an organization might hesitate to fully support. Additional time may also be required to provide the coaching and consultation needed to solidify newly acquired practices and may raise the fee beyond the reach of an individual trainee or an organization (especially when considered together with the cost of the trainee's time). As specialization of the practice increases (either because of the prerequisite training required of trainees or the decreased need among providers), the investment per trainee increases even more.

Some of this support may also be important in helping to establish the new or expand the existing programs needed to scale up training. As outlined in Chapter 3, several principles can help guide new training programs to become successful. I have found that few professionals working in isolation can effectively develop and disseminate a moderately or highly specialized training in a specific topic. Engaging a person knowledgeable in the specific topic of training is necessary to developing a training program but rarely sufficient: The design and delivery of an effective training program is itself a skill that few acquire quickly, easily, or naturally, without the support of colleagues or a program with experience in other kinds of training. Second, there is currently a lack of professionals capable of undertaking such training, and a training center can not only coordinate such training but can also help a new generation of trainers to emerge. Third, the development of such a program can take years, and only after establishing momentum with multiple, related training endeavors, especially for postdoctoral training programs. Finally, such a program is more likely to bring together people from multiple disciplines, domains, and agencies and begin to break traditional silos down. In most cases, such programs would reside most naturally in a university setting, preferably in centers such as the UCEDDs or programs such as LEND that promote the multidisciplinary, research-based, family-focused, community-centered, and culturally sensitive models of care that can address disparities in access. The programs offered by the CDC (Chapter 12) and NPDC (Chapter 13) illustrate many of the principles described earlier.

Even practices that require less intensive training (e.g., disseminated by workshop[s] or a single 3-credit course without a specific training infrastructure) will benefit from a more coordinated program of implementation, especially as the number of potential trainees or training sites increase. Most presenters will hesitate to do more than prepare core elements (e.g., slides and perhaps a reference list) for a workshop that they might give once or twice. When multiple workshops are given in order to reach providers over a broad region, presenters can commit to enhance these core elements: Adapt the workshop based on ongoing feedback, collect relevant videos, evaluate which practices meet the threshold as evidence-based, develop an annotated bibliography or resource guide, create pre- and posttests, or integrate case studies or practice opportunities with fidelity checklists. When similar workshops are given in different states, or different regions of one state, then a state- or federally funded program can bring potential workshop leaders together to share in the development of these enhancements. Examples of topics that would benefit from this coordinated approach because of the large number of potential providers include screening, paraprofessional support, child care providers, summer camps, training in resource utilization, and dental care (see Figure 14.4).

State and National Policies and Programs to Increase Services Must Include Specific Plans to Engage Local and Regional Providers in the Adoption of New Practices Even training programs that are developed with state and federal support may fail to change practice if they do not dedicate adequate time and resources to the final steps of engagement and dissemination. The first step— delivering the training—is usually complicated by the lack of a training network or infrastructure. Except for college courses, most training events occur outside of a preexisting training program in which the availability of trainees, a venue, and a date is already assured. In most cases, trainers must themselves identify and reach the pool of potential trainees, find a venue that will accommodate the anticipated number of trainees, and choose dates that do not conflict with other events. Those new to the challenge of providing training invariably underestimate the difficulty of completing even these steps: Every time I have created training events that are repeated one or more times a year, the second such event is much easier to organize once the parameters of the training have been established.

The second step involves ensuring a dialogue with providers within the targeted agency regarding potential barriers to implementing practice. In most cases, the practice being disseminated will require small but important changes to existing practices within the agency or an investment or reallocation of resources: For example, the adoption of a new assessment procedure may require the purchase of materials, the replacement of an existing protocol with which others are familiar, and an additional time commitment on the part of the professional or the person with ASD. In some cases, the practice being disseminated will require a larger change in the institutional culture: For example, the adoption of positive behavior supports in a school requires a fundamental shift away from a reactive model that relies on visits to the principal's office, suspensions, and expulsions to change student behavior. Many of these barriers can be anticipated by a thoughtful and experienced trainer, though the exact nature and extent of each of these barriers—and their corresponding solutions—can vary significantly from setting to setting. Sometimes all that is needed is to provide additional opportunities during the training itself for trainees to brainstorm with each other or the trainer regarding potential barriers and their solutions. Other times, training may require additional steps: a meeting with decision makers to review potential barriers and to ensure their support for the anticipated changes, and presentations to others in the community to generate interest in the potential changes in practice. Although both steps are important in providing information to other stakeholders, the opportunity to specifically solicit and respond to the concerns of stakeholders is itself invaluable to ensuring their full support.

Completion of the first and second steps sometimes sets the stage for the third; the creation of local leaders for change within an agency or across a region. New practices are often implemented gradually, over a period of months or even years, and the momentum created by the initial training event and attempts to engage the broader community may quickly fade. Barriers may only emerge later on, new parents or staff may join the agency at a later date, or the new practice may engender so much interest that new resources must be sought to meet emerging demands. In these cases, the training and associated activities in these first two steps can help create a local "champion" who is capable of both demonstrating the practice and generating enthusiasm for it and thus who can help maintain the momentum for change.

Sometimes changes in practice require a fourth step: improved coordination across individuals or agencies or with other training initiatives. A significant proportion of practices benefit from, if not depend upon, collaboration with others. Improving specialized identification of ASD across a region may require, for example, that a hospital-based diagnostic clinic link up with various agencies: 1) community-based pediatricians, early intervention providers, and school districts for potential referrals; 2) advocacy groups to help generate interest in the new service among parents; and 3) a screening for ASD initiative sponsored by the state department of public welfare. Sometimes the champion can serve formally or informally as a regional leader and resource for those outside of the agency, and sometimes the champion's agency or organization can serve as the hub for the network. In either case, an important first step for a training program could include an initial meeting, or the creation of an advisory board, consisting of stakeholders from multiple agencies.

Different Approaches to Developing More Specialized Training Programs Offer a Range of Ways to Build Capacity and Mobilize Change   The programs described in this kind of book illustrate several different approaches to the challenges discussed earlier. Most of the programs act as more traditional regional or statewide centers, often university-based, that address a broad range of training topics over a multiyear period, with the support of various state and federal grants. Some are led by a state agency, perhaps in partnership with a hospital- or university-based program. Some of the training offered

might be more specialized, and other training might be intended to reach a broad audience. This kind of center-based model may offer several advantages: 1) it can respond more flexibly to new or emerging need for training, because the infrastructure is already established; 2) over time, it can establish the center as a hub for services and expertise and help it to become a trusted resources for the community; and 3) it can become a magnet for related research and policy initiatives, especially those that build upon ongoing evaluation of services. The greatest challenge is ensuring the continuity of core staff and leadership through overlapping 1–3 year grants, unless a state agency can provide a 3- to 5-year funding commitment for at least a base level of service. Perhaps the most effective combination is a stable, state-funded entity that has the flexibility to bring in other partners for specific needs.

The range of training programs in Pennsylvania illustrates some options available via a center-based approach (see Chapter 6). As a state agency, the Bureau of Autism Services (BAS) has enjoyed a limited but relatively stable level of base support. This allows it to develop a range of initiatives and training programs across the state with its own staff. BAS also leads the oversight of the Autism Services, Education, Research, and Training (ASERT) regional collaboratives. The three ASERT collaboratives, each under the leadership of a single university or hospital with established programs for ASD, allows BAS to leverage other agencies to increase the potential training expertise available and ensure a better response to local needs.

As a branch of the Pennsylvania Department of Education, the Pennsylvania Training and Technical Assistance Network (PaTTAN) has enjoyed the continued support needed to develop and deliver a range of training programs across the state using its own staff. Because it is not a university-based or private center but part of the state network of services, PaTTAN has been able to connect much more readily with the public school system (e.g., to create model classrooms across the state). PaTTAN has also leveraged other sources of expertise, most notably to host the highly successful annual National Autism Conference with Penn State.

Another approach entails a more time-limited focus on a specific set of training goals, such as teacher training or identification of ASD. This topic-based approach appears to have other advantages: 1) it may help to develop capacity more quickly within a specific area of need, 2) the focus on a specific topic may make it easier to build bridges between agencies and disciplines, 3) the time-limited nature of the initiative may help to quickly build momentum among a community of stakeholders who otherwise might not remain engaged over a longer time frame, and 4) it can establish a template for program development and growth that can be applied to other regions or states. Together, these factors make such programs attractive to policy makers wary of long-term funding commitments but open to a specific grant competition. The more focused and time-limited approach also means that leaders must carefully demarcate the goals and scope or risk diffusing effort and should consider whether they can transition leadership of the initiative to another center or agency at the end of the initial funding period.

The Learn the Signs. Act Early. initiative (Chapter 12) and the NPDC (Chapter 13) are examples of topic-centered approaches that illustrate all of the advantages listed earlier, including how to develop local capacity for at least services and training, if not research and policy. All too often, ambitious training initiatives result in the creation of a series of workshops, a web site, and other supporting materials, but provide no guarantee that services are actually increased or made more accessible. Both of these initiatives, however, have creatively and dynamically involved local advocates and providers in the design of state and national policy initiatives intended to directly improve the lives of people living with ASD.

REFERENCES

Bureau of Autism Services, Pennsylvania Department of Public Welfare. (2011a). *Pennsylvania Autism Needs Assessment: A survey of individuals and families living with autism: Barriers and limitations to accessing services.* Retrieved from http://www.paautism.org/asert/ASERT_Barriers_August%202011.pdf

Bureau of Autism Services, Pennsylvania Department of Public Welfare. (2011b). *Pennsylvania Autism Needs Assessment: A survey of individuals and families living with autism: Family impact.* Retrieved from http://www.paautism.org/asert/ASERT%20Family impact_August%202011.pdf

Bureau of Autism Services, Pennsylvania Department of Public Welfare. (2011c). *Pennsylvania Autism Needs Assessment: A survey of individuals and families living with autism: Getting an autism diagnosis and follow-up care.* Retrieved from http://www.paautism.org/asert/ASERT_Diagnosis_August%202011.pdf

Bureau of Autism Services, Pennsylvania Department of Public Welfare. (2011d). *Pennsylvania Autism Needs Assessment: A survey of individuals and families living with autism: Statewide summary.* Retrieved from http://www.paautism.org/asert/ASERT_Statewide%20Summary%20August%202011.pdf

Burgess, A.F., & Gutstein, S.E. (2007). Quality of life for people with autism: Raising the standard for evaluating successful outcomes. *Child and Adolescent Mental Health, 12*(2), 80–86.

Committee on Educational Interventions for Children with Autism. (2001). *Educating children with autism.* Washington, DC: National Academies Press.

de Bildt, A., Sytema, S., Ketelaars, C., Kraijer, D., Mulder, E., Volkmar, F., Minderaa, R., et al. (2004). Interrelationship between *Autism Diagnostic Observation Schedule-Generic (ADOS-G), Autism Diagnostic Interview-Revised (ADI-R),* and the *Diagnostic and Statistical Manual of Mental Disorders (DSM-IV-TR)* classification in children and adolescents with mental retardation. *Journal of Autism and Developmental Disorders, 34*(2), 129–137.

Doehring, P., Wagner, B., Ruhe-Lesko, L., Peters, K., Abel, J., & Myers, K. (2008). *Where are the data? Publication profiles of articles on autism in JABA, JADD, and JPBI.* Atlanta, GA: Association for Behavior Analysis.

Glessner, J.T., Wang, K., Cai, G.Q., Korvatska, O., Kim, C.E., Wood, S., et al. (2009). Autism genome-wide copy number variation reveals ubiquitin and neuronal genes. *Nature, 459*(7246), 569–573.

Ingram, K., Lewis-Palmer, T., & Sugai, G. (2005). Function-based intervention planning: Comparing the effectiveness of FBA function-based and non-function-based intervention plans. *Journal of Positive Behavior Interventions, 7*(4), 224–236.

Jacobson, J.W., & Mulick, J.A. (2000). System and cost research issues in treatments for people with autistic disorders. *Journal of Autism and Developmental Disorders, 30*(6), 585–593.

Lawer, L., & Mandel, D.S. (2009). *Pennsylvania Autism Census Project: Final report.* Harrisburg: Bureau of Autism Services, Pennsylvania Department of Public Welfare.

Leaf, R., & McEachin, J. (1999). *A work in progress: Behavior management strategies and a curriculum for intensive behavioral treatment of autism.* New York, NY: DRL Books.

Lovaas, O.I. (1987). Behavioral treatment and normal educational and intellectual functioning in young autistic children. *Journal of Consulting and Clinical Psychology, 55*(1), 3–9.

Mandell, D.S. (2008). Psychiatric hospitalization among children with autism spectrum disorders. *Journal of Autism and Developmental Disorders, 38*(6), 1059–1065.

Maurice, C., Green, G., & Luce, S.C. (1996). *Behavioral intervention for young children with autism: A manual for parents and professionals.* Austin, TX: PRO-ED.

McEachin, J.J., & Lovaas, O.I. (1993). Long-term outcome for children with autism who received early intensive behavioral treatment. *American Journal on Mental Retardation, 97*(4), 359–372.

National Autism Center. (2009). *The National Standards Project: Addressing the need for evidence based practice guidelines for autism spectrum disorders.* Randolph, MA: Author.

Reichow, B., Doehring, P., Cicchetti, D.V., & Volkmar, F.R. (2011). *Evidence-based practices and treatments for children with autism.* New York, NY: Springer.

Volkmar, F.R., Reichow, B., & Doehring, P. (2011). Evidence-based practices in autism: Where we are now and where we need to go. In B. Reichow, P. Doehring, D.V. Cicchetti, & F.R. Volkmar (Eds.), *Evidence-based practices and treatments for children with autism* (pp. 365–391). New York, NY: Springer.

Wang, K., Zhang, H.T., Ma, D.Q., Bucan, M., Glessner, J.T., Abrahams, B.S., . . . Hakonarson, H. (2009). Common genetic variants on 5p14.1 associate with autism spectrum disorders. *Nature, 459*(7246), 528–533.

15

Where We Can Start

Immediate Opportunities for Improving the Lives of People with Autism Spectrum Disorder

Peter Doehring

As described in Chapter 1, this book was originally conceived as simply a collection of model programs for children with ASD, from which professionals and parents might identify examples to apply to their own organization or region. It soon became apparent that professionals and parents might lack the breadth of perspective to recognize the most pressing needs and then to choose the type of program most likely to meet these: Section I seeks to provide that perspective. In the course of assembling this information, specific gaps and opportunities emerged within and across the network of services, training, research, and policy. These may help to identify where professionals might begin to build capacity and provide the vision and the confidence to face autism at the local, regional, state, and even national levels. Before recommending specific examples of the kinds of programs that can begin to build a truly integrated network, it may be helpful to summarize some of the principles presented earlier.

Professionals may be intimidated by the complexity of the spectrum of ASD across the life span and discouraged by the lack of a cure for ASD. Professionals and agencies may respond to this complexity by narrowing their focus to invest in developing specific areas of expertise over a period of years. As a result, they may overlook real and immediate opportunities to help people with ASD by ensuring that simple but effective interventions are implemented consistently and intensively and basic but important services are easily accessible. Professionals and agencies may also overlook real and immediate opportunities to help people with ASD by addressing co-occurring conditions (i.e., intellectual disability [ID], problem behaviors, other medical and psychiatric disorders) that can sometimes be as debilitating as the ASD itself. For those specifically with ASD and ID, collaborating with the broader ID community can help to establish the critical mass of need required to develop new service and training programs.

The direct impact on the health and well-being of caregivers is underestimated, especially considering that they may act as the primary advocates, case managers, direct service providers, and/or agents of generalization (see Chapter 14). Yet these roles suggest that information, services, and supports provided to caregivers will magnify other interventions provided directly to the person with ASD. A well-informed and well-supported caregiver

297

may have greater impact than any single agency and/or professional. For caregivers affected by poverty, isolation, or other factors, efforts to improve access to services and supports can have an immediate impact.

Professionals and agencies might become discouraged by the challenge of translating ideas into real improvements for people living with ASD. Because the impact of training, research, and policy initiatives is almost always mediated by associated improvements in services, most initiatives will require active coordination with service providers. In this context, pivotal services are especially important, facilitating access to and coordination with other critical services (see Chapter 2). Refocusing on truly meaningful outcomes for individuals with ASD, their caregivers, and the system of services can also help to reenergize initiatives.

The lack of trainers and training programs is often cited as one of the biggest barriers to scaling up capacity. This volume offers examples of programs that have demonstrated how to use training to build capacity at the state level (see Chapters 12 and 13), outlines a comprehensive and integrated approach to training (see Chapter 3), and describes principles for scaling up capacity by considering the extent of the need, the intensity of the training, and the level of specialization required (see Chapter 14).

Advocates and professionals become discouraged because research findings that initially suggest major breakthroughs rarely translate into real and immediate improvements in services and outcomes, but new trends in research may begin to convert the growing understanding of ASD into action (see Chapter 3). By recognizing the contribution of single case and other types of research designs, and systematically evaluating the quality of the research, those in the field can more confidently designate certain practices as evidence-based and thus provide clear direction to practitioners and policy makers. A small but growing body of research testing how to translate research into practice, together with a greater understanding of specific service needs and barriers for the entire population, can also help program leaders to better target resources.

Advocates for ASD are increasingly seeking to expand services, training, and research through policy changes. Over time, advocates have become more strategic in the methods they chose, and more ambitious in the outcomes they seek, and have learned that poorly conceived policy can fall far short of expectations. As outlined in Chapter 3, by first raising awareness and creating momentum for other changes, and then building on a careful and ongoing assessment of current understanding and resources, policy can promote the convergence of scientific, ethical, and legal standards and oversight to drive services and training.

As described in Chapter 4, the infrastructure supporting services, training, research, and policy for ASD is a patchwork of agencies and organizations. In most cases, the elements of this ad hoc network were neither developed originally nor mandated specifically to address the needs of people with ASD. Nonetheless, the programs described in this volume reveal the potential for leadership and innovation everywhere: through agencies at the state level (in Pennsylvania) and at the federal level (at the Centers for the Disease Control and Prevention and through programs funded by the U.S. Department of Education); in hospitals (in Utah and Ontario), in public school programs (in Delaware), and of course in universities (in Indiana, West Virginia, Kansas, North Carolina). In each of these cases, the success of these programs ultimately depended on the ability of leaders to nurture partnerships with other agencies and build bridges across elements (e.g., integrating services, training, research, and/or policy) and levels (e.g., with local, regional, state, or national organizations).

FIRST STEPS: A COORDINATED NETWORK FOR THE IDENTIFICATION OF AUTISM SPECTRUM DISORDER

A review of the information provided in previous chapters regarding screening for ASD and diagnosis reveals why it is perhaps the best strategy for a region or state to get started with, especially one with a relatively underdeveloped service system. This review also reveals specific barriers to be overcome and suggests which solutions might be possible.

Services

As described in Chapter 2, identification of ASD is pivotal because it is the gateway to all other services, and the early intervention it can lead to is recognized as one of the most important contributors to positive outcomes. Many of the procedures needed to ensure accurate identification have been developed and validated, and standards for their use have been outlined by multiple organizations. As a service needed by everyone living with ASD, investments in improving identification of ASD will yield broad benefits. The identification of ASD is also a cost-effective service that builds on an existing pool of professionals and agencies. Screening for ASD can be completed quickly and easily by primary care practitioners, if not by other community-based professionals (see later in the chapter); in many cases, an accurate diagnosis can be achieved within one to three visits, with a community-based professional (e.g., a pediatrician, a psychologist) or via more specialized professionals or clinics. Given the services, training, research, and policy outlined in this volume, there is no reason why most children with ASD cannot be identified by 36 months of age and why almost all cannot be identified by the time they enter kindergarten.

The identification of ASD illustrates how the lack of awareness or coordination across agencies and domains can create delays and yield findings that are confusing and contradictory for parents. Consider the many professionals and agencies potentially involved in each stage of identification (see Figure 15.1) in one of the first projects from the Pennsylvania Autism Services, Education, Resources, and Training (ASERT) Centers (Chapter 5), described in more detail further on. Screening and surveillance (Stage 1 and 2) can be provided at the local level by primary care practitioners, teachers, and a wide range of agencies and other professionals. Additional assessments (Stage 6a) or multidisciplinary evaluations (Stage 3) can occur through local hospitals, schools, or other community-based providers. Basic diagnostic assessments (Stage 4) and the response to intervention (Stage 6a) and other assessments can involve local, community-based practitioners, while assessments of comorbidities (Stage 6a) or more specialized diagnostic assessments (Stage 6b) might be provided by professionals at the regional level (e.g., in specialized clinics or hospitals).

There is the expectation that many children could ultimately be diagnosed with ASD following the primary steps recommended by the American Academic of Pediatrics (AAP) (represented in Figure 15.1 by solid arrows). As professionals and agencies acquire a shared understanding of the steps involved inidentification of ASD and begin to connect with other providers, however, alternate and potentially more efficient routes to identification can emerge (represented in Figure 15.1 by outlined arrows). For example, the AAP guidelines acknowledge that some children might be referred following surveillance immediately for multidisciplinary evaluation or even for a diagnostic evaluation. When professionals and agencies understand ASD and the steps involved in its identification and are familiar with other providers in the region, rapid and accurate

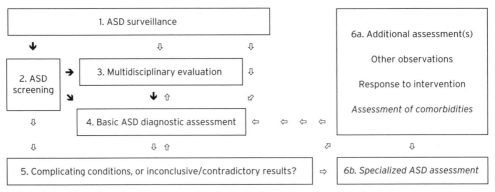

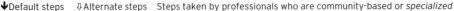

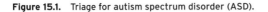

Figure 15.1. Triage for autism spectrum disorder (ASD).

diagnosis can be achieved by coordination of all of these steps across agencies. A breakdown at any point in this network can, however, create significant inefficiencies and delays.

One strategy to easily increase the capacity for rapid and accurate ASD identification is to target specific bottlenecks in the network—for example, the lack of a diagnostic protocol that is both efficient *and* effective for community-based professionals working at the local level (e.g., psychologists or pediatricians working independently or in nonspecialized clinics). On the one hand, assessment tools developed for specialized clinics and research purposes require too much time to administer, too much training to master for most diagnosticians, and are perhaps unnecessary in less complex cases. On the other hand, brief checklists may not be powerful enough to disentangle ASD from other complicating conditions. As a result, community-based diagnosticians at the local level must sometimes choose between undertaking evaluations that yield inconclusive or contradictory results or referring families to specialized professionals or clinics at the regional level where they may encounter 12–24 month waiting lists.

My colleagues and I undertook to address this bottleneck in one of the first Pennsylvania ASERT initiatives (see Chapter 6), and captured in Figure 15.1. We began by proposing a two-tiered model of diagnostic evaluation that distinguished a basic diagnostic assessment protocol (e.g., a combination of simple checklists and observations selected to yield converging evidence of specific *Diagnostic and Statistical Manual of Mental Disorders, Fourth Edition, Text Revision* [*DSM-IV-TR*; American Psychiatric Association, 2000] symptoms) from a specialized diagnostic protocol (e.g., use of the Autism Diagnostic Observation Schedule [ADOS; Lord, Rutter, DiLavore, & Risi, 1999] and/or the Autism Diagnostic Interview–Revised [ADI-R; Lord, Rutter, & Le Couteur, 1994]). We proposed specific criteria to help local, community-based diagnosticians decide if they could use a basic assessment to confidently diagnose ASD in one or two visits by themselves (Stage 4) or if they should take additional steps. For example, we recommended that local diagnosticians consider seeking additional assessments (Stage 6a) or pursue a more specialized assessment for ASD (Stage 6b) if the results obtained via a basic assessment were inconclusive or contradicted previous diagnoses. We also suggested that local diagnosticians may pursue a more specialized assessment for ASD in lieu of a basic assessment under some conditions (e.g., for a child younger than 24 months of age, when profound ID or sensory impairments are diagnosed or suspected) and under other conditions when these occur in combination with each other (e.g., when there is a clear history of behavioral regression, a sibling diagnosed with ASD, when English is the second language for the child or the family). We also suggested that local diagnosticians may also first pursue additional assessments for a child suspected of neurological conditions (e.g., seizure disorder; abnormal magnetic resonance imaging, electroencephalogram, or computed tomography findings), co-occurring psychiatric disorders (attention-deficit/hyperactivity disorder, anxiety), or genetic conditions (e.g., fragile X, Down syndrome, tuberous sclerosis). Finally, we recommended that local diagnosticians consider taking other steps, such as conducting additional observations to gather converging evidence or forestalling diagnosis pending an evaluation of the response to 6 months of more specialized intervention, when initial results were inconclusive or contradictory. Based on the results obtained following the options outlined earlier, a local diagnostician may still decide on a diagnosis or pursue a specialized assessment for ASD at the regional level. For states with significantly underserved regions, this could include the use of traveling assessment teams, as used successfully in Utah (see Chapter 10).

There are other sources of inefficiency that represent opportunities for improvement. For example, professionals working individually (or even as a part of a team) conduct detailed assessments that rarely reference the results of colleagues. In general, these can leave parents and professionals swamped with recommendations (sometimes that contradict each other), without clear priorities. A coordinated, multidisciplinary evaluation for ASD can help to gather converging evidence to support or refute specific symptoms of ASD, allowing the diagnostician to approach the task with greater confidence. In addition, the adoption of the two-tiered model of diagnostic evaluation described earlier may help broaden the range of professionals involved in diagnosis. For example, I have developed successful training programs in ASD diagnosis for school psychologists (see Chapter 7) and nurse practitioners, effectively increasing diagnostic capacity while ensuring that a more specialized diagnostic assessment is available as needed. Finally, initiatives to promote screening for ASD must reach beyond primary care physicians to include any professional working closely with young children (see Chapter 12).

Training

Many tools and models of training in identification of ASD referenced in earlier chapters makes it more realistic to implement a program of training in identification of ASD. For example, training protocols for many of the most commonly used assessment tools are well established and readily available, and models for disseminating this training regionally and statewide to a wide range of providers are described in this volume (see Chapters 8, 12, and 13). Given the structure of programs leading to initial licensure as described in Chapter 4, training in screening for ASD is best incorporated into all master's level training curricula and/or practica, whereas training in diagnosis of ASD can be best provided in the context of postdoctoral residencies and internships. Regional and statewide agencies may also consider training in the use of a two-tiered model of diagnosis of ASD similar to that described earlier. When training includes a road map for services (see later in the chapter), local professionals can make best use of other specialized and regional resources.

Screening for ASD offers great potential as a strategy to quickly scale up capacity because it requires relatively little training and utilizes an existing infrastructure (local physicians and other professionals). I believe that it is realistic to efficiently provide training in screening via 3- to 6-hour workshops or online, under the leadership of a state-level team as created by an Act Early State Team (see Chapter 12) or under the leadership of a state agency (see Chapter 6). Another immediate opportunity is creation of a more coordinated training program using the principles outlined and the example provided in Chapter 3. Although individual training activities can be assembled by separate agencies for local practitioners, the training and coaching needed by more specialized teams dealing with more complex cases requires an ongoing program of professional development under the leadership of a regional "expert." Such experts can be created from intelligent and ambitious diagnosticians, with the proper guidance and support as described in Chapter 3 and through programs funded and/or overseen at the state level.

Research

As described in earlier chapters, considerable research has already been conducted to identify the features of ASD critical to their effective screening and diagnosis. A shift in research may emphasize disparities in the identification of ASD, barriers to screening and diagnosis, and the evaluation of methods and procedures that would increase the efficiency and accuracy of community-based diagnosis. The needs assessments conducted in Pennsylvania (see Chapter 6) offer a powerful tool for precisely targeting other service and training initiatives; these can identify specific regions requiring additional services and training, specific groups that are underserved, and specific bottlenecks in the network of services while also establishing a baseline against which progress can be closely tracked.

Policy

As described in Chapter 4 and elsewhere, policy surrounding ASD builds awareness, creates momentum, supports data-based decision making, drives the development and implementation of standards, allocates resources, and promotes cross-agency coordination through integrated programs. The Act Early Program (Chapter 12) is a model for addressing many of these components, especially awareness, momentum, and cross-agency coordination. Policy surrounding ASD can help to designate and support a lead agency for promoting improved identification of ASD within the state, assuring the continuity of funding needed to lead the implementation of practice standards through training and oversight. Although guidelines for identification of ASD have been identified by many states and organizations and coordinated training programs can be extremely effective in promoting change, the failure to promulgate these as standards when appropriate will ultimately limit improvement. For example, many guidelines begin with a definition of autism or ASD drawn from the *DSM-IV-TR*, but some states and agencies rely on outdated or incomplete definitions that effectively exclude significant proportions of the autism spectrum. An immediate opportunity is to revise state laws and agency regulations to align operational definitions of ASD with the *DSM-IV-TR* (see Chapter 7). Guidelines promoting specific screening and assessment protocols must be accompanied by policy supporting appropriate reimbursement for these activities. Policy changes may also be needed to allow other allied other professionals (e.g., nurse practitioners, school psychologists) to act as diagnosticians.

NEXT STEPS: USING ROAD MAPS AND CASE MANAGEMENT TO BETTER UTILIZE EXISTING SERVICES

What might be other priorities for agencies, regions, states, and countries that have established mechanisms for assuring reasonably accurate and rapid identification of ASD? Other areas of critical need come to mind but do not always offer the same potential to address highly prevalent needs, immediately affect broad and narrow outcomes (see Chapter 14), promote cross-agency and cross-domain coordination, and ultimately begin to build a truly integrated network of services, training, research, and policy at the local, regional state, and national level. Public school programs (see Chapter 7) and early intervention programs (see Chapter 10) certainly address highly prevalent needs and so are worthy targets but perhaps require too great an investment to deliver immediate returns. One strategy more likely to result in immediate improvement involves making better use of the services and service systems that are already in place and especially those that harness the tremendous knowledge, energy, and commitment of caregivers and self-advocates. This strategy precludes the need to lobby for significantly more resources to support new services or service providers and their associated training programs. For example, this might include initiatives that improve timely access to existing services, prevent duplication of services, and help to precisely target new areas of growth to documented areas of need. I have already argued that limited access to services is a challenge in ASD (see Chapter 4) and presents an immediately opportunity to improve outcomes (see Chapter 14). The review in Chapter 3 reveals many agencies that potentially duplicate services: the identification of ASD, assessment of cognitive and adaptive functioning, behavior support, case management, and so forth. The initiatives described next take advantage of these opportunities.

Providing Caregivers with Road Maps for Pivotal Services and Decisions

Although most agree that the needs of people with ASD vary greatly from one person to another and across their lifetime, there are nonetheless questions raised by many if not all people concerned with ASD: Does my child have ASD? How do I get help once he or she is diagnosed? How do I get help for behavior problems? How do I plan for adulthood? Some of the general information needed for each of these answers does not significantly vary from one person to another, although the specific agencies and service systems involved will vary from one state or region to another. Many states and regions have devoted considerable energy to developing resource centers that provide critical guidance to families (see Indiana; Chapter 8). A road map can help provide the information to at least guide caregivers and professionals through these kinds of decisions, and, when accompanied by a directory, can help to identify some of the professionals and agencies who might help. Simple web-based road maps and accompanying materials can be created to guide caregivers seeking to determine if their child has ASD, to identify how to initiate early intervention services, to begin to address behavior problems, and to plan for the transition to adult services. A well-constructed road map can help a caregiver take charge of the construction and oversight of his or her child's plan of care across agencies.

The need for such road maps is perhaps illustrated by the number of caregivers I encounter who do not receive medical assistance. Medical assistance is intended to be universally available and readily accessible: It is a federally driven program that can provide many important benefits to many people with ASD, regardless of their level of income. In some states, completion of the application for medical assistance is necessary to gain access to other important services. Therefore, there should be many incentives and no barriers to applying for medical assistance. Nonetheless, I have found that caregivers are confused by important state-to-state variations in the range of services offered, the means to access these services, and the agencies designated to administer these services. As a result, I continue to encounter families whose access to critical services is delayed because they never applied for medical assistance.

Cross-Domain Road Maps and Related Information   The first step is to develop a cross-domain road map that takes advantage of other relevant information that may already be available in written or electronic form and transform it to actively guide caregivers and professionals toward important decisions. A pamphlet, web site, or book may provide many accurate and relevant facts for a parent concerned about his or her child but still leaves caregivers wondering what step to actually take next. This is especially true for caregivers who may be struggling to accept the difficulties their child might be facing or who are already intimidated by the bewildering system of care. This problem might be solved by organizing the information around a series of questions caregivers might ask when deciding if and how to act on a concern and presenting it in a web site that gives caregivers the option of clicking links to learn more. Parents seeking a simple answer can find the information they need quickly, with additional background information only a click away for those seeking more. Oftentimes the general information published by a specific agency is confusing to caregivers because it is relevant only to the services which that agency offers, whereas a road map can be organized to answer critical questions that might be addressed by multiple agencies (e.g., seeking ASD identification through education and health care services). A web-based road map paired with a glossary can also help to work around the baffling terms used by professionals. For example, I have developed sample web sites in which a simple definition of a term (*screening, Medicaid*) appears when the cursor hovers over that term, with the option of reading even more about that term by clicking on it. Conscious efforts must also be taken to eliminate anything that might dissuade a caregiver from probing further. In many respects, the information developed by the Learn the Signs. Act Early. campaign (see Chapter 12) serves as a model for this approach, as do the toolkits developed by Autism Speaks.

Online Directories of Service Providers   The second step is to tie the road map and glossary into a web-based cross-domain directory of local resources. Many agencies and organizations have valiantly undertaken to develop lists of relevant services and providers. Lists published in print format can be difficult to search, are a tremendous challenge to maintain, and are out of date almost immediately; web-based lists can be searchable by any number of variables (and even linked to maps) and updated continuously by the providers themselves. Lists that are not accompanied by an explanation of what the services are, why they might be important, and when they should be sought are of little use to many caregivers; aligning a web-based directory to a road map helps to ensure that the services sought are relevant to the caregiver's concerns. Lists developed by one agency or organization focus on a more limited range of services: Those tied to a road map as described earlier can draw on a greater range of services and perhaps help caregivers to avoid duplicating services. Lists developed by national organizations cannot capture important state-to-state differences in the range of services available; whereas the broad framework of a directory might be developed by a national organization, the directory and the accompanying road map may be tailored to each state.

A web-based road map with an accompanying glossary and resource directory can support other important initiatives. First, it can become the springboard for caregiver and professional training. I have found that many professionals are equally confused by the role of other agencies and professionals; a road map and directory also help them direct caregivers to relevant resources. The framework provided by the web site—that is, the translation of general information about ASD into a series of questions and terms understood by caregivers—provides a much better structure around which a workshop can be organized and prepares participants to make best use of the road map and directory. Second, the development of the road map and directory can spur efforts to improve access to services. Feedback from users can help to identify barriers to access created at specific decision points and highlight specific service gaps in specific regions.

Case Management

As described throughout this volume, many people with ASD require the involvement of many different professionals from many different agencies, and the lack of access to and coordination of these multiple services leads to frustration and potential duplication. Thus, case management was designated as a pivotal service in Chapter 3. Although the case studies presented in Chapter 1 illustrated how many different professionals can formally or informally act as case managers, these sometimes occurred only because the professional was willing to stretch his or her traditional role in various ways. Before any of these or other case management activities can be considered, individual professionals must generally recognize and appropriately value the ways in which other services might complement their own. Although appropriate training prior to licensure can help professionals generally recognize the role of others, I have found that over time professionals tend to overvalue their own contribution and to undervalue the contribution of others, unless the importance of cross-disciplinary collaboration is heavily emphasized in their initial training (see later in the chapter) and current work. What are the steps that professionals and agencies might take to continue to evolve and incrementally expand case management to better help the people they serve? What changes in individual practice, and associated training, research, and policy at the agency, regional, and state levels, might be needed to take each of these steps?

Promoting Awareness of Other Local and Regional Services for People with Autism Spectrum Disorder   General training regarding the role of other professionals that may be provided during initial licensure may not include the level of detail needed to understand all of the needs specific to people with ASD and which agencies in the region might provide such services. Professionals can acquire more specific knowledge regarding the needs of people with ASD through any variety of general workshops and books; in this regard, road maps and associated training activities described earlier are particularly relevant. Because the specific agencies and organizations providing these services can vary from region to region and state to state, professionals might have to explore agency-specific web sites for information about specific services, unless state-specific road maps, regional directories, and associated training are available. The additional time needed to begin to promote awareness is otherwise minimal. Perhaps the greatest change in practice at this stage will be the inclusion of recommendations in evaluation reports and treatment summaries regarding other services.

Supporting Access to Other Local and Regional Services   Professionals and agencies who build on initiatives to promote awareness by helping the family to obtain other relevant services may encounter different barriers. First, professionals or agencies might not accept this responsibility (even those who are quick to blame others for the lack of progress). A solution might require setting a professional or an agency standard—that is, any professional who relies on services provided by another type of agency or professional must help caregivers to gain access to these services by providing the necessary forms, preparing relevant information to support the application, and either coaching the parents or directing them to appropriate coaching to complete the process. Second, it may be very unclear—even for a professional—how to gain access to these services, in which case changes to the service itself might be required. Third, this kind of simple support can itself take time, especially when multiplied across many clients in an already busy practice. Agencies must themselves consider this when planning and distributing resources, taking the amount of time into account when allocating workloads, designating other personnel to assume this responsibility (e.g., shifting these responsibilities from a pediatrician to a nurse practitioner in a pediatric practice), and recognizing these as billable activities. Finally, the agency and professional might consider how to change their practice to facilitate referrals to other services and taking the first real steps toward creating a seamless network (see later in the chapter). For example, a school that recognizes that respite funded through a state intellectual disabilities program is important to families, and that applications to these programs requires an up-to-date estimate of intelligence quotient (IQ), might use the periodic reassessment of IQ as an opportunity to encourage families to apply for these services.

Actively Coordinating Intervention Across Multiple Providers for Specific Needs

Professionals and agencies may build on initiatives to support gaining access by adjusting their ongoing intervention based on interventions obtained elsewhere. An enhanced professional or an agency standard may be helpful here: Any professional providing a service for which progress depends on other services delivered to the child (e.g., a Board Certified Behavior Analyst [BCBA] who believes that improved behaviors will also depend on the pediatrician's medication management) should be obligated to communicate with the other professional regarding treatment. Initiating a multidisciplinary team meeting is an excellent first step: Information is at least shared. Better yet, a consensus might be established about intervention goals and time lines. Ideally, treatment decisions might be adjusted based on the feedback from others. Sometimes agencies can expand upon existing, multidisciplinary case management activities; for example, a school-based individualized education program (IEP) team can decide to invite the physician prescribing psychotropic medication to a key meeting to describe behavior support needs. Each of these steps will require a plan to increase resources in a manner similar to that described earlier. The amount of resources required for ongoing case management may be prohibitive at this point, in which active coordination of intervention may be time limited or focused on specific questions or need. For example, a coordinated meeting might be needed to review the services and supports needed to initiate in-home behavioral support or to justify a recommendation for a residential program.

Proactive and/or Ongoing Case Management

Active coordination of intervention at a specific point in time can be an effective response to a short- or medium-term need. An agency that is committed to addressing an array of needs over a significant span of the person's lifetime, however, will begin to recognize that it is more efficient to anticipate those needs requiring active case coordination, especially whenever service gaps or bottlenecks are known to jeopardize progress. By anticipating these needs, agencies can develop mechanisms for training, research, and oversight to establish standards, push through these barriers, and improve overall quality. For example, almost all states have developed programs of training and oversight for the transition from education-based services to those provided by adult agencies. The result is that such transition planning has evolved to often become more parent friendly and person centered, to include a variety of training activities to orient all participants to their respective roles in transition planning, and to result in a comprehensive written plan to guide services. The Family Focused Positive Behavior Support (FFPBS) project in West Virginia (see Chapter 5) provides an excellent model for how to take a similar approach for a subset of children—those with significant behavior support needs.

Toward Services that Are Need, Not Agency, Driven   These incremental improvements in case management illustrate why it is necessary to look beyond the services that one professional or agency might provide to one individual living with an ASD. With the increased prevalence of ASD, large organizations, and especially those at the regional and state level, can no longer feign surprise when they encounter gaps and barriers in service needs that span multiple agencies. They can anticipate these gaps and barriers by developing training and policy, perhaps through specific programs such as FFPBS. Over time, this may lead agencies to consider the final step: the metamorphosis from a agency-driven program (e.g., in which independent agencies each control separate service functions blended on a case-by-case basis into a single plan) to a needs-driven program (e.g., in which a team receives a voucher that they can use to purchase different services as needed).

An Interim Solution: Supporting Caregivers as Case Managers   I have outlined steps that agencies and organizations at the local, regional, and state level might take to improve case management, but service professionals should frankly acknowledge the strong possibility that caregivers are likely to be the only people positioned to provide case management, at least in the short term (see Chapter 14). This is especially likely in regions with poorly organized services or for groups that lack intensive support (e.g., adults with ASD and significant ID). The development of road maps and service directories, especially paired with training, will help caregivers make specific transitions and decisions. Caregivers will also benefit from more active coaching, training, and direct support in their role as case managers. Many local and regional advocacy organizations and parent information centers already provide many of these services, and so expansion might simply require the development of train-the-trainer programs and/or funding for caregiver-coaches. Programs involving caregiver-coaches can capitalize on an excellent source of personnel: caregivers who have already acted successfully in this role.

NEXT STEPS: TOWARD A
COORDINATED NETWORK OF BEHAVIOR SUPPORT

For agencies and regions that have already established programs for identification of ASD and that are more ambitious, another excellent opportunity is the development of a coordinated network directly and indirectly addressing behavior support. By behavior support, I am referring to a wide range of assessment and intervention activities, services intended to address problem behaviors that prevent the person with an ASD from remaining at home or gaining access to school, work, or community settings (see Chapter 2). In general, behavior support is an excellent focus for the development of an integrated network: It can be provided in any of these settings, problem behaviors are one of the most common barriers to gaining access to these settings, problem behaviors are a major source of stress for caregivers, and a wide range of evidenced-based practices and training programs are already in place.

Services

As described in Chapter 3, behavior support potentially encompasses a wide range of activities. Although the task of assessing behavior and developing a behavior plan often falls to a relatively restricted range of professionals (e.g., behavior therapists, BCBAs, psychologists), the successful implementation of a plan often depends on the involvement of many different professionals and agencies. Consider Evan, whose journey was summarized in Chapter 4. His primary care practitioner addressed sleep problems and ear infections thought to contribute to his tantrums and referred him for evaluations to address comingled anxiety; his ID case manager helped his parents to gain access to support to address related toileting problems; implementation of the behavior plan was guided in school by his teacher and in the home by his community-based behavioral specialist. Evan's case also illustrated how problem behavior limited access to many key services, like primary and emergency medical care, school-based services, and the after-school care needed so that his parents could return to work.

A coordinated service network of behavior support builds on many existing systems. The positive behavior support (PBS) movement and the number of behavior specialists have both continued to grow, with the result that behavior support is available in an increasing number of private and public education and behavior health agencies at the local and regional level. These services take advantage of the expanding body of evidence supporting behavioral interventions, which, with the increasing sophistication of social skills training, self-management, and cognitive-behavior therapy (CBT) (see later in the chapter) can begin to more effectively address the needs of people living with Asperger syndrome. A range of community-based and more specialized physicians more comfortable with medication management and is sensitive to the impact of co-occurring conditions such as anxiety, depression, sleep disorders, and other problems that can complicate behavior support. When behavior problems arise because of specific skill deficits and the failure to implement specific accommodations, and/or are exacerbated by specific conditions, a competent multidisciplinary team can act quickly on the insights gained through a functional behavioral assessment. Given the services, training, research, and policy outlined in this volume, it can be expected that most children with ASD should be able to gain access to relevant support for behavior problems from school, community, or health care providers.

When the kinds of aforementioned case management helps to coordinate behavior support across settings, progress is accelerated and magnified to include the kinds of broad outcomes for both the person with an ASD and his or her caregivers, as described in Chapter 14. A case coordinator—or even a professional who assumes elements of that role (e.g., a special education teacher)—can help align school- and community-based plans to ensure they are complementary and not contradictory and create an intensity and consistency of treatment that accelerates progress. Too often, practitioners also fail to appreciate how many places and activities families avoid because of problem behavior, with the result that families can become prisoners to their child's increasingly narrow and unsatisfying routines. Practitioners also adopt a "train and hope" model of generalization and assume that gains demonstrated in one setting will transfer easily to others. But those practitioners who embrace the need to pursue broad outcomes pertaining to quality of life, for both the person with an ASD and his or her caregivers, can aggressively pursue generalization by providing training and support to ensure that problem behaviors are not a barrier to gaining access to any settings or activities, getting primary medical and dental care, gaining access to after-school care or respite, participating in community-based recreation and leisure, or just going to a restaurant or movie. In effect, coordinated behavior support can help people living with ASD begin to take back their lives.

Closer examination of the network of behavior support also reveals specific and critical gaps in the many levels of care potentially required. Basic interventions are more likely to be available, ranging from schoolwide PBS (e.g., a shift from emphasizing how the majority of children are playing well at recess instead of focusing on the few who are acting out) to relatively generic individual behavior plans targeting relatively mild behaviors. The more specialized interventions needed by a smaller proportion of people with ASD, but that have a greater impact on outcomes, are more likely to be lacking. For example, supports needed for very challenging behaviors that pose an immediate danger to others (e.g., significant aggression, self-injury) that require the use of extraordinary measures such as physical restraint or result in suspension (e.g., major tantrums, property destruction) may at best result in a team meeting, the increased involvement of the behavior specialist, or result in the assignment of one-to-one support. Little else might be considered because caregivers do not understand what else might be available, because clinicians lack the necessary expertise and because program leaders do not know where to get additional support and are locked into inflexible funding mechanisms. Clinicians and leaders focused on local needs may encounter relatively few such cases each year, may consider these to be "exceptions," and so may lack the impetus to plan proactively. Yet these conditions can act as a trigger for additional services, support, and oversight, as offered in Delaware (see Chapter 7). In this way, more specialized and costly service options can be ready to employ at the regional level (e.g., across multiple counties or school districts) and represent a more cost-effective option in the long term.

Another level of specialized care that is conspicuously lacking is inpatient behavioral stabilization designed for people with ASD (see Chapter 2). People with ASD in behavioral crises not only place themselves or others in immediate and significant danger but place tremendous stresses on the system of care; schools required to ensure a free and appropriate education struggle to meet this need; general emergency rooms and crisis centers can find themselves obligated to accommodate individuals they are barely equipped to handle, sometimes for days at a time until another placement is identified; and others might end up in police custody. The fact that perhaps a dozen specialized inpatient behavioral stabilization programs are scattered across the United States does not reflect the level of need but rather the tremendous challenges involved with setting up and maintaining such programs. Given the prevalence of ASD, the likelihood of hospitalization for behavioral or psychiatric reasons, the stress created on systems of case management, and probability that inpatient stabilization will forestall if not prevent long-term residential placement, every state and many regions should identify ways to support the creation of such programs.

Throughout this volume, I have emphasized that the apparent presence or absence of ASD is sometimes irrelevant when planning for the needs of people with significant ID;

this is especially true when addressing problem behaviors. People with significant ID can present with the same behaviors and respond to the same interventions whether or not they have a formal diagnosis of ASD. Given that the population of people with significant ID but not ASD is likely to outnumber those with ASD and ID, it is easier to create the critical mass needed to support more specialized behavior support programs that span these populations.

Training

Some important components of training are already in place. A number of different professionals already involved in behavior support receive specific training in behavior management as part of their initial certification and sometimes also in the context of internships and practica: Most teachers receive instruction in at least classroom-wide behavior management, psychologists receive training in behavior support and in the identification and treatment of co-occurring conditions, psychiatrists receive training in medication management, and so forth. Of course, training provided to behavior analysts is much more relevant and extensive, and, when it entails exposure to models of PBS, also promotes the broader perspectives of multidisciplinary teamwork and person-centered planning central to the interventions emphasized in this volume. Perhaps the biggest gap in initial licensure will continue to occur as long as broadly defined "behavior specialists" act in place of professionals with more extensive and relevant training, such as behavior analysts and psychologists. Continued expansion of the number of states that recognize and fund BCBAs will be essential. Additional training and certification programs, including those recently adopted in Pennsylvania as part of its autism insurance legislation (described in Chapter 3), can help also close this gap.

Targeted expansion of PBS will also be important. Many of the programs have made important first steps in shifting the emphasis from reaction and punishment to prevention and have begun to create primary change at the schoolwide level across a range of populations. These programs must place equal weight on promoting change at the secondary and tertiary level to promote individual behavior support plans and more creative programming in the case of children with very intensive behavioral needs. PBS can also be expanded to community settings—child care, in-home behavioral support, residential programs—as part of the coordinated case management approach described earlier (and in Chapter 5 in West Virginia's FFPBS). Consistent with the comprehensive training approach described in Chapter 3, this emphasis on prevention and skill-building can become the shared vision promoted across professionals and environments. Too often, professionals also seem to assume that behavior plans fail because they identified the wrong function or selected the wrong intervention, instead of recognizing that many simple interventions can be extremely effective if they are applied with high levels of intensity and fidelity. In this context, cross-systems training in a core set of simple but effective positive and preventative interventions can help assure the intensity and fidelity needed.

Training will also be critical to supporting the more specialized behavior support services described earlier and in Chapter 3. These additional training resources can include ongoing professional development intended to build the expertise of psychologists and behavior analysts over a period of years, as well as targeted coaching and consultation for specific cases that improve services to the children involved *and* provide unparalleled training. This kind of training program can be a cost-effective way for a local or regional agency to develop a partnership with experts and programs that otherwise might have little opportunity or incentive to work intensively at the local level.

Research

Behavior support can already benefit from many evidence-based practices, a significant proportion of which are derived from single case design. As described in Chapter 3, evidence-based practice standards still fall short of meeting the day-to-day needs of most clinicians, who must tailor interventions according to very specific targets, in the light of specific characteristics and prerequisite skills demonstrated by that particular individual with an ASD. Behavior support may therefore represent the best testing ground for demonstrating how to distill research findings into recommendations for a given child. This could entail an expansion of the National Autism Center's (2009) summary of findings according to treatment target and diagnosis to include the function of behavior and functioning level and married with the evidence-based practice briefs and videos offered by the National Professional Development Center (NPDC) (see Chapter 13).

The increasing recognition that antecedent conditions can greatly influence the intensity if not the direction of problem behaviors offers other promising avenue of research. Just as I have argued that co-occurring conditions may be more amenable to treatment than the ASD itself, some of the co-occurring conditions associated with problem behaviors (e.g., disorders of sleep, mood, seizure) may also be good initial targets. Research that begins by grouping children with problem behaviors, according to the presence or absence of a specific co-occurring condition, may help to clarify the role of these conditions.

One of the greatest contradictions in the research and practice in ASD is the continued reliance on various medications as a primary form of behavior management for a wide range of behavior targets, despite the lack of convincing scientific evidence of their effectiveness. This could reflect that there are specific instances in which medication is clearly effective but that are difficult to capture in treatment designs or simply that caregivers and professionals will choose medication when it is more readily available than competent behavior support. These possibilities will remain difficult to disentangle as long as different interventions are evaluated using different research designs: Although it appears that the vast majority of research examining problem behaviors to date is based on single case design, most research on the effectiveness of medication is based on group comparisons. Studies that bridge this divide—for example, single case designs that include medication trials and group designs that consider the relative impact of medications and positive/preventative techniques—may help to better elucidate the unique role of medications in behavior support.

Policy

Some of the policy changes needed to take advantage of the opportunities to improve service, training, and research described earlier are relatively straightforward, whereas others are more complex. Policy changes at multiple levels (e.g., state, county/school district) will be important to supporting the more intense and specialized supports needed for those people with ASD presenting with highly problematic behaviors, as described earlier. The range and impact of policy changes are, however, much more variable. Consider how changes to autism insurance legislation might facilitate some of the recommendations regarding behavior support. On the one hand, caregivers and providers would likely concur that the design and supervision of insurance-funded behavior support should fall to properly trained personnel, such as BCBAs and psychologists, or, at the very least, professionals from a related field training who have completed specialized training. This may lead to more universal recognition of BCBAs as a critical license. On the other hand, legislation that expands the amount of funding available or broadens the traditional definitions of behavioral rehabilitation applicable to one group will surely raise questions of parity. How is it that insurance-funded services are so much more intensive and comprehensive than those available to others? Why is it that the amount and kinds of services funded for people with ID but not ASD are so different from those for people with ASD, when many of these needs are comparable?

OTHER KEY SERVICES, RESEARCH, TRAINING, AND POLICY

There are clearly so many opportunities to improve services and training through research and policy at the local, regional, state, and national level. I have highlighted a handful of these that address specific gaps or that represent specific and immediate opportunities to increase capacity and to begin to create an integrated network by coordinating across levels and elements.

Key Services

Specialized After-School Care and Respite   As described in Chapter 2, the lack of specialized after-school child care is a significant barrier to many parents returning to work. Respite is also important, providing a welcome or necessary break from the pressure of ongoing care. Most families living with ASD can only dream of taking a family vacation or an outing in the community or to visit friends; even the simple task of shopping for food requires as much planning as launching a major military campaign. For some families, this situation improves over time, but for others—for example, single-parent families, those in poverty—these difficulties persist throughout the person's lifetime. Existing service providers might begin by extending their current services. For example, a school might provide after-school care using school facilities and school personnel (but administered privately), offer child care for after-school parent trainings or meetings, or offer a Friday night out for parents once a month.

- *Training:* Those seeking to create an after-school program or more formal network of respite providers should consider establishing minimum training standards (e.g., a standard 1-day workshop). Programs might compensate by recruiting potential providers from relevant groups (e.g., paraprofessionals) or settings (e.g., specialized schools).

- *Policy:* Increasing funding for respite will certainly help to increase respite and spur the development of new resources, although the impact may only become apparent over time, because families may initially hesitate to use respite, or because a provider network has not been created. For specialized after-school care, policy makers may also consider providing a supplemental rate for such care. In both cases, policy that creates new funding, ideally tied to training and other standards, may also increase capacity.

- *Infrastructure:* Hotlines and online directories (see earlier in the chapter) can help to connect families to respite providers, managed by a lead agency at the regional or state level (together with a source of funding for start-up and ongoing maintenance).

Training in Advocacy for Self-Advocates   Just as caregivers can be educated and equipped to act as case managers for their children, those living with ASD are naturally positioned to advocate for themselves, with the proper training. For college students with ASD, this training can draw on the support of peer mentors (as used in West Virginia—see Chapter 5) and can be a natural extension of social skills training. This training can also be incorporated into a post-21 transition planning program for high school students and therefore reach even those who are not college bound. An added benefit is that self-advocates can take a proper seat at the table to shape local, regional, state, and national policy with other decision makers.

- *Training:* Given that such programs are just beginning to emerge, a train-the-trainer program funded at the state or national level can help new programs to emerge.

- *Policy and infrastructure:* Wherever peer mentors are involved, colleges should consider designating these as an opportunity for course credit or a recognized practicum/community-service experience. Agencies at all levels will also have to determine where and how to provide self-advocates with a seat at any committees that set policy.

Other Key Services   *A synthesis of CBT and social skills training:* As described in Chapter 2, CBT is a very promising practice that is only being slowly adopted in ASD. By broadening CBT to include verbally mediated interventions that address cognitions (Wood, Fujii, & Renno, 2011), service professionals might take better advantage of techniques well established for CBT and apply these techniques to social skills training. This might encourage CBT techniques to spread beyond doctoral level clinicians conducting individual therapy.

Key Training

Paraprofessional Training   As described in Chapter 3, paraprofessionals are the direct-care staff (e.g., teaching assistants, residential assistants, mental health technicians, child care/after-school assistants, camp counselors, health aides, job coaches, in-home assistants providing intensive early intervention or wraparound services, peer mentors) who provide intensive day-to-day support. Regardless of the setting, paraprofessionals spend more time in direct contact with people with ASD than anyone save the caregivers themselves. They constitute the most commonly used, most underappreciated sector of intervention, but because they usually receive little training, their potential as agents of intervention is largely untapped.

It is necessary to improve training by defining a core set of competencies relevant to most or all of these settings and across the ASD spectrum; a general understanding of the needs of people with ASD, techniques derived from positive behavior supports, an understanding the experiences of people living with ASD (see later in the chapter). Given the high number of people potentially benefiting from such training, it is cost effective for state agencies or large organizations to invest in a regional or statewide training strategy. One option might include a series of live or online seminars consisting of a minimum of 12 hours but potentially extending up to 40 hours or more if it includes supplemental training in specific techniques. A second option can include incorporation of this training into a certificate program offered at a community or technical college. Each of these options can then be supplemented by agency-specific training. The investment may spur even more individuals to seek more advanced training as teachers, nurses, behavior specialists and help to funnel those who otherwise might have initially hesitated to pursue such training (e.g., high school graduates who did not immediately enter college, parents returning to the workforce).

- *Research:* I believe that the most cost-effective way to immediately improve services is to ensure that simple but effective teaching techniques are used frequently and consistently. Improvements in paraprofessional services can be guided by research that defines the optimal intensity and fidelity of intervention (see later in the chapter).

- *Policy and infrastructure:* Policy that sets minimum standards for training at the agency level or at the state level can help to drive training. Policy can also support the creation of specialized certificates (such as West Virginia's Autism Mentor program described in Chapter 5) or a work-study program to help paraprofessionals seeking an undergraduate degree (such as Delaware's program described in Chapter 7).

Training for Primary Medical and Dental Practitioners   Given the contribution of co-occurring conditions to the problem behaviors of people with ASD, and the barriers to essential medical and dental care created by these behaviors, training directed to community-based medical and dental practitioners can yield great benefits if it is appropriately targeted. One strategy is to develop specific treatment algorithms to help primary care practitioners provide support for common co-occurring conditions and guide referrals to specialists. The work of the Autism Treatment Networks for gastrointestinal and sleep disorders provides one example, which perhaps can be extended to other important topics, such as medication management. Another strategy is to ensure that such practitioners understand when and how to refer to nonmedical providers for early intervention services, school-based services, caregiver support, case management, advocacy, and so forth. A third strategy is to develop other toolkits, such as the Autism Speaks Dental Professionals Tool Kit, that identify accommodations that practitioners can use to facilitate care for their patients. And, of course, training programs should continue to support the emergence of new medical homes (see Utah's programs described in Chapter 10). Whenever possible, such programs should target support staff (e.g., dental hygienists, nursing assistants), who may have more flexibility in participating in training.

- *Research:* Additional research to clarify the prevalence of co-occurring conditions and to identify simple and powerful intervention strategies will help target training.

- *Policy and infrastructure:* Training may need to be paired with policy changes to appropriate reimburse medical and dental practitioners for the increased time required to provide the necessary consultation and case management. Translating these practices into formal professional guidelines may help to speed their adoption. Grants to fund the development of such programs will also be important and can take advantage of the existing state professional organizations (e.g., state chapters of the AAP).

Other Key Training   *Living with ASD:* Many books have provided first-person accounts of people living with ASD, and a number of national organizations have sought to convey this experience through web sites, videos, and other materials. Although such efforts have certainly raised awareness in the general population, I continue to find that many professionals lack this perspective. It is therefore important to ensure that professionals receive training in the experiences of people living with ASD soon after they begin to work with this population. Such training can promote a person- and family-centered perspective, convey the challenge each faces in the course of his or her journey (especially for those from traditionally underserved populations), and address the common sources of miscommunication between professionals and people living with ASD. A general module can be supplemented by modules for specific groups and agencies that address their own unique role.

Developing trainers and leaders: Whether addressing services, training, research, or policy, almost every major review of the future of programs serving people with ASD has lamented the lack of program leaders. In many cases, program leaders appear to have emerged from the ranks of people working directly in the field as educators, clinicians, academics, and/or researchers and shift (or are thrust) into significant positions of leadership and responsibility with little training in program development and a relatively narrow domain of experience from which to draw upon. Because ASD is relatively specialized, agencies and organizational entities (e.g., a program within a hospital, center within a university) that focus on this population tend to be too small to have layers of leadership, and so there is limited opportunity for leaders to move up through the ranks within an organization. Instead, they are more likely to move from leadership positions in smaller entities to a position of greater responsibility within a different organization. This convoluted career path is further complicated by the lack of natural opportunities to network with and learn from peers who are also ASD leaders. This has begun to change, with a number of regional and national conferences targeting autism leaders.

Key Research

As described in Chapter 4, it cannot be assumed that basic research findings will naturally trickle down into improvements in services delivered daily across the country; specific efforts will be needed to identify new evidence-based practices and remove barriers to their implementation so that as many people as possible can benefit immediately from new research in ASD. One of the most significant barriers to projecting the cost of scaling up services is the lack of data on optimal treatment intensity. As described in Chapter 3, the lack of critical information akin to a dose–response ratio—for example, the number of hours of group or individual intervention needed to attain a given outcome (Volkmar, Reichow, & Doehring, 2011)—makes it very difficult for leaders to determine the resources needed to implement a program or to estimate the rate of progress. Given that salary support for direct care staff often constitutes the most significant expense for service delivery programs and that programs for people with ASD are often more expensive to run than other programs, program leaders will remain under constant pressure to deliver results with inadequate resources until such research is conducted.

A related gap is the contribution of treatment fidelity to program implementation and outcomes. Although treatment fidelity is recognized as a critical characteristic of high-quality research (Reichow & Volkmar, 2011), its importance to training and service delivery is underappreciated. Achieving treatment fidelity requires the development of a more comprehensive training program (e.g., those described in Chapter 3) and so directly facilitates more widespread adoption of the practice. Demonstrating treatment fidelity, especially in a community-based setting, is necessary before the cost of scaling up the practice can be justified and helps to establish who can be trained, how much training is required, and so forth. I have found that practitioners often conclude prematurely that a practice is ineffective, without first confirming that it was implemented with the necessary fidelity and/or intensity. This can lead to the constant pursuit of other, more complex interventions when a simple evidence-based intervention can be effective if it is applied intensively and consistently.

The census and statewide needs assessments conducted in Pennsylvania (Chapters 3, 4, 6, and 14) are other ways that research can directly inform policy. Although the methodology used may limit the scientific precision of the results finally obtained, it nonetheless can reveal actual and perceived gaps that are impossible to ignore. For example, variations in the services across different regions and different populations can generate specific goals for state agencies seeking to improve access. This sets the stage for the next step needed to face ASD across the entire country; the shift from demonstrating pockets of service excellence in programs accessible to a privileged few to ensuring that everyone can benefit from the advances in training and research in ASD.

Key Policy and Infrastructure: Integrated Networks that Build Local and Regional Expertise

Decision makers at the highest levels are increasingly aware of the needs and ambitions of people living with ASD, because of the increasingly articulate and ardent community of advocates. Economic downturns, political movements to shrink the role of government, and examples of programs that fall far short of their goals make it harder for advocates to build support for new investments within the public sector for services, training, and research. What might be the most strategic changes to policies and infrastructure to pursue in this climate? As described next, I would focus on developing networks that integrate existing services, training, research, and policy across traditional service domains, with the immediate goal of increasing capacity for high-quality services and supports at the local and regional level.

Invest in People, Not Facilities   Every week, somewhere in the United States, a collection of program leaders, advocates, and funders cuts a ribbon to open a building: A photo appears in a local paper or company newsletter, and everyone celebrates the creation of a new center for ASD. Although the effort required to design and build a new center should not be underestimated, this celebration is nonetheless premature. Over time, the investment in bricks and mortar is far, far outweighed by the investment in people who will make the center come alive. Moreover, this must often include a substantial investment in training over many years (e.g., that I would estimate to be equivalent to 5%–10% of total labor costs) to compensate for the fact that many service providers, trainers, researchers, and leaders only acquire the necessary expertise long after they have completed their initial certification, especially for more specialized programs. Unfortunately, no photo opportunity exists to celebrate the moment when a well-trained team becomes effective.

Develop Networks, Not Stand-Alone Centers   A focus on new centers also perpetuates another myth that drives ambitious program leaders and developers; that the answer to ASD will be found by the work of a single center or program. Despite the desires of advocates desperate for change and of well-heeled supporters ready to support new programs, no single program, center, or agency will ever be in a position to meet all—or even a substantial proportion—of the needs of people living with ASD or the professionals seeking to help them.

Require All Programs to Demonstrate Some Immediate and Tangible Outcomes Some of the research and training initiatives described in this volume will require years of effort, but there are many pivotal services that professionals already know how to provide, that contribute to critical outcomes, that build bridges across disciplines, and that can be scaled up quickly—for example, identification, case management, behavior support, training in information, and advocacy. policy for ASD should be structured to yield some immediate benefits in these or other services.

Strategically Scale up Local and Regional Capacity by Considering the Extent of the Need, the Intensity of the Training, and the Level of Specialization Required It is unrealistic to expect that changes in policy and infrastructure will immediately affect all services equally quickly, but incremental improvements are possible if some of the principles outlined in the last chapter are followed. It may help to first target essential services needed to ensure access (e.g., programs for the early and accurate screening and identification of ASD) or provide training and support relevant to the majority of people with ASD (e.g., core training for educators and early intervention providers, the availability of information about resources for ASD, specialized child care for families), especially when guidelines and/or evidence-based standards have already been established. Only then might professionals target services or training that are so highly specialized or so rarely needed that they could simply never be provided locally (e.g., specialized medical evaluation, inpatient behavioral stabilization) (see also examples described in Chapter 14).

Promote Cross-Element, Cross-Domain, and Cross-Population Collaboration from the Beginning Integrated networks must span multiple elements (services, training, research, and policy) and/or domains (health, education, community supports) and encompass the interests of people living with ASD and the professionals who seek to help them. Such networks should also begin to build bridges with services, training, and research conducted with other populations (e.g., those with ID) whenever possible and appropriate. This will help to counteract the pressure toward increasing specialization and isolation and promote the balance and cross-fertilization needed to scale up services most efficiently. Programs like the Leadership Education in Neurodevelopmental and related Disorders (LEND) and many University Centers of Excellence on Developmental Disabilities (UCEDDs) referenced at various points in this volume strive to provide multidisciplinary, culturally sensitive, family-centered, and community-focused training to new clinicians in service delivery, research, and policy. Many LENDs and UCEDDs promote interdisciplinary programs of study by bringing together professors from multiple departments and schools. The push toward increased specialization and the perpetuation of service- and discipline-specific silos may ultimately begin to subside, however, only when it is recognized that the best care almost always requires collaboration across individuals, agencies, and disciplines, and when this challenge is approached with the humility of a team who assumes a shared responsibility, instead of the arrogance of the expert who assumes that he or she alone holds the keys.

Recognize that Many Agencies and Organizations Can Provide Leadership This volume offers examples of different kinds of "networks." State programs have supported specialized networks for ongoing training that are based in universities, public agencies, or combinations of the two (as in the case of West Virginia, Pennsylvania, Delaware, Indiana, Kansas, Utah, and Ontario). Universities are still best positioned to act as leaders.

They naturally blend training and research, they shape services by providing the training to practitioners who will lead them, they can also leverage funding from a variety of sources to develop pilot programs, and those with a center of emphasis on disabilities are also more likely to venture into public policy and play an important advisory role in local and state government. But, with some exceptions discussed in this volume, universities have not successfully scaled up services to reach a broad clientele, nor do they always properly value the development of such services as compared to fueling academic discussion and research about (at times esoteric) topics less likely to immediately improve outcomes. For these reasons, other public agencies and advocacy organization such as Autism Speaks will play an increasingly important role.

Programs Can Provide Models for Developing Leaders, Building Local Capacity, and Promoting Collaboration   Various programs described in this volume such as Learn the Signs. Act Early. (Chapter 12), the NPDC (Chapter 13), and Pennsylvania's ASERT collaborative (Chapter 6) are explicitly focused on the rapid dissemination of knowledge and practice and on building local expertise. They also provide an invaluable opportunity for leaders in ASD to work together to establish common goals and learn from one another. Although many trainees have some experience in the particular practice being disseminated, this is often the first time they have been provided guidance in the development of training programs, including the principles and practices of implementation science. Grant competitions themselves can be structured so as to reward agencies with a track record of collaboration and require the development of in-state networks.

REFERENCES

American Psychiatric Association. (2000). *Diagnostic and statistical manual of mental disorders* (4th ed., text rev.). Washington, DC: Author.

Lord, C., Rutter, M., DiLavore, P.C., & Risi, S. (1999). *Autism Diagnostic Observation Schedule (ADOS).* Los Angeles, CA: Western Psychological Services.

Lord, C., Rutter, M., & Le Couteur, A. (1994). Autism Diagnostic Interview-Revised: A revised version of a diagnostic interview for caregivers of individuals with possible pervasive developmental disorders. *Journal of Autism and Developmental Disorders, 24*(5), 659–685.

National Autism Center. (2009). *The National Standards Project: Addressing the need for evidence based practice guidelines for autism spectrum disorders.* Randolph, MA: Author.

Reichow, B., & Volkmar, F.R. (2011). Evidence-based practices in autism: Where we started. In B. Reichow, P. Doehring, D.V. Cicchetti, & F.R. Volkmar (Eds.), *Evidence-based practices and treatments for children with autism* (pp. 3–24). New York, NY: Springer.

Volkmar, F.R., Reichow, B., & Doehring, P. (2011). Evidence-based practices in autism: Where we are now and where we need to go. In B. Reichow, P. Doehring, D.V. Cicchetti, & F.R. Volkmar (Eds.), *Evidence-based practices and treatments for children with autism* (pp. 365–391). New York, NY: Springer.

Wood, J.J., Fujii, C., & Renno, P. (2011). Cognitive behavioral therapy in high-functioning autism: Review and recommendations for treatment development. In B. Reichow, P. Doehring, D.V. Cicchetti, & F.R. Volkmar (Eds.), *Evidence-based practices and treatments for children with autism* (pp. 197–230). New York, NY: Springer.

Index

....

References to tables, figures, and footnotes are indicated with *t*, *f*, and *n*, respectively.